Reimagining a Child's Heart

Thomas J. Kulik • Macdonald Dick

# Reimagining a Child's Heart

## The Lone Pines of Congenital Cardiology

Springer

Thomas J. Kulik
Boston Children's Hospital
Harvard Medical School
Boston, MA, USA

Macdonald Dick
C.S. Mott Children's Hospital
University of Michigan
Ann Arbor, MI, USA

ISBN 978-3-031-88607-2 ISBN 978-3-031-88608-9 (eBook)
https://doi.org/10.1007/978-3-031-88608-9



This Springer imprint is published by the registered company Springer Nature Switzerland AG
The registered company address is: Gewerbestrasse 11, 6330 Cham, Switzerland

*In memory of Thomas J Kulik - Beloved Clinician, Teacher, Researcher, Colleague, and Friend*

# Foreword

On January 6, 2021, Thomas J. Kulik, MD, a renowned pediatric cardiac Intensivist, cardiologist to many devoted patients, basic science researcher in pulmonary hypertension, scholar, teacher, and leader, came home from work at Boston Children's Hospital in the late afternoon, donned his sweat suit, and jumped on his stationary bike. After he completed his workout, he returned to the kitchen and suddenly collapsed to the floor. His wife, Linda, returned home a little later and found him there. He could not be resuscitated. Tom had distinguished sequential academic careers on the faculties of the University of the Minnesota Medical School, the Harvard Medical School, the University of Michigan Medical School, the University of Cincinnati Medical School, and then again the Harvard Medical School.

Tom, since medical school days, had been thinking deeply (Tom rarely, if ever, thought superficially regarding anything) about congenital heart disease, and eventually the last frontier of congenital heart disease confounding surgical therapy—the hypoplastic left heart syndrome (HLHS) (see Fig 9.7 in Chap. 9). He developed a keen and deep interest in medical history, especially related to congenital heart disease. He also was fascinated by the similarities and differences between medical innovation and engineering innovation. He planned to put his musings and writings into a book; this is that book. Tom and I discussed his planned book a number of times as he did with others;[1] I also had the pleasure and privilege of reviewing his chapters as he was putting them together. He was very close to reaching his goal. After he was gone, I, with deliberate restraint and allegiance to his voice and with the approval of Linda, undertook finishing his project.

Tom has a primary theme that runs through all the chapters. He was interested in the people who contributed to the development of therapy for congenital heart disease. The characteristics he was seeking in these individuals were those who "thought differently," those who were tenacious, those with imagination—thinking out-of-the-box—and those who were "all in" in their commitment to solving the

[1]Aldo R. Castanẽda, Giovanni Stellin, Barbara Carlon, Stephen P. Sanders, Michael D. Freed, Robert Truog, John J. Lamberti, Peter Lang, Edward L. Bove, Roberta G. Williams, Flavio Coceani, Richard Van Praagh, and Robert H. Anderson.

problem. He called these individuals "Lone Pines," those who stood out on the tundra alone, independent, and motivated by their own internal impulses rather than the "noise" around them.

You will learn much about them, though most of the names are not unfamiliar to those in the field. New stories will be told and old ones retold, all with Tom's wry interpretation and insight. You will also come across cathedrals, aqueducts, steam pumps, steam engines, mining, art, ocean navigation, fish physiology, mountain climbing, hypothermia, hibernation, and aviation. You will encounter the ancients in medicine as well as the Renaissance and Enlightenment giants—Harvey and Lavoisier—along with the nineteenth-century chroniclers of congenital heart disease. You will read about early operations (no anesthesia) such as amputations, hernia repair, kidney stones, bone setting, cataract removal, tonsillectomies, tracheostomies, not to mention the unfolding of cardiac surgery. In telling this story I changed very few words; this is Tom's voice—breathing life into each of the many major characters and with a profound attachment to the story. Like his teaching, Tom's voice is conversational but candid; witty, yet scholarly, richly annotated and referenced. Be sure to read the footnotes. Like all good writers, his word usage is original with an idiomatic, idiosyncratic choice of words and phrases. He takes an ordinary verb and maybe an unusual verb and using it in a wry, unique way that may cause you to smile but also will cause you to see his point more clearly.

Tom notes in his introduction that his telling of the story of congenital heart disease is his alone and that he left some important players and institutions out. We too acknowledge that there are many contributors to this story who are not included; our apologies.

There are a few editorial changes that I did make with Linda's permission. First Tom's musing about engineering and medical innovations were originally interspersed among the history chapters about congenital heart disease, Linda and I agreed that they disrupted the flow of that story so I put them at the end as Appendices. We think they stand alone as a window into Tom's fascination with medical and engineering innovation. Second, Tom did not come up with a title that he settled on. He tried "Beautiful Palliation," "Beautiful Rescue," and "Lone Pines" that are in his notes. We settled on "Reimagining a Child's Heart—The Lone Pines of Congenital Cardiology."[2] These, we thought, emphasized two of his criteria—requirement for imagination and for thinking differently, i.e., "Lone Pines." The final alteration was creating two new chapters out of his long chapter about the Norwood operation. I moved the prostaglandin story to its own chapter as well as the stories of four twentieth-century cardiac pathologists. Tom felt that these stories were close but not quite at the "Lone Pines" level. You can make your own decision. However, I moved them not in disagreement but because they were different stories and seemed to need their own space. I hope Tom will forgive me.

---

[2] Tom came up with this term—congenital cardiology—to combine pediatric cardiology and pediatric cardiovascular surgery; I have encountered it elsewhere so I am not sure that it is original with him.

One never takes on a project like this alone. Linda was a constant support and force, reviewing each and every word at least three times along with checking for copyrights. Tom's administrative assistant, Lynne Patkin, gathered notes, computer files and guided us to access to copyrighted photos. Myles Clarke lent his critical eye to the references and footnotes. Thanks to all.

Fame is fleeting as the saying goes and Tom addresses it in his conclusion in Chap. 11. To understand the past is to prepare for the future. And in the end as mentioned in one of his last lectures that I heard him give (via Zoom, of course), he, a basic scientist at heart, looked for these future "Lone Pines" to emerge from basic science fields such as genetics and molecular biology. Enjoy.

C.S. Mott Children's Hospital
University of Michigan
Ann Arbor, MI, USA

Macdonald Dick

# Introduction

In the unlit hollow where life organizes itself, a miniscule tube transforms into an exquisite pump. This process is convoluted, despite taking place on a tiny scale: in an embryo less than 2 mm long the primitive heart is a straight tube, less than half a pencil-lead wide. Yet as it grows, this tube bends and twists, effecting an elegant origami as it transforms it into four complex chambers.[1] Rapidly multiplying cells thicken the walls in some sections of the developing heart. In others, cells die and disappear, leaving behind gossamer leaves of one-way valves, a creation by subtraction no sculptor has equaled. Cables of myocardial cells with special electrical inclinations—to control the rhythm of the heart—are laid in precise corridors. As if this feat of bio-fabrication weren't miracle enough, the half-formed heart begins pumping when the embryo is just 4 mm from crown to rump—nature's equivalent of cooking Thanksgiving dinner while renovating the kitchen. Its design is pretty much complete by 8 weeks, when the heart spans only about 3 mm (Fig. 1).

At birth, this tiny human engine is gorgeous. Walnut-sized, glistening pink and etched with finely serrated bands of muscle and tiny arteries, two or three times a second it swells almost imperceptibly, then wrings out the blood so accepted, as relentless as the balance wheel of a Swiss watch. This pump is as complex as it is exquisite. In a book describing the development of the Boeing 777, the enormous plane is referred to as "4,000,000 parts all moving in close formation."[2] If so, it comes a poor second to the newborn human heart, with nearly two billion cells beating in close formation.[3]

[1] Davis (1927, pp. 245–284).

[2] Sabbagh (1996, p. 40).

[3] Rakusan (1984, p. 146).

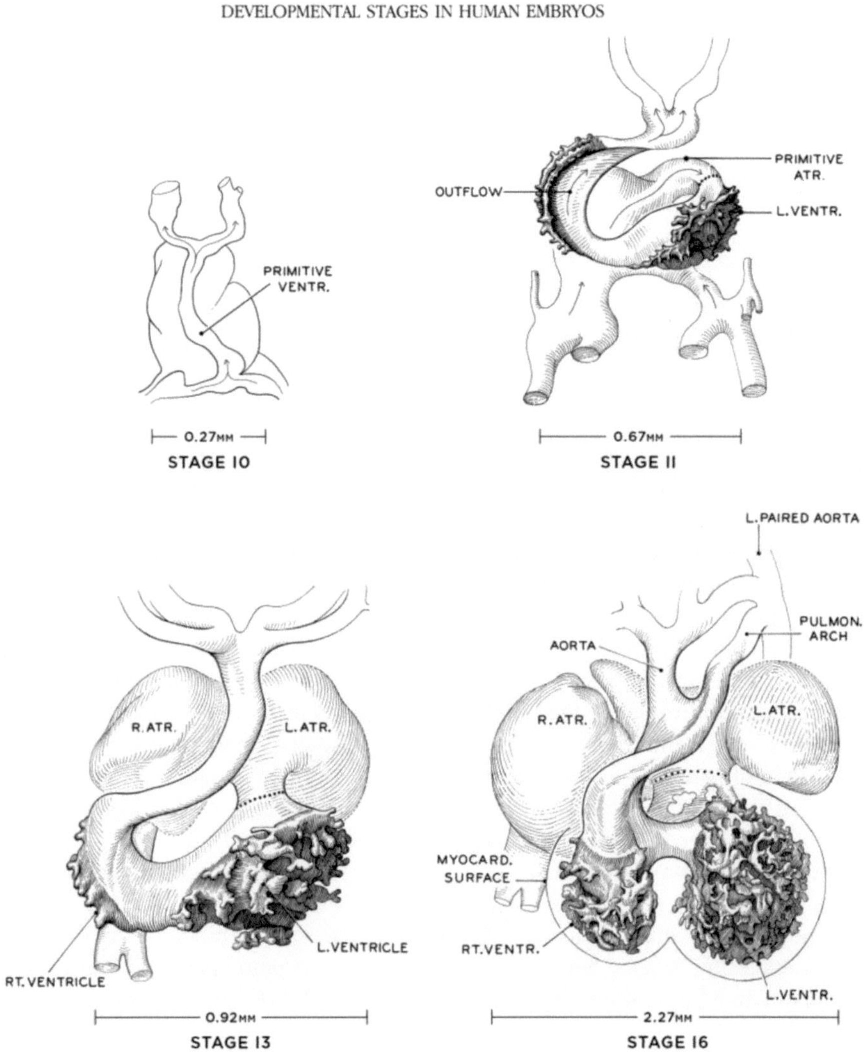


**Fig. 1** Diagram of early cardiac embryonal development. (With permission from O'Rahilly and Muller (1987))

The embryo accurately crafts this vital muscle over 99 times out of a 100,[4] but its shape can go awry at many turns: Valves are misshapen and do not open or close properly, or even have gone missing; a hole between the chambers permits abnormal blood flow inside the heart; blood vessels connecting with the heart link up to the wrong chamber.[5] Not uncommonly, multiple defects are combined. Conceptually, the heart is deceptively simple—four chambers, four valves, and a few attached blood vessels—and small; an adult's heart can be squeezed into a 12 ounce soda can. Its major features are few and its size trifling, but cardiac defects are of such perplexing variety that the world's most famous cardiac pathologists have been squabbling for decades over how to think about and describe congenital anomalies in these few cubic inches of organic real estate. Some of these malformations may be of little consequence and the individual, unaware, lives a normal lifetime, but a few so critically compromise cardiac function that life ends before it really starts.

Of the many varieties of cardiac anomalies, "single ventricle" malformations have commanded the most attention for the past several decades. Variations on this theme are legion, the common denominator being that the heart has only one, rather than the usual two pumping chambers (ventricles), and other abnormalities (usually of the valves or blood vessels) are also almost always present. While this might seem untenable for the developing fetus, in utero development is usually otherwise substantially normal.[6] William Harvey, the seventeenth-century English physician who first described the circulation of blood, in some sense anticipated this centuries before it could assume clinical relevance: "In embryos, while the lungs are still inactive and perform no function, as if they are not even present, nature uses the two ventricles of the heart as if they formed (only) one for the transmission of the blood."[7] While that's not exactly true, it's true enough—inside the womb's singular environment, the requirements for cardiovascular function are very different than outside.

There is occasionally a grace period for a baby with a single ventricle, though it usually runs out well before her first true smile. The problem is always one of blood

[4]Actually, the embryo's batting average for producing a normal heart is imprecisely known, and estimates of the prevalence of congenital heart disease in newborn babies vary. The Baltimore-Washington Infant Study found 4.9/1000 newborns to have a congenital heart defect (Ferencz et al. 1993, p. 42). In a review of 62 published reports, Hoffman and Kaplan (2002) found the incidence of congenital heart defects to vary widely but concluded that about 5.5/1000 live births will have a heart defect requiring therapy in childhood. Also, about 15% of pregnancies spontaneously terminate between the 3rd (when the heart is just beginning to form) and the 26th week of fetal life (Harlap in Porter and Hook (1980, pp. 145–158)). Some of these spontaneous terminations are presumably due to severe maldevelopment of the heart.

[5]For a summary of congenital heart defects, their characteristics and treatment, see Allen et al. (2016).

[6]In utero brain development is often abnormal in some patients with some forms of single ventricle (Licht et al. 2009; Matthiesen et al. 2016; Hansen et al. 2017), possibly due to abnormal hemodynamics associated with the cardiac malformation. A significant fraction of these patients also have other congenital abnormalities (Patel et al. 2016).

[7]Harvey (Carty), *de Motu*, p. 39.

flow, depending upon the malformation's geometry. In some cases, the body's circulation is reduced to a trickle. With other malformations, too little blood reaches the lungs. Hypoxia—insufficient oxygen in the blood—sets in, starving especially the heart and brain of the element most acutely needed for energy generation. In yet others, *excess* blood flow to the lungs forces the heart to pump more than it is designed to handle, ultimately debilitating the baby. Untreated, survival outside the first few weeks or months is rare.[8]

Even so, untreated single ventricles[9] do occasionally eke their way well into adulthood.[10] Early observers (before modern therapy) documented survival out to the third or fourth decade—one paper reported a death at the age 56 years—with some souls having few symptoms until shortly before dying.[11] And untreated survivors still surface now and again. Early in my career, I saw a Mexican boy several years old who had somehow found his way to the University of Minnesota Hospitals. Otherwise looking much like other kids his age, his cyanosis (the blue skin color seen with certain cardiac malformations) was the only tip-off that he had a heart defect. I can still picture the angiograms (radiologic movies of the heart) that told the story: His left ventricle was tiny, and only the right ventricle pumped blood. "Hypoplastic left heart syndrome" is ordinarily lethal in infancy, but in his case a blood vessel (the ductus arteriosus) which normally closes shortly after birth didn't, providing an avenue for his right ventricle to send blood to his lungs and body. This, combined with lungs which accepted blood less readily than usual, summed up to three wrongs making a right. And later in my fellowship, I was paged to the emergency room at the Hospitals to see a gangling teenage boy with a pounding solo ventricle. He had gone into atrial flutter, an abnormal heart rhythm often afflicting such patients. As apparently healthy as any of his friends, he had spent little time in the company of cardiology until that night. His malformation (of a different type than the other boy's) had been diagnosed years ago, but there seemed insufficient reason to subject him to surgery that, in the 1970s, had a sobering risk of mortality and an unknown long-term outcome. I don't know what became of either of these fellows, although they may have enjoyed many more years before losing much steam.

Although lengthy natural survival is anecdotal rather than typical, it offered doctors a vital clue: It's not the missing ventricle that is rate-limiting, at least over a run of many years.[12] The vascular connections between the heart and body and lungs,

---

[8] For example, as of 1978, before the advent of effective therapy, of 72 neonates with hypoplastic left heart syndrome (the most common type of single ventricle) at a large pediatric hospital, only 18% were alive at 1 week of age and all had succumbed by 7 months (Keith et al. 1978, pp. 544, 547).

[9] For the sake of reducing word clutter, I sometimes use "single ventricle" as shorthand for a *person* with this malformation (in the same way that "diabetic" substitutes for a person with diabetes). For this I apologize, recognizing that people are not their medical condition.

[10] Taussig (1947, pp. 96, 292, appendices I and II), Nadas (1957, pp. 337–339), and Dick et al. (1975).

[11] Peacock (1858, pp. 16–18), Abbott (1908, p. 363), Jordan and Sanders (1966), and Keith et al. (1978, pp. 535–536).

[12] Rychik et al. (2019).

and how the lungs regulate their blood flow, largely determine the patient's fate. Very occasionally, as for the boys described above, a single ventricle has a fortuitous combination of derangements that, in effect, balance each other out, and are compatible with a relatively long life.[13] For the majority not so lucky, one ventricle is quite enough if the cardiovascular system is *surgically* reshaped. That's game-changing, since growing a second ventricle isn't possible, neither now nor for the foreseeable future.

Starting in the mid-1940s, ingenious operations were devised as workarounds, directing blood flow to provide a functional, if hardly normal, circulation. One reads about *repair* of the single ventricle; indeed, two of the landmark papers in the history of these therapies flaunt "repair" in their title.[14] But that's using the word far too generously. Doctors cannot craft a normal circulatory system for the single ventricle; our treatments are *palliative*. Current therapies sustain life beyond what nature, unmodified, usually offers, but cannot produce a circulation as efficient, dynamic, or resilient as normal. People with a single ventricle require surgery, medicines, and close medical follow-up. Their maximum exercise capacity is less than their two-ventricle peers, as is their life expectancy. Pregnancy, while often possible, carries a substantial risk of serious complications and fetal mortality. And, like my Minnesota patient, they may suffer heart-related complications and hospital stays. Life with a single ventricle is a different journey than most of us take, with speed bumps and detours that a second ventricle would have avoided.

But surgical treatment is still beautiful palliation. Class plays, diploma walks, dirt bike races, soccer games, friendships, happy marriages, and uncountable other experiences have been added to the calendar of people who would have otherwise perished shy of diaper graduation. People enjoy family lives and raise families of their own. They drive trucks, sell real estate, doctor, lawyer, teach, and build businesses. "Heck, I jumped out of a plane, I should be able to do anything"—so blogged a vital and eloquent woman with a single ventricle—"but sometimes the superhero gets scared too. So, after a good cry, I put back on my big girl cape and do me as long as I can. When I see the little CHD (congenital heart disease) patients I care for (as a pediatric cardiac intensive care nurse), I realize I work in a field I love. I travel, I play violin in an orchestra, I'm learning to swim, I have a rabbit and a bird, a family that loves me, and my parents are still with me. You know, I've lived almost a

[13] This course is rarely enjoyed by few people my colleagues or I have encountered with a single ventricle heart (Pickup et al. 2017). But they also face many special challenges. Formal academic studies differ in design, methodology, and patients surveyed, and their findings are therefore inconsistent, but most have found that quality of life in adolescents and adults with a single ventricle heart is often reduced relative to those without chronic illness. The reasons for this primarily relate to physical activity limitations, symptoms, and cognitive and psychosocial difficulties (Uzark et al. 2016; Overgaard et al. 2011, 2014; Pike et al. 2011, 2012; Idorn et al. 2013; Saliba et al. 2001). But studies have also reported an amazing resilience among single ventricle heart patients, who develop strong coping strategies, a feeling of being comfortable with their heart, and satisfaction with life experiences (Berghammer et al. 2015; Zahmacioglu et al. 2011).

[14] Fontan and Baudet (1971) and Norwood et al. (1983).

half century with half a heart! I have been blessed!" (my parentheses).[15] The creation of effective, if imperfect, therapies—"single ventricle rescue" is my shorthand for this suite of treatments—proudly stands as a major landmark in *congenital cardiology*, my condensation of pediatric cardiology and cardiac surgery.

Activity in this space is mushrooming. It's no exaggeration to say that we live in the day of the single ventricle, stretching out as far as the eye can see. Strenuous efforts to improve current therapy are partly responsible: Academic centers join in outcomes research, where survival, quality of life, and complications are captured and analyzed; clinical trials investigate possibly useful medications; computer modeling of cardiovascular flow patterns will—we hope—inform more efficient surgical reconfigurations. Organisms as diverse as mice, fish, and flies, and their constituent cells, are interrogated in basic science labs, searching for biological insights transformable into new drugs.[16] Careers have been and are being built in the single ventricle factory, as practitioners develop novel therapies and cardiac surgeons apply existing and innovative techniques ever more cleverly.

The single ventricle's impact is also a matter of demographics. Each year, roughly 3000 single ventricle babies are born in the United States, and over 1000 Fontan operations (discussed later) are performed; by 2018, about 50,000 to 70,000 people, worldwide, had had this operation.[17] Nothing better attests to the success of current therapy than the ever-expanding population of patients growing ever older, which translates into an increasing demand for medical services. Single ventricle rescue accounts for much of congenital cardiology's many-fold growth since the 1980s, reverberating throughout the field more forcefully than any development since open heart surgery's invention in the early 1950s.

*Reimagining a Child's Heart* explores the invention of pivotal therapies, which amplify life's quantity and quality for people with a single ventricle. It is, in other words, a creation story of single ventricle rescue. While there are many ways to fashion its history, I'm inclined to share it from 10,000 feet rather than ground level, staying mostly big picture and out of the weeds. High altitude, of course, implies focusing on the most substantial features on the landscape, concentrating the juices

---

[15] Grasty (2016).

[16] For me, "science" connotes an activity that generates knowledge and ideas about how the natural world works, and which is grounded in empirical observations (Fores 1971, p. 624). Thus, the goal of science is to understand how nature works in general and fundamental ways. The term *basic science* is sometimes used to distinguish this search for fundamental knowledge from a related but distinct activity: utilizing the methods employed by basic science (e.g., careful study design, experimental verification of hypotheses, obtaining quantitative data) to answer practical *clinical* questions. For example, studying the effect of a drug on blood pressure and its adverse effects in a sample of people is needed to determine the utility of such therapy, but may reveal little about human biology. These investigations sometimes contribute to our understanding of how nature works, but that is not their primary goal. Most of the "science" in "scientific" medicine refers to this sort of activity. I mean *basic* science when I say that science is only a fraction of what goes into therapy creation. However, even if science is more broadly construed, that still leaves it the flour in the chocolate cake—other key ingredients are still required.

[17] Hoffman and Kaplan (2002), Akintoye et al. (2019), and Rychik et al. (2019).

of therapy creation and avoiding the tedium of unproductive detail. (I say more about this later.) My second aim is to tightly link new therapies with their authors. The human element is the most engaging piece of many narratives, but it enriches in another way: Unlike a painting or novel, one need know nothing about a therapy's creator to understand the creation but considering both in our case yields invaluable lessons about what spins invention's gears. We, therefore, will explore *major, seminal developments and their creators*—Lone Pines, as one might think of them, standing distinct from the rest of the landscape. Our story encompasses much more than the single ventricle: Because these treatments are tightly interwoven with those for other cardiac defects, single ventricle rescue affords an opportunity to examine therapy invention across much of congenital cardiology. Indeed, it provides a perspective onto medical innovation extending beyond congenital heart disease.[18]

*Ancient* therapy for congenital heart disease—medicines of limited efficacy (or worse) and activity prescriptions—fades back hundreds of years, at least. Patients were made to bleed, puke, poop, and blister, and were exposed to various toxins. There was some value, if only placebo, in these "treatments," but none modified the pathology of the heart defects. *Modern* therapy is primarily surgical or interventional catheter-based procedures, complemented by medical interventions. Reconfiguring tissue *does* improve cardiovascular function, sometimes even normalizing a severely deranged circulation. Using the power of available therapies as the indicator of its state of the art, I think of congenital cardiology as unfolding over *three eras*.[19] During its multi-millennial *Early Days*, people advanced from knowing nearly nothing about the body to almost enough for successful surgical interventions. Knowledge and craft accumulated slowly at first, then more rapidly in the early twentieth century, with the first successful cardiac surgery being performed in 1938. The *New Dawn* of congenital cardiology, with its first truly effective therapy, was the first of its two major disruptions. The surgery was limited in scope and applicable to only a fraction of people with defects, but the discipline was galloping along now, and this era lasted only about 15 years. During congenital cardiology's *Modern* era, it was radically transformed again, this time by the invention of open heart surgery in the early 1950s. Heart defects previously unapproachable, or whose ill effects could be only alleviated, were now repaired. This breakthrough and more sophisticated physiology eventually culminated in the apogee of single ventricle rescue, the Fontan operation. In one sense a strange operation, out of physiological step with other cardiac procedures (as we later see), the Fontan—and all of single ventricle rescue—is nevertheless of a piece with the whole of congenital cardiology.

One cannot usefully discuss therapy creation without a few words on its basics. Threaded through congenital cardiology's evolution (and most therapy invention) is what can be thought of as the *fabric* of therapy creation. Its strands include *knowledge, ideas,* and *craft*.

[18] I leave largely or completely untouched many factors (organizational, financial, ethical, legal, educational) impacting medical creation.

[19] Congenital cardiology's evolution can be construed in other ways; for example, see Neill and Clark (1995).

Two types of knowledge course through the cloth. The first is derived from *scientific* investigations, usually carried out in the laboratory, although occasionally in the clinical domain. Medical innovation has so often revolved around the axle of science that the "art and science of medicine" sums up its essence for many, including notable scholars.[20] Claude Bernard was under no illusion (in 1865) that medicine was scientifically well-grounded, but envisioned it maturing into an "*exact science* based on experimental determinism" (my emphasis).[21] Eighty years hence, Richard H. Shryock, in *The Development of Modern Medicine* (1947), described how science and medicine have pulled each other along since the fifteenth century. Mightily impressed with the advances in scientific medicine, Shryock wondered whether "the spectacular progress made in (medical) science during the past century" hadn't even led the public to expect too much of medicine.[22] More recently, Roy Porter married science and medicine in his *The Greatest Benefit to Mankind: A Medical History of Humanity* (1997). After reciting the scientific provenance of a string of milestone advances, he concluded that "Basic research, clinical science and technology working with one another have characterized the cutting edge of modern medicine."[23]

Medicine's predilection to look to basic science for the grist of new treatments is most concretely—literally—conveyed by a visit to most academic medical centers and taking in edifices packed with basic science labs. Whom the National Institutes of Health employs in its intramural research program is also revealing; the vast majority of its roughly 1200 researchers have a PhD (with or without an MD).[24] Unlike medical training, aimed primarily at producing practicing physicians, basic scientists are the goal of PhD training. This is not to say that MDs are never basic science researchers—indeed there are many—but the predominance of PhDs reveals an inclination to rely upon investigators with the most strenuous science backgrounds for treatment-animating discoveries. Congenital cardiology, like other disciplines, has advanced on the back of science, in ways both obvious and not. Consider, for example, the iconic Norwood operation. In the late 1970s, Bill Norwood finally cracked the nut of neonatal hypoplastic left heart rescue when he crafted a technical tour-de-force which made him famous, at least in the world of congenital cardiology. Less widely appreciated is the fact that his operation's impact would be puny had it not been for the work of two relatively little-known physicians working in Toronto; the "prostaglandin $E_1$" they spirited from the laboratory to the intensive care unit proved as vital to the success of the Norwood as a runway is for

[20] Bing (1999, p. xiii).

[21] Bernard (1865/1927, p. 140).

[22] Shryock (1947, p. 431).

[23] Porter (1997, p. 595).

[24] National Institutes of Health, Physician-Scientist Workforce Working Group (2014, p. 16).

an airliner.[25] Whether palpable or obscure (mostly the latter), scientific discovery has been indispensable for single ventricle rescue.

But thinking of therapy for congenital defects—or any medical innovation—as purely an expression of applied science is a hopelessly *incomplete* way of understanding its genesis.[26] While laboratory discoveries periodically urge the field forward, much of what is central to therapy creation isn't "science." In Chap. 5 I suggest that the first successful intracardiac surgery may have been as much *delayed* as facilitated by laboratory exertions, and that it owed its eventual development—at least in the hands of Charles Bailey—more to a pretty homely variety of knowledge. Bailey, a primary inventor of early mitral valve surgery, cited his previous experience selling ladies lingerie—not experiments—as pivotal for developing his operation.

And so we come to the second species of knowledge, *clinically derived information*. Acquired in the course of treating people, not experimental dogs or cats, nor derived from clinical trials or other formal studies, its laboratory is the hospital, the clinic, or even phone calls with patients. If we had perfect animal models, applicable to all clinical scenarios, human observation could be supplanted by lab investigations. Unfortunately, such models are usually lacking and often unreliable when available. "Scientific" clinical trials are the gold standard for evaluating medications, but many drugs have never been so studied, or formally assessed in the context of some specific uses. Congenital cardiac operations are rarely rigorously studied;[27] efficacy is more commonly assessed through workaday observations and retrospective reviews. Doctors have learned, and continue to learn, much of what works, and what doesn't, through clinical experience. It tells us how to safely and effectively apply available concepts and interventions, and also *provides new ideas* for therapy. One idea from congenital cardiology's most esteemed pioneers grew directly from unstructured clinical observations made by a highly perceptive and esteemed cardiologist.

*Ideas* suggest ways to extract new knowledge and transforming existing knowledge into a concept or theory, or to a practical end. Their significance needs no elaboration.

*Craft*, as I use the word, is done with the hands. It is the capacity to make physical transformations with one's hands (tools are usually involved), and it implies something more than rudimentary skills. And more than manual dexterity is required. The Italian word *designo*, as applied in the context of art, is perhaps better, as it specifies both the skill to transform materials *and* the ability to design the transformation.[28] For many types of therapy creation—developing new medicines, for example—craft plays little if any role, but for congenital cardiology, advancing the

---

[25] Olley and Coceani (1976) and Elliott et al. (1975). Other investigators were involved as well, as discussed in Chap. 10.

[26] Weisse (1991).

[27] For an example, see the rare example of a prospective trial for a congenital cardiac surgical procedure, Ohye et al. (2010).

[28] Bambach (2017, p. 21).

craft *can be* inventing therapy. The manual expertise needed for cardiac interventions is not innate; individuals must learn how to manipulate tissues. When they teach others how to do the same, the craft is diffused throughout the field. Craft can be developed in the lab, but not always. Surgeons learned a lot about manipulating tissues using animals, but lacking such models for most defects, technique was mostly developed in the clinical arena.

Finally, I use "fabric of therapy creation" to splice the above elements with the *human qualities* needed to generate them. The centrality of the human element in medical—and all—invention is, of course, old news. Richard Bing emphasized this in *Cardiology: The Evolution of the Science and the Art*. "This editor has lived through three phases of cardiology: a purely clinical phase … a period … where some cardiac diseases were explained on a purely hemodynamic basis … and, finally, a time when invasive procedures together with biochemistry, biophysics, and molecular biology became the primary influence. The common denominator in this rapidly changing field has been the *human factor*. … Without the human element, history becomes a colorless recitation of facts. This is even more true when dealing with medical science, which has as its final goal the application of science to human beings" (italics mine).[29] Sherwin Nuland's lyrical *Doctors: The Biography of Medicine* takes precisely this tack; doctors are the warp and weft of his account of medicine's evolution.[30] Allen Weisse's *Medical Odysseys*, though organized around specific discoveries and developments, is centered more on innovators than technical details.[31]

The pioneers who rescued the single ventricle, and their qualities and inclinations, permeate *Reimagining a Child's Heart*. They were reasonably smart, of course, and typically worked hard. All were curious, but in varying degrees and to different ends. A few burned to know for knowing's sake, while others sought understanding chiefly to achieve a practical end. And they were almost (but not quite) always "all in," sustained by a bone-deep belief in their work. All are important qualities, but not their most salient. Three characteristics, recurring with monotonous regularity, strike me as the most potent drivers of these pioneers' extraordinary contributions: capacious *imagination* and its progeny, a proclivity for *thinking differently*, and extraordinary *tenacity*. We see later that science and clinical observations revealed the nature of cyanosis, but that imagination was the driver of its first effective therapy. Cardiology's core discovery was made by a man thinking differently while gnawing away on a puzzle-bone for several years. And an early aficionado mustered congenital cardiology's critical mass by laying more and more bricks into a structure that others had long since been satisfied to declare complete. Time and again, whether the quest was to gain new knowledge, hone the craft, or transform them into therapy, what strikes me most—to paraphrase Edison—was that the perspiration, rather than inspiration, paid out. Of these three innovation-powering

[29] Bing (1999, p. xiii).

[30] Nuland (1989).

[31] Weisse (1991).

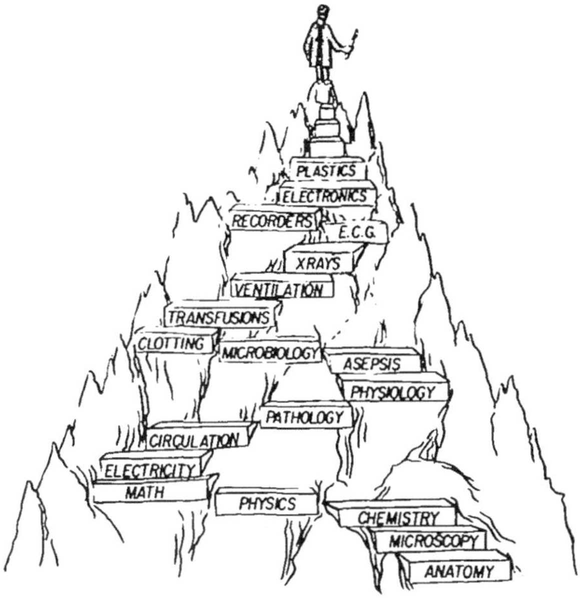


**Fig. 2** Comroe and Dripps diagram. (Comroe Jr and Dripps (1974) (Fig. 2 from that paper). Permission granted by Circulation Research (footnote in article). Comroe and Dripps pointed out that an accumulation of many scientific advances was required to culminate in the ability to conduct open heart surgery)

characteristics, history shows that tenacity is the most potent: Congenital cardiology advanced not by a hundred chicks pecking once at their shell, but by a handful of chicks pecking hundreds of times.

That is not to say that other human attributes have not bent rescue's trajectory. Charles Bailey, who made the cover of *TIME* magazine in 1957, recalled his state of mind while pursuing mitral valve work after his early fatal failures jeopardized his medical license: "Finally, however, you have to face the 'moment of truth,' and the poignancy is so great that I can't really express it. You know that almost all the world is against it; you know that you have a great personal stake and might even lose your medical license, or at least your hospital privileges if you persist. In fact, the thought crosses your mind that maybe you really *are* crazy. And yet you feel that it has to be done and it must be right."[32]

If the single ventricle story must be an amalgam of inventions and inventors, the question is, which ones? In 1974, Julius Comroe and Robert Dripps articulated the knowledge required for developing open heart surgery.[33] After identifying 25 essential bodies of knowledge (e.g., diagnostic skills and blood transfusion expertise), they listed a raft of developments populating these bodies (Fig. 2). And this is a gross over-simplification—a complete accounting would reveal that each step on the mountain rests on a previous one, and that perhaps even those granite chunks are supported by yet others. This list concerns only open heart surgery, while our story encompasses much more; a thorough archeological reconstruction would involve undoing numberless skeins of developments. So what goes in and what stays out?

[32] Weisse (2002, p. 77).

[33] Comroe Jr and Dripps (1974).

I constructed this history with two things in mind. First, I wanted to write a book for the reader who prefers a jewel-studded crown to a large sack of gems; that is, someone hoping to enjoy the most beautiful and important jewels, arranged in a coherent pattern, rather than every loose stone in history's sack. This book is for those curious about congenital heart disease (and therapy creation), many nonmedical people, for whom every jot and tittle become a distraction. Second, some developments and people in this story clearly eclipse others, and the less significant should not distract attention from the most. This strategy mostly (though not entirely) ignores the discipline's many operational advances, the landscape anchoring the pioneers. For example, learning how to make a diagnosis and the best use of various medications and procedures are largely passed over, as important as they are. But their provenance is usually diverse, multiple, and often obscure, so it is hard to extract a story and useful lessons. Signal developments are not the whole history, but they comprise the most concentrated and vibrant chapters.

The pioneers are therefore the spine of our story. I've used three criteria to select them: First, these are major, discipline-changing contributions, linked with names and sometimes dates, and often major awards. A thought experiment characterizes them: How would single ventricle rescue (and congenital cardiology) be different if the advancement had never been made? If the answer is that the field would be a mere shadow of what it is today, that suggests pioneers. The contributions selected come down to judgment and personal inclinations, of course, but I am a bit buoyed by a recent survey of practitioners who were asked to suggest the outstanding people or seminal contributions in congenital cardiology. Of the eight most often mentioned, I had (independently) chosen six. Second, with a few exceptions (especially in the first two chapters), they are specific to congenital cardiology, or closely adjacent fields (such as non-congenital heart surgery). Medicine-wide inventions (as crucial as they have been) such as X-ray, pharmacology, anesthesiology, and ultrasound imaging are not covered; their development was diffuse and not congenital cardiology-specific. Finally then, pioneers have definable temporal margins. While the knowledge and craft underlying them may have accreted slowly, they abruptly changed the scenery, via publication of a book or papers, or a first successful operation. Much of congenital cardiology's operational landscape—for example, how it decided which holes in the heart to close, and when—evolved too gradually and without a definite point of resolution to make much of a story—at least a very interesting one for the non-cardiologist.

The pioneers selected are described below. Even if theirs are not congenital cardiology's only significant advances, none exceed them. With a few exceptions, they have been previously chronicled, and for some (e.g., Harvey's circulation and the Blalock-Taussig-Thomas shunt[34]), many times. I think that there are good reasons to

[34] For many years this iconic operation was known as the Blalock-Taussig shunt; more recently recognition of Vivian Thomas's major contribution has resulted in renaming it the Blalock-Taussig-Thomas shunt. Tom did not know of this prior to his writing this chapter but he clearly recognized it as his Chap. 6 about the shunt demonstrates. Thus we have updated the B-T shunt to the B-T-T shunt.

revisit them. First, their stories have been often incompletely told: Interesting and provocative aspects of inventions and their creators have gone unexplored, or never placed in revealing context. For example: Breakthroughs often ride in on the back of new technology; new tools (e.g., the microscope or a means of measuring the amount of oxygen in the blood) enable the discovery of the previously undiscoverable. While the profound significance of Harvey's discovery of the circulation has often been (correctly) stressed, it is little noted that he made it using the *very same tools* as were available for over 1400 years. And another: Robert Gross, congenital cardiology's primogenitor surgeon, had invented a novel operation, but when a cardiologist from Johns Hopkins suggested that he apply it to desperately sick humans he summarily declined. Why? And a third: Vivien Thomas, laboratory technician for Alfred Blalock, a great American surgeon, is widely lauded for his role in developing congenital cardiology's single most important operation. I found a trove of new angles to history long since told, and I try to cast a raking light on rather shop-worn stories so that we can see, and think about them, differently.

The second justification for my strategy is *pattern*. Patterns and themes emerge when multiple inventions and inventors are explored in depth that otherwise never see the light of day. The near invariance of tenaciousness as a prime enabler of innovation is one example. But an even more indelible motif is the no rules rule: Components of creation's fabric have been—for one pioneer or another—culled from nearly the entire register of human characteristics and motivations. Chicks pecking many times is a near constant, but how they work the shell, and why, runs the gamut. And another pattern: Accounts of medical invention have highlighted how creators found proof of principle, and sometimes even perfected therapies, in the animal lab. But the more subtle but truer pattern is that animal models are often unavailable or fickle. They get ignored, sometimes with salutary results, sometimes not. Though the image of a pioneer suggests anything but a pattern, by considering many of them, over a long span of time, interesting themes ultimately emerge.

This book is arranged in three parts, each covering one era. Its *Early Days* was chockablock with new knowledge and ideas, especially from the sixteenth century on, when ingenious investigators tremendously expanded biology and medicine's foundational folio. Anatomists demonstrated new details of our corporeal architecture, and physiologists probed organ function and the body's uncanny talent for adjusting its internal milieu to accommodate ever-changing conditions. Microscopes and special stains revealed that tissues are an association of many individual cells, a discovery of transcendent significance for biology. Pharmacologists defined the cellular actions of ancient medicines and added new remedies. Embryologists surveilled developing organisms and (just) scratched the surface of the miracle of embryogenesis. Any of these advances, or yet others, could have been woven into the story. I chose instead two achievements that, while suffusing all of medicine, are especially germane for congenital cardiology: the discovery of the blood's circulation, and the uncovering of the body's scheme for energy generation. The cardiovascular system and lungs subserve multiple functions but energy production is the biggie (Chap. 2). The stuff of cellular energy generation (*cellular respiration*)—oxygen and fuels, mostly sugars and fats—must be continuously supplied to all sectors of the body, or the cell's machinery abruptly collapses. This is as basic as biology gets—of all the lines and curves on physiology's blueprint, none are more fundamental. In fact, boiled down, the problem of heart disease is one of reduced oxygen and fuel delivery; too little blood is pumped (or its quantity cannot be augmented with exercise), or the blood contains too little oxygen, or both. How Harvey traced the blood's path through the body, a quintessential, perhaps unequalled, demonstration of persistence and thinking differently, is Chapter One's main task. And as conceptually complete as his theory was, one piece he unavoidably left missing—the invisible connections between miniscule arteries and the cognate veins. This region of circulation's map was filled in by an Italian who, unlike Harvey, had more than tenacity going for him—new technology enabled his discovery.

How oxygen and fuel are delivered to the cells is Chapter One's charge, what happens once they get there is Chapter Two's. Spending only a little time with the chemical pathways and reactions involved, we are largely occupied with the puzzle of *air*: The ancients knew that life was hinged upon it but hadn't a clue why. Intensely curious and tenacious "natural philosophers" solved this puzzle, mostly powered by raw ingenuity. Science has always required measurements, made today using complex machines with inscrutable innards. It's hard to imagine it, but chemistry's foundation was laid using blown glass flasks, tubes, and brass balances. Early chemists separated air into its component parts, learned the basics of combustion followed by a glimmering notion of how the body burns fuel, using simple tools (including animals as chemical sensors) and a handful of chemicals. We touch on several pioneers responsible for unpacking cellular respiration, dwelling longest on a husband and wife team, tragically severed by the French Revolution, to whom chemistry—and, eventually, single ventricle rescue—are forever indebted.

In *Early Days*' last chapter, I paint a picture of what physicians grappled with on the threshold of congenital cardiology's *New Dawn*, as they ministered to their cardiac patients. Medicine had long substituted imagination and folk discovery for science, generating a formidable variety of drugs. A few could bring some relief to those suffering from heart defects. But most were of dubious benefit, and the fact is, with structural defects, there is no real substitute for structural remedy. Though not apparent at the time, heart surgery was on the near horizon, thanks partly to surgical craft developed over literally millennia. We briefly survey medicine's anodyne. *State of the Art* also explores how basic science and clinically derived knowledge joined to produce the first congenital cardiology-specific conceptual breakthrough, resolution of the puzzle of cyanosis, *the* iconic sign of congenital heart disease.

In *New Dawn*, we examine how an advance in the *craft* of cardiac surgery and a *growing understanding* of anatomy, physiology, and their clinical correlates twisted together to culminate in the *first congenital heart operations*. The invention of open heart surgery—which served as the poster child for hi-tech medicine until gene therapy and editing came along—was the biggest news in *Modern Era*. But advancing single ventricle rescue also required probing the *limits of cardiovascular physiology* in the laboratory, leading to the invention of the *Fontan operation*, this epoch's third fiber.

We settle into the *New Dawn* epoch as *Mens et Manus* describes how surgeons advanced into the heart's domain. Technical, as opposed to scientific, developments, as well as the strong personalities which spawned them, are these chapters' themes. Maude Abbott, our preoccupation in *Collector of Hearts*, was a most unusual woman and the author of what I think of as the Periodic Table of Congenital Cardiology. Her role in nascent congenital cardiology was vital; in fact, one imagines that the field might have only barely poked along for years without her infusion of energy and enthusiasm. The Blalock-Taussig-Thomas shunt operation was the first major breakthrough in single ventricle therapy; *Collaboration* dips into its technical aspects, but mostly lays eyes on the team that worked the problem. Human inclinations aplenty color this swatch of our tapestry, as does the invisible human infrastructure that fashioned it.

The *Modern Era,* third and last, commences with Chap. 7, *Dry Hearts—Breaching the Wall.* The invention of open heart surgery vastly expanded the healing repertoire of congenital cardiology and set the table for our most effective single ventricle rescue. *Strange Operation*, Chap. 9, describes how doctors invented a new circulation, known as the Fontan procedure. Very different in root concept than other therapies occupying the medical terrain, the Fontan currently occupies the apex of single ventricle rescue. For the vast majority of patients with a single ventricle, the Fontan is the most physiologically efficient form of palliation and the final goal of today's multi-stage treatment program. We also meet the Norwood procedure in our last chapter, a long-elusive surgery which extended single ventricle rescue to many babies formerly left out.

Single ventricles are so unusual that only a relatively few practitioners have a refined idea of the anatomy and physiology involved. But the meat and potatoes of the heart and vascular system, including most congenital malformations, is surprisingly straightforward. My aim is to present the basics, not arcane details, but enough so that even the uninitiated will be equipped to fully understand and enjoy this book. My goal: Those who turn a few pages will develop an understanding and appreciation of the essence of congenital heart disease.

Those with a curiosity for Tom's thinking about engineering and medical innovation, their similarities and differences, should check out his Appendices at a time of their own choosing.

## References

Abbott ME (1908) Chapter IX: Congenital cardiac disease. In: Osler W (ed) Modern medicine: its theory and practice, vol IV. Lea Brothers & Co., Philadelphia, pp 323–425

Akintoye E, Miranda WR, Veldtman GR, Connolly HM, Egbe AC (2019) National trends in Fontan operation and in-hospital outcomes in the USA. Heart 105:708–714

Allen HD, Shaddy RE, Penny DJ, Feltes TF, Cetta F (2016) Moss and Adams, heart disease in infants, children, and adolescents. Wolters Kluwer, Philadelphia

Bambach CC, Barry C, Caglioti F, Elam C, Marongiu M, Mussolin M (2017) Michelangelo: divine draftsman and designer. Metropolitan Museum of Art, New York

Berghammer MD, Brink E, Rydberg AM et al (2015) Committed to life: adolescents' and young adults' experiences of living with Fontan circulation. Congenit Heart Dis 10:403–412
Bernard C (1865/1927) An introduction to the study of experimental medicine (trans: Green HC). Macmillan Co., New York
Bing RJ (1999) Cardiology: the evolution of the science and the art, 2nd edn. Rutgers University Press, New Brunswick
Comroe JH Jr, Dripps RD (1974) Ben Franklin and open heart surgery. Circ Res 35:661–669
Davis CL (1927) Development of the human heart from its first appearance to the stage found in embryos of twenty paired somites. Contrib Embryol Carneg Inst 19:245–284
Dick M, Fyler DC, Nadas AA (1975) Tricuspid atresia: clinical course on 101 patients. Am J Cardiol 36:327–337
Elliott RB, Starling MB, Neutze JM (1975) Medical manipulation of the ductus arteriosus. Lancet 1(7899):140–142
Ferencz C, Rubin JD, Loffredo C, Magee CA (1993) Epidemiology of congenital heart disease: the Baltimore-Washington Infant Study, 1981–1989. Futura Publishing Co., Inc., Mount Kisco
Fontan F, Baudet E (1971) Surgical repair of tricuspid atresia. Thorax 26(3):240–248
Fores M (1971) Price, technology, and the paper model. Technol Cult 12:621–627
Grasty T (2016) Half a century with half a heart, 28 January 2016. https://www.achaheart.org/blog/2016/half-a-century-with-half-a-heart/. Accessed 2 Oct 2024
Hansen T, Henriksen TB, Bach CC, Matthiesen N (2017) Congenital heart defects and measures of prenatal brain growth: a systematic review. Pediatr Neurol 72:7–18
Harvey W (1628/2016) Exercitatio anatomica de motu cordis et sanguinis in animalibus [On the motion of the heart and blood in animals] (Carty JA ed, trans: Willis R). Resource Publications, Eugene
Hoffman JIE, Kaplan S (2002) The incidence of congenital heart disease. J Am Coll Cardiol 39:1890–1900
Idorn L, Jensen AS, Juul K et al (2013) Quality of life and cognitive function in Fontan patients, a population-based study. Int J Cardiol 168:3230–3235
Jordan JC, Sanders CA (1966) Tricuspid atresia with prolonged survival. Am J Cardiol 18:112–119
Keith JD, Rowe RD, Vlad P (1978) Heart disease in infancy and childhood, 3rd edn. Macmillan Publishing Co., Inc., New York
Licht DJ, Shera DM, Clancy RR, Weronvsky G, Montenegro LM, Nicolson SC et al (2009) Brain maturation is delayed in infants with complex congenital heart defects. J Thorac Cardiovasc Surg 137:529–536
Matthiesen NB, Henriksen TB, Gaynor JW et al (2016) Congenital heart defects and indices of fetal cerebral growth in a nationwide cohort of 924422 liveborn infants. Circulation 133:566–575
Nadas AS (1957) Pediatric cardiology. W.B. Saunders Co., Philadelphia
National Institutes of Health (2014) Physician-Scientist Workforce Working Group report, June 2014. https://acd.od.nih.gov/documents/reports/PSW_Report_ACD_06042014.pdf. Accessed 3 Oct 2024
Neill CA, Clark EB (1995) The developing heart: a history of pediatric cardiology. Kluwer Academic Publishers, Dordrecht
Norwood WI, Lang P, Hansen DD (1983) Physiologic repair of aortic atresia-hypoplastic left heart syndrome. N Engl J Med 308:23–26
Nuland SB (1989) Doctors: the biography of medicine. Knopf, New York
Ohye RG, Sleeper LA, Mahony L et al (2010) Comparison of shunt types in the Norwood procedure for single-ventricle lesions. N Engl J Med 362(21):1980–1992
Olley PM, Coceani F (1976) E-type prostaglandins: a new emergency therapy for certain cyanotic congenital heart malformations. Circulation 53:728–731
O'Rahilly R, Muller F (1987) Developmental stages in human embryos, vol 637. Carnegie Institution of Washington, Publication pp 100, 180
Overgaard D, Schrader A-M, Lisby KH et al (2011) Patient-reported outcomes in adult survivors with single-ventricle physiology. Cardiology 120:36–42

Overgaard D, Schrader A-M, Lisby KH et al (2014) Substance use, dental hygiene, and physical activity in adult patients with single ventricle physiology. Congenit Heart Dis 9:75–82

Patel A, Costello JM, Backer CL et al (2016) Prevalence of noncardiac and genetic abnormalities in neonates undergoing cardiac operations: analysis of the Society of Thoracic Surgeons congenital heart surgery database. Ann Thorac Surg 102:1607–1614

Peacock TB (1858) On malformations, &c., of the human heart. John Churchill, London. Reprinted in The Classics of Medicine Library. Gryphon Editions, Ltd, Birmingham; 1981

Pickup L, Gaffey T, Clift P et al (2017) Employment characteristics of a complex adult disease cohort. Occup Med 67(6):453–455

Pike NA, Evangelista LS, Doering LV et al (2011) Clinical profile of the adolescent/adult Fontan survivor. Congenit Heart Dis 6:9–17

Pike NA, Evangelista LS, Doering LV et al (2012) Quality of life, health status, and depression: a comparison between adolescents and adults after Fontan procedure with health counterparts. J Cardiovasc Nurs 26:539–546

Porter R (1997) The greatest benefit to mankind: a medical history of humanity. W.W. Norton & Co., New York

Porter IH, Hook EB (1980) Human embryonic and fetal death. Academic, New York

Rakusan K (1984) Cardiac growth, maturation, and aging. In: Zak R (ed) Growth of the heart in health and disease. Raven Press, New York, pp 131–164

Rychik J, Atz A, Celermajer DS, Deal B, Gatzoulis MA, Gewillig MH et al (2019) Evaluation and management of the child and adult with Fontan circulation. Circulation 140:e234–e284

Sabbagh K (1996) Twenty-first-century jet: the making and marketing of the Boeing 777. Scribner, New York

Saliba Z, Butera G, Bonhoeffer P et al (2001) Quality of life and perceived health status in surviving adults with univentricular heart. Heart 86:69–73

Shryock RH (1947) The development of modern medicine. Knopf, New York

Taussig HB (1947) Congenital malformations of the heart. The Commonwealth Fund, New York

Uzark K, Zak V, Shrader P et al (2016) Assessment of quality of life in young patients with single ventricle after the Fontan operation. J Pediatr 170:166–172

Weisse AB (1991) Medical odysseys: the different and sometimes unexpected pathways to twentieth-century medical discoveries. Rutgers University Press, New Brunswick

Weisse AB (2002) Heart to heart: the twentieth century battle against cardiac disease—an oral history. Rutgers University Press, New Brunswick

Zahmacioglu O, Iidiz CE, Koca B et al (2011) Coming from behind to win: a qualitative research about psychological conditions of adolescents who have undergone open-heart surgery for single ventricle between the ages 0–5. J Cardiothorac Surg 6:155

# Contents

# Part I
# Early Days

# Chapter 1
# Transport and Distribution—The Circulation

> Finally, upon reflecting on every part of medicine, physiology, pathology, semiotics, and therapeutics, I now see how many questions can be answered, how many doubts resolved, and how much obscurity can be illuminated by the truth we have declared and the light we have made to shine (the discovery that blood circulates).
>
> – William Harvey, *De Motu Cordis* (1628).[1]

The cardiovascular system is in the transport and distribution business. It's three chief compartments by design—indefatigable muscle, myriad tubes of widely-ranging diameter,[2] and 25 trillion miniscule yet capacious boxcars—are few in number but exquisite in their execution. This maestro of delivery needs stuff to deliver, and for oxygen it works hand-in-glove with the lungs, the body's chief agents of exchange: Oxygen is exchanged for carbon dioxide in the lungs, the reverse in the tissues. Supplied also by nutrition-procuring and processing systems and organs such as the gut and liver, it provides a continuous bounty of the materials of respiration to every district in the body. (And it also does the reverse: metabolic waste products are evacuated from the tissues to the lungs and kidneys for disposal.) The heart does the pumping—over 2000 gallons a day—and the blood vessels actively distribute blood to areas of greatest need. More blood goes to exercising muscles than those relaxed; flow to the gut increases after eating. When the heart's output is compromised, the heart and brain are the first hogs at the trough, and less critical areas, such as the skin and gut, get less. The design of the blood is every bit as clever as the heart and its conduits. Hemoglobin, cunningly packaged in red blood cells, gives this mandatory fluid its iconic color and sufficient capacity to transport oxygen to the tissues and carbon dioxide to the lungs. It's not for nothing that "boxcars" rather than, say, "wheelbarrows" is the metaphor that physicians sometimes use for the red blood cells when discussing oxygen delivery: Hemoglobin can carry 67 times as much oxygen as can be dissolved in water (at atmospheric

[1] Harvey, *De Motu Cordis* (trans. Carty), p. 83.

[2] Milnor, "Cardiovascular System," in Mountcastle (1980), p. 954.





T. J. Kulik, M. Dick, *Reimagining a Child's Heart*,
https://doi.org/10.1007/978-3-031-88608-9_1

pressure).[3] Without this vital protein, our cardiovascular system could move only a fraction of the required volume of oxygen and carbon dioxide.

Our personal transport and distribution network is the most seamlessly efficient in the world. But despite this most elegant system's manifest presence, people came surprisingly late to apprehend its dynamic layout: The heart pumps blood, which then traces a circuit from the arteries through the capillaries to the veins, and back again to the heart, in an endless loop. In this chapter, we explore how an extraordinary Englishman—William Harvey—showed that blood circulates, one of the most profound discoveries in all of science and medicine. Since effective treatment for many diseases, not just cardiac, hinges upon knowing the cardiovascular system's operating characteristics, this physiological blueprint constitutes the footings of modern medicine *and* the bedrock underneath. How Harvey came to his foundational and long a-coming insight is an invaluable lesson regarding the nature of scientific discovery.

> I long ago realized that if the Muses themselves were to write a book it would still not win more renown than the outpourings of complete imbeciles, and so never had any ambition that my works might be valued among men.
>
> – Galen, *The Order of My Own Books*[4]

We set the stage for Harvey with Galen of Pergamon (ca. 129–200 CE; Fig. 1.1), though we could have cast back further; obsession with the cardiovascular system long preceded this legendary physician. Aristotle (384–322 BCE), for example, first clearly outlined the branching of the blood vessels, and Praxagoras of kos (b. ca. 340 BCE) had distinguished arteries from veins half a millennium before Galen.[5] Erasistratus (304–250 BCE) formulated a complex and comprehensive theory of the cardiovascular and pulmonary systems.[6] Galen's physiology built upon and then displaced Erasistratus' and was the canonical view from the *second* to the *seventeenth* century, a run far longer than any competing description. Galen and Hippocrates were the most persuasive medical authorities, but Galen emerged as the reigning physiologist during the first centuries of the CE.[7] Alexander of Aprodisias, a Greek philosopher and contemporary of Galen, situated him alongside Plato and Aristotle as a "man of repute,"[8] and the encomiums multiplied over the years. Michael Servetus (of whom more later) wrote that "the birth and rebirth of Galen was granted as a kind of divine gift for the assistance of various mortal needs."[9]

---

[3] Hemoglobin's molecular design is ingenious: Oxygen is taken up in areas of high oxygen partial pressure (the lungs), but ejected from hemoglobin in regions of low oxygen (the tissues). The biconcave discs which cradle the hemoglobin and other enabling proteins are elegant and flexible, shape changing as they squeeze and jostle through the capillaries.

[4] Singer (1997), p. 23.

[5] Wilson (1959).

[6] Dobson (1927); Wilson (1959).

[7] Temkin (1973) pp. 1, 191–192; Singer (1997), p. vii; Nutton (2002).

[8] Nutton (1984).

[9] Temkin (1973), p. 126.

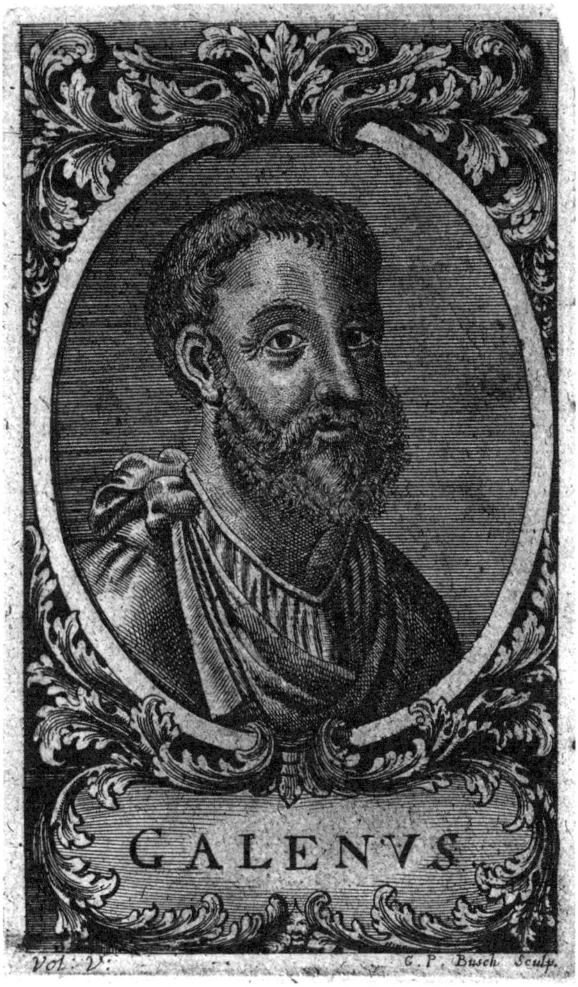


**Fig. 1.1** Portrait of Galen, G.P. Busch. From the Wellcome Collection, free to use with attribution

Physician and anatomist Jacobus Sylvius (1478–1555)—admittedly a fan—wrote that "After Apollo and Aesculapius [Hippocrates and Galen] were the greatest powers in medicine, most perfect in every respect, and they had never written anything in physiology or other parts of medicine that was not entirely true."[10] Even Ioannes Argenterius (1513–1672), a strenuous critic of Galen, allowed that he was "extremely gifted" and that "we owe him more than to all the others who have hitherto written on medicine."[11] Non-medical people also knew of Galen: Shakespeare, for example,

[10] Temkin (1973), p. 126.

[11] Temkin (1973), p. 151.

mentioned him,[12] and in the *Inferno*, Dante assigned Galen—along with the likes of Socrates, Plato, Euclid, and Hippocrates—to the first circle of hell.[13]

Born in Pergamum, a provincial city in the Roman empire (now western Turkey), Galen's luck with his parents was mixed. His father, a well-to-do architect, was "extremely slow to anger, as well as extremely just, decent, and generous." His mother, on the other hand, was quarrelsome, treated her husband shabbily, and was so ill-tempered that she occasionally bit the maids. Not surprisingly, Galen shunned the distaff side of his parents, and apparently happily complied when his father, "persuaded by clear dreams," directed him to study medicine and philosophy.[14] His studies took him to Smyrna, Corinth, and Alexandria, but he returned to Pergamum for several years, later moving to Rome where he spent most of his career. Emperor Marcus Aurelius was one of his patients,[15] but Galen was not nattily attired, well-modulated celebrity doctor. He was a surgeon to the slashed, punctured, and fractured gladiators in Pergamum. For those who had suffered "dissolution of continuity," bandages and stitches re-approximated the tissue ("But it is Nature that closes the wound up and restores the original unity"). Foreign missiles were removed, wounds cauterized, abscesses drained, gangrene excised. He set broken bones using chalkstone bound around the break to form a circle. Gangrene was plastered and cellulitis, olive oiled. Ruptured tendons were stitched together, and for abdominal wounds, protruding intestine was stuffed back inside and the rent sutured. Shards of bone were chiseled out of skull fractures.[16]

Physician *and* philosopher, Galen was deeply steeped in classical Greek thinkers and philosophy. He wore his erudition and fame on his sleeve, claiming that Marcus Aurelius declared him to be "first among doctors, but the *only* philosopher."[17] Galen argued that "The best doctor is also a philosopher" (although he knew that few physicians could pull this off),[18] and put great stock in melding experience with rational analysis. Academic department chairs prize faculty members who are a "triple-threat"—the unusual physician who is highly accomplished in all three key aspects of the trade (patient care, research, and teaching); Galen was that and much more—a thought-leader of a magnitude and persistence that we will surely never see again.

Galen's research was anatomical and physiological. Human cadavers were unavailable to him, so he dissected innumerable animals, alive and dead. His anatomical exertions were later superseded by human dissections, most notably

[12] Temkin (1973) p. 125.

[13] This circle is for virtuous pagans, good people born without the opportunity to know the Savior; they are not tormented but cannot aspire to paradise. Dante Alighieri, *The Divine Comedy*, canto IV (John Ciardi, translator).

[14] Singer (1997), pp. 27–28, 119; most background on Galen is from Temkin (1973) and Singer (1997).

[15] Temkin (1973), p. 46.

[16] Galen, *The Art of Medicine*, in Singer (1997), pp. 383–384; Toledo-Pereyra (1973).

[17] Singer (1997), p. xvi.

[18] Singer (1997), pp. 30–31; Temkin (1973), p. 38.

Vesalius', but his anatomic studies informed his physiology.[19] For example: Galen's conception of cardiovascular physiology differed from Erasistratus' partly because the latter thought that pneuma—derived from inspired air—occupied the left ventricle and arteries, which contained no blood. Galen taught that the arteries carried blood, demonstrating that lacerating an artery is not followed by any escape of pneuma; knifing the beating heart, or inserting a quill, immediately delivered blood, not pneuma. Discerning blood in mesenteric arteries (the mesentery being the thin, transparent membrane attached to the bowels), not pneuma, was another argument Galen adduced for rejecting Erasistratus' theory.[20] But, like the rest of us, he could veer off course. Interposing a tube between the cut ends of an artery, Galen found that the distal vessel no longer pulsated, suggesting to him that the pulse was not caused by the impulse of the blood, but rather a force traveling in the wall of the artery itself (more on this later).[21]

Galen's curiosity was manifest as an obsessive yearning for the *truth,* which runs incessantly through his writing.[22] Also shot through his surviving text (of which there are roughly 12,000 pages)[23] is arrogance, impatience, dismissiveness, and raw disdain of his rivals. Not caring much for athletes, he opined that they are "unable to contemplate anything clearly, mindless as beasts without reason… . Their life is thus like that of pigs—except that pigs do not over-exert or force-feed themselves."[24] And Galen didn't brook much give-and-take. When arguing the importance of philosophy for medical doctors, he wrote that "I hope that no one is going to quibble over words and come out with some nonsense just for the sake of arguing … . This would be to agree on the factual issue, but shamelessly concoct a disagreement on a purely semantic basis. We do not have time for this sort of thing. You would be better to return to common sense, and not to quarrel with your fellow over mere sounds, like a jackdaw or raven."[25] Phrases like the following liberally punctuate his writings: "[T]hey are like asses listening to music"; "It is quite possible that the utterly ignorant will have no idea of what I am referring to. I shall try to make it clearer for them"; "[A]mong those who claim to be practitioners of philosophy there are many with whom I do not even consider it worth having a discussion."[26] I've obviously selected these fragments, but they are typical of Galen's disposition[27]; if you tape a page of his text from P.N. Singer's *Galen, Selected Works* on the wall and launch a dart at it, there is a good chance of its finding a phrase or passage of self-praise, pungent pedantry, or acidulous contempt. But so over the top that you may—like

[19] Temkin (1973), pp. 134–135.

[20] Wilson (1959).

[21] Harris (1973), pp. 378–380.

[22] Temkin (1973), p. 36.

[23] Temkin (1973), p. 5.

[24] Singer (1997), p. 47.

[25] Singer (1997), p. 34.

[26] Singer (1997), pp. 130–136.

[27] Temkin (1973), pp. 6–7; Poynter and Keele (1961), p. 21.

me—find yourself laughing out loud, while forming an image of a famously cranky grandfather who nevertheless commands great respect for all that he has done to enrich the family.

But we are here not to raze or praise Galen. Our main interest is his physiology, which is difficult. It's unsettling partly because his conception of the cardiovascular-pulmonary system is complex and so disconnected from reality that it almost seems a concoction out of a fantasy novel. He was not beyond ambiguity and self-contradiction; his theories changed over time, and his explication demands a fine understanding of context and a certain willingness to indulge in interpolation and extrapolation. Not surprisingly, scholars disagree on multiple aspects of Galen's physiology.[28] I offer the following summary (see Fig. 1.2) to give a sense of what the standard thinking was prior to Harvey, with the caveat that some details have been left out, and that not all scholars agree on everything.[29]

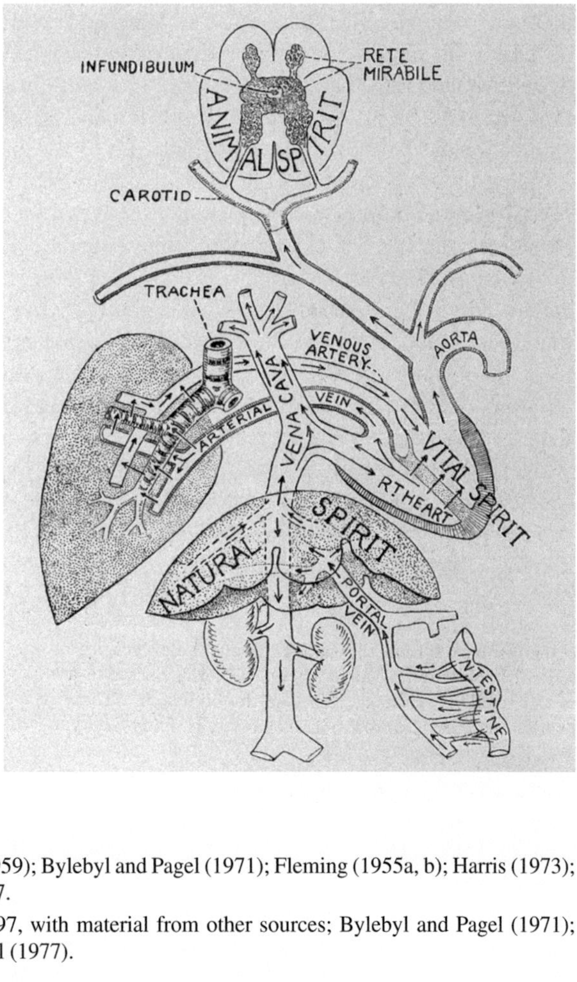


**Fig. 1.2** From the Wellcome Collection, free to use with attribution

[28] See Boylan (2007); Wilson (1959); Bylebyl and Pagel (1971); Fleming (1955a, b); Harris (1973); and Temkin (1973), pp. 156–157.

[29] See Harris (1973), pp. 267–397, with material from other sources; Bylebyl and Pagel (1971); Fleming (1955a, b); and Bylebyl (1977).

By Galen's lights, nutriment (chyle) passes from the intestines and stomach through the portal vein to the liver, where it is transformed into blood. This blood is conducted by the *veins* (starting with the vena cavae) peripherally, where it is absorbed. Blood is not pumped—rather, it is *attracted to the tissues by the tissues*, with gravity and *horror vacui* also playing a role. Although the blood mostly moves outwards, because the kidneys and spleen cleanse it there must be some back-and-forth movement.[30] Some venous blood flows into the right ventricle, where it is further refined, and from there through the pulmonary artery to provide nutriment to the lungs. Perhaps a very small amount of blood passes through the lungs into the pulmonary veins, although it is not clear if it enters the left ventricle. Some quantity of blood moves, through pores too fine to see in the interventricular septum, from the right ventricle into the left. It is the movement of the chest, rather than the right ventricle, which moves blood into the lungs. In fact, *neither the right nor left ventricle actually do much pumping*. For Galen, the principal function of the heart and arteries is to supply innate heat, not to pump blood. Active dilation of the arteries, more than contraction of the left ventricle, are what moves arterial blood.[31]

The lungs' very small airways connect with the pulmonary veins, which serve as ducts through which the left ventricle takes in cooling air during diastole, the principal function of the air being to cool excess heat of the heart. But the left ventricle also needs air to generate heat, and it discharges heated air and sooty vapors through the pulmonary veins (assuming the mitral valve to be leaky) into the airways for exhalation. Air is also converted into *pneuma* in the left ventricle and the arteries, which is distributed peripherally. It's not clear exactly what form the pneuma takes in the left ventricle and arteries; is it dissolved in the blood, or run alongside the blood? Pneuma and the vapors of the blood are converted into spirits—psychic (or animal) spirit in the brain, natural spirit in the liver, and vital spirit in the left ventricle. (It is uncertain whether Galen believed that there were two or three spirits.)[32]

The arterial pulse originates in the heart, but *not* from blood propelled into arteries from the heart; contraction and relaxation of arteries is energized by the heart and transmitted distally through the arterial walls. The pulse distributes innate heat, and when arteries relax (dilate) they draw in air through the skin and produce "pneumatiferous" blood. The arteries interchange air and blood with the veins via invisible and extremely fine anastomoses (connections).

Even if you allow that, in some ways, Galen anticipated true anatomy and physiology (for example, transit of a little blood across the lung, air contributing to heat generation, minute anastomoses connecting arteries and veins), his edifice blatantly defies actual physiology (and physics). But he was surely a genius, perceptive, and deadly serious. He performed many experiments on living animals and must have developed some appreciation of blood flow dynamics from injured gladiators. How could he have gotten this so wrong?

---

[30] Harris (1973), pp. 330–331.

[31] Bylebyl (1973), p. 431.

[32] Harris (1973), p. 351.

Perhaps Galen did not divine the true nature of the circulation, as historian C.R.S. Harris observed, because "he was for all his gifts essentially a conservative … his temperament was that of a synthesizer, an eclectic who tried to reconcile as far as he could the often irreconcilable doctrines of the great masters of the past. Hippocrates was God, and Galen was his prophet."[33] But another expert, Owsei Temkin, argued that Galen's aim was to understand the fundamentals of how food, drink, and air interact with the body, not the movement of blood; he thinks that the term "cardiovascular system" is inappropriate in the context of Galen's physiology.[34] Galen scholar Jerome Bylebyl elaborated on this notion, observing that the ancient's "basic view is that food is transformed into blood in some central organ, and that the blood then moves slowly outward to be assimilated and ultimately lost through invisible emanation… . This assumed link between the movement of the blood and the nutritive process was one of the greatest obstacles to any conception of the circulation, in which the blood had to endlessly retrace the same pathway rather than simply distributed on a one-time basis."[35] Bylebyl also pointed out that there was a widely held notion that blood could "flux" to particular localities in response to various stimuli. This supposed property offered alternative explanation for observations which would otherwise suggest circulation of blood.[36] Temkin also notes that the ancients conceived of the animate and inanimate, air, and warmth, differently than moderns.[37] As we will see in the next chapter, anything like modern chemistry was non-existent, and everyday concepts such as heat and vacuum were little understood in Galen's time. If one thing learned leads to another, the message is: You need to learn certain things before you can learn others. It has also been pointed out that Galen's writing was partly driven by his desire to gain debating points against Erasistratus and his physiology, with some statements aimed more at gaining argumentative advantage than necessarily reflecting actual observations.[38] Finally, Galen utilized general explanatory principles, such as the four humors, which muddied his perspective.

How could this deeply flawed construct have persisted for as long as it did? Galen's reign outlasted 47 English monarchs, and his catechism survived 220 popes; the tissue of his physiology remained intact roughly seven times as long as the United States is old. One answer is the force of *authority*, which was immeasurably more powerful then than now. People clung to the ideas of giants such as Hippocrates and Galen in a way we can hardly imagine today. And were it easy to spot the cracks in the foundation of classical ideas, surely ancient teachers and their notions would have soon yielded to fresh perspective. But it was not. As we will see, the English physician who finally formulated a good and true picture of the cardiovascular

[33] Harris (1973), p. 267.

[34] Temkin (1973), pp. 154–157.

[35] Bylebyl (1977).

[36] Bylebyl (1978).

[37] Temkin (1973), p. 156–157.

[38] Wilson (1959); Boylan (2007).

circulatory scheme in the early seventeenth century found his task nearly impossible. If something beats nothing every time, absent concocting a whole new foundation, a few cracks were hardly reason to bulldoze a useful structure, especially lacking a better replacement.[39]

Perhaps Daniel Kahneman cut close to the quick of this question in *Thinking Fast and Slow*. In 1737, Swiss scientist Daniel Bernoulli constructed a model of "expected utility" which was widely accepted and is still alive and well, despite being seriously flawed in a pretty obvious way. Asking why this model could have survived for nearly 300 years, Kahneman, a Nobel Prize-winning psychologist, suggested that its longevity can be explained by "a weakness of the scholarly mind" which he calls "theory-induced blindness"; accepting a theory, and using it, makes ditching it very difficult. You assume that any problems with the construct that you come across must have been noticed and resolved by others, that you are simply missing something. Kahneman quotes psychologist Daniel Gilbert as observing that "disbelieving is hard work."[40] Indeed it is. Cutting successfully against the received grain requires deeply understanding and pondering that plank of wood, a chore that few will pursue.

The overcast stretch from Galen to William Harvey was pierced by a few precious shafts of illumination. With the fall of Rome, nearly all Greek science was lost to the West, although the Byzantine Empire retained a considerable residue. Ibn al-Nafis, a thirteenth-century Arab physician born in Damascus, speculated that blood traverses the lungs. In his *Commentary of the Anatomy of Avicenna's Cannon* he offered that "blood, after having been refined (in the right ventricle) must rise in the arteriosus vein (pulmonary artery) to the lung in order to expand in its volume and to be mixed with air so that its finest part may be clarified and may reach the venous artery (pulmonary vein) in which it is transmitted to the left cavity of the heart." But his notion was based primarily upon theoretical considerations, and al-Nafis adduced no experimental evidence to support it. He did not conceive that the entire volume of blood passes through the lungs, but only a fraction of it, and thought that the right heart has no active movement. His theory was little disseminated and likely had no influence in Europe. Only in 1922 did Egyptian medical student Muhyi ad-Din at-Tatawi unearth the *Commentary* in the Prussian State Library and discuss it 2 years later in his doctoral thesis.[41]

Michael Servetus, a Spanish physician and theologian, was the first in Western Christendom to question Galen's teaching that blood transited the interventricular septum via invisible pores. In *Christianismi Restitutio* (1553), he pointed out that the pulmonary artery is too large merely to send nourishment to the lungs, and also that the interventricular septum is, in fact, imperforate, asserting that right ventricular blood passes through the lungs, where it picks up air, and then into the left

[39] Schultz (2002).

[40] Kahneman (2011), pp. 272–277.

[41] See Meyerhof (1935); Temkin (1940); and Cournand in Fishman and Richards (1964), pp. 15–16.

ventricle.[42] It is unclear what experimental observations supported this idea,[43] although Servetus was a skilled dissector, and his observing that the color of the blood changes after pulmonary passage suggests that his views had at least some empirical basis. But his idea had little or no circulation, and he ran afoul of religious authorities, was branded a heretic, and perished at the stake in 1553. His books suffered the same fate, and few survived. Of one thousand books printed in 1553, only three authentic copies remain (two complete). It re-surfaced only in 1694 when William Wotton obtained a transcription from an English surgeon.[44] Also, like al-Nafis, Servetus did not posit a complete circulation, apparently believing that blood mostly moved, as Galen supposed, centrifugally in the veins.[45]

Far more influential were the observations of Realdo Columbo, an Italian anatomist and surgeon. Assistant to Vesalius at the University of Padova, and later physician for Michelangelo and Pope Julius III, he dissected countless human corpses and live animals, observing that the pulmonary veins contain blood, not air. Combined with his conviction that the heart's valves permit only one-way flow of blood, and that the interventricular septum was too dense to permit passage of blood, he wrote in *De Re Anatomica* (1559) that "the blood is carried through the pulmonary artery to the lung and is there attenuated; then it is carried, along with air, through the pulmonary vein to the left ventricle of the heart." Although slow to spread[46] his book did not dead-end; Harvey appropriated Columbo's observations in formulating his own theory of the circulation. Not all scholars agree that Harvey was influenced by Colombo regarding transpulmonary transit.[47] But like Servetus, Columbo subscribed to Galen's centrifugal venous flow. A few commentators have suggested that a pupil of Columbo's (in Pisa), Andreas Caesalpinus, discovered the circulation before Harvey. While he may have appreciated the transpulmonary passage of blood (perhaps because of his association with Columbo), Caesalpinus did not demonstrate the circulation, and was inconsistent in his writings on the subject. Harvey was unaware of his work before publishing *De Motu Cordis*.[48]

> When I first turned my attentions to … discovering the motions and functions of the heart … I found the task so truly arduous, so full of difficulties, that I was tempted to think, with Fracastorius, that the motion of the heart was only to be comprehended by God.
> – William Harvey, *De Motu Cordis* (1628).[49]

If you've read much history of medicine or science, *The Universita Degli Studi di Padova* has likely caught your eye. Planted in a modest town 25 miles west of Venice, the University was founded in the fall of 1222 when a crowd of disgruntled

[42] See Cournand in Fishman and Richards (1964), pp. 18–23; and Blainton (1951).

[43] Young (1940), pt. 1.

[44] Cournand in Fishman and Richards (1964), pp. 20–22.

[45] Blainton (1951).

[46] Wilson (1960).

[47] See Coppola (1957); Whitteridge (1971), pp. 49, 92; and French (1994), p. 82).

[48] See Whitteridge (1971), pp. 65–68, 102; Keynes (1966), pp. 107, 172; and Singer (1946).

[49] Harvey, *De Motu Cardis* (ed. Carty), p. 17.

students and professors—suffering too little scholastic freedom—migrated from the Studium of Bologna to Padova. Medicine was first taught at the University about 1250, and it matured into one of a baby's handful of elite European medical schools, along with Paris, Montpellier, and Bologna.[50] Would-be physicians trekked many leagues to arrive Padova, including (in addition to Italians) Flemish, Belgians, Dutch, Swiss, Silesians, Poles, Russians, Hungarians, Spaniards, French, and British.[51] Anatomy, medicine, surgery, pharmacology, pathology, epidemiology, and teratology—all of these and more were areas of study at Padova by the seventeenth century.[52] The medical school is famous for Europe's first permanent anatomical theatre constructed in 1594,[53] where anatomists dissected bodies of animals and humans while students peered down from narrow carved wooden tiers (Fig. 1.4). Beautiful in a hoary way today, in the sixteenth century, the theater certified the university's preeminence in anatomical research and teaching students what lies under the skin and muscles, the cutting-edge preoccupations at the time.

But this university owes its special place in history not to wood and stone, but to flesh and blood. The inventory of distinguished physicians and scientists who trained or taught at Padova is remarkable.[54] Nicholas Copernicus was a student there, and Galileo was on faculty. Some of the most venerable names in Western medicine—Vesalius, Columbo, Falloppia, Fabricius, Morgagni—strolled through its ancient courtyard and pontificated behind its lecterns. It was onto this intellectually vital campus that a "small, swarthy man with an alert and eager manner, interested in everything around him, observant, (and) intelligent"[55] strode in early 1600, destined to achieve fame as one of Padova's, and the world's, most famous physician-scientists.

Born on April Fool's Day, 1578, in a "faire-built stone house" in Folkestone, situated in Kent's chalk uplands, William Harvey (Fig. 1.3) chose his parents more wisely than Galen. Thomas Harvey achieved enviable success in business and raising a large and successful brood (nine children). William's mother Joan was "Deere to her Husband: Reverenced of her Children: Beloved of her Neighbors: Elected of God."[56] They raised William well. Leaving aside his nearly unmatched professional vita, one of his best known (and admittedly sympathetic) biographers offered that "Even if we wished to do so, it would be difficult, from the evidence in our possession, to find any serious flaw in Harvey's character."[57] That may go too far, but he enjoyed the warm regard of the fellows of the College of Physicians, and he earned

---

[50] See Gallo, "The Medieval Period," and Ongaro, "Medicine," in Negro (2001–2003); and Whitteridge (1971), p. 9.

[51] Whitteridge (1971), p. 13.

[52] Ongaro, "Medicine," in Negro (2001–2003).

[53] Keynes (1966), p. 25.

[54] Ongaro, "Medicine," in Negro (2001–2003).

[55] Keynes (1966), p. 423.

[56] Keynes (1966), pp. 5–6.

[57] Keynes (1966), p. 422; see also pp. 420–426 and Singer (1946).

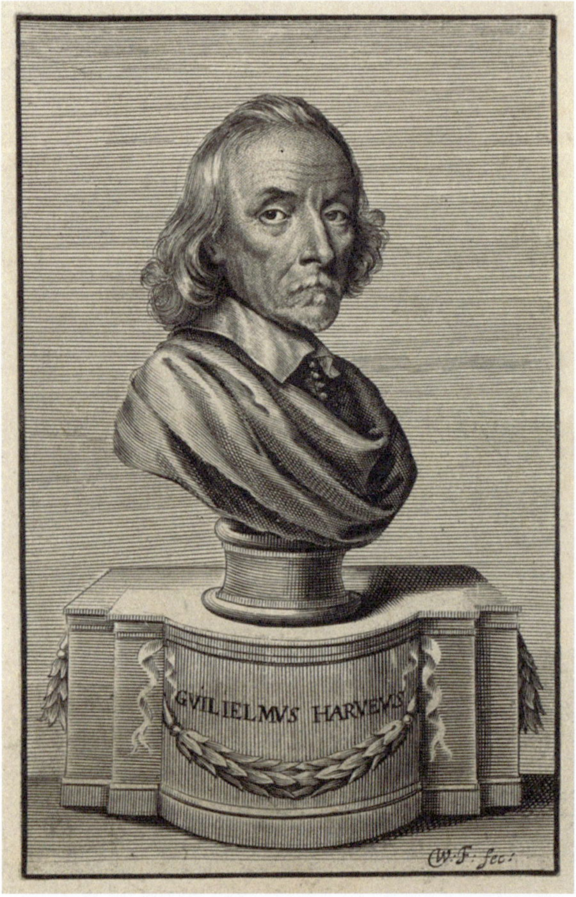


**Fig. 1.3** William Harvey, line drawing by W. Faithhorne, 1653. From the Wellcome Collection, free to use with attribution

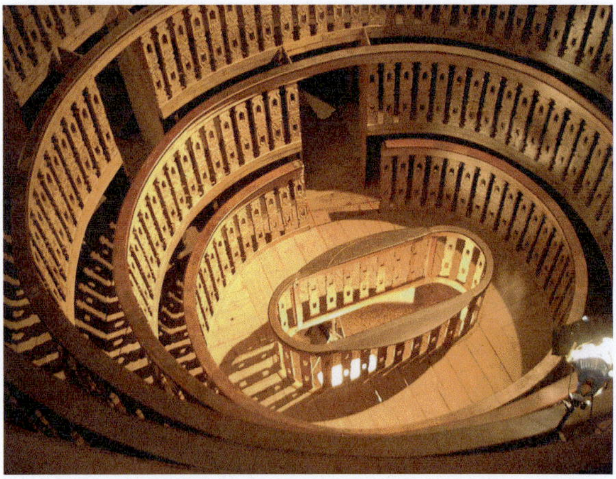

**Fig. 1.4** Anatomical theatre, University of Padua. In the public domain

the respect of two English kings (James I and Charles I) and the likes of Francis Bacon, Robert Boyle, and Thomas Hobbes. He was said to be generous and courteous, invariably honest, and had the highest ethical standards. Despite having amassed considerable wealth,[58] his taste in dress and food was simple.[59] Harvey revealed little of his take on religion; though he apparently revered divine authority, it is unlikely that he subscribed to any organized faith. He could be privately cynical and bitter, but gracious in his public life. For example, when Parisian physician Jean Riolan penned a ludicrous criticism of *De Motu Cordis*, Harvey offered an unyielding defense of his theory while demonstrating extravagant respect for Riolan, referring to him as "the learned gentleman," and congratulated him on having written a "learned, polished and concise book of unsurpassed elegance."[60] (Galen would have shredded the faulty logic *and* the critic.)

Of what shaped Harvey into a gentleman disrupter, we have few clues. There being no school in Folkestone, his very early education was presumably via itinerant teachers. At about age ten he enrolled in King's School at Canterbury. His undergraduate years were endured at Gonville and Caius College, Cambridge. Ambling about the college, students passed through the Gates of Humility, Virtue, Wisdom, and Honour, which gave good indication of the tenor of the place, whose daily schedule would attract few if any subscribers today: Compulsory chapel at 5:00 AM; four hours of lectures starting at 6:10; dinner at 10 or 11:00 AM, consisting of meat, broth, bread and salt. And "After thys slender dinner they be either teachynge or learnynge untyll v. of the clocke in the evenynge, when as they have a supper not much better than theyr dyner. Immediatelye after the whyche, they go ethyer to reasonyng in problemes or unto some other studye untyll it be nyne or tenne of the clocke, and there being without fyre are fayne to walk or runne up and downe halfe an houre, to get a heate on their feete whan they go to bed."[61] Caius wasn't for everyone, perhaps not even the studious Harvey. As far as we know, he never gave any sign of gratitude or fond remembrance of his undergraduate institution.[62] Harvey took his B.A. in 1597 but was still in residence at Cambridge until sometime in 1599, when he departed England for Italy.

Harvey's medical alma mater was a little rough around the edges during his tenure there. Politically motivated fights broke out among rival gangs at Padova, and Harvey took to wearing a dagger for self-protection.[63] When shortages of cadavers curtailed the ever-popular anatomy demonstrations, students resorted to grave

[58] Keynes (1966), p. 423.

[59] The value of Harvey's estate was estimated as £20,000, or $4.46 M in 2019 US dollars (Nye, *Pounds Sterling to Dollars: Historical Conversion of Currency*, accessed January 31, 2019, http://www.uwyo.edu/numimage/currency.htm), and he had previously contributed generously to The Royal College of Physicians (Shackelford 2003, p. 124).

[60] Keynes (1966), p. 324.

[61] Keynes (1966), p. 19.

[62] Keynes (1966), p. 20.

[63] Keynes (1966), p. 24.

robbing until severe penalties put a crimp in this practice.[64] (Executed prisoners were the sanctioned source of bodies for dissection.) We know few details of Harvey's life in Italy. The fact that he was elected *Consiliarius* for the English Nation suggests that he may have enjoyed considerable respect and trust in medical school; an alternate view could be that his election was more likely due to a paucity of enrolled Englishmen.[65] The professor who most influenced Harvey at Padova was Girolamo Fabrizi d'Acquapendente (Fabricius), a famous physician and anatomist. It seems that Harvey spent considerable time with Fabricius, although the exact outlines of their relationship are fuzzy.[66] There were at least two ways his influence likely contributed to Harvey's later work. Fabricius was the first to establish comparative anatomy as a field; Harvey would later build his case for the circulation in part using observations from a variety of different animal species. And Fabricius likely demonstrated the venous valves to his students. Although neither teacher nor student initially understood their function or significance, Harvey would later recognize that the one-way flow of venous blood towards the heart that these structures enforced was incompatible with the Galenic notion of centrifugal flow (towards the periphery) of venous blood.

Leaving Padova soon after taking his doctorate in April 1602, Harvey moved to London. Having passed the customary oral exams, he was granted permission to practice medicine in 1603 and was fully licensed (and married) in 1604. Elected a fellow of the College of Physicians in 1607, he secured an appointment to St. Bartholomew's hospital 2 years later. Harvey had myriad interests and responsibilities. In addition to research, he had a private practice and clinical duties at St. Bart's, and he ministered to two kings (James I and Charles I), including undertaking various official duties attached to serving Charles I.[67] Most notably, he was was appointed as Lumleian Lecturer in August of 1615. Surgery and anatomy were covered in twice weekly talks over 6 years in this lecture series aimed at improving London's then woefully poor surgery.[68] While we have no record of Harvey's talks, his *prelectiones* (lecture notes) survive and provide clues regarding the evolution of his theory.

The *prelectiones* indicate that, by 1616, he agreed with Columbo regarding the transpulmonary transit of blood, and he had deduced both that it is the heart that moves the blood, and that the pulse is due to ejected blood, not active pulsation of the artery wall.[69] Harvey knew that the heart receives blood from the vena cava and sends it through the lungs to the left ventricle, then to the aorta, but he persisted in the idea that some blood reaches the periphery via the veins. He did not fully

[64] Whitteridge (1971), p. 19.

[65] Keynes (1966), p. 23; Whitteridge (1971), p. 10.

[66] Keynes (1966), pp. 27–28.

[67] Whitteridge (1971), p. 201.

[68] Keynes (1966), p. 85.

[69] Bylebyl (1973).

formulate his concept of the circulation until sometime between about 1619 and 1625.[70] *Exercitatio Anatomica De Motu Cordis et Sanguinis in Animalibus* (On the Motion of the Heart and Blood in Animals) announced Harvey's profound rethinking of physiology (1628). Summarizing his findings in Chap. 14, Harvey ripped ancient physiology's recalcitrant fabric beyond hope of patching: "[T]he blood passes through the lungs and heart by the force of the ventricles and is distributed to all parts of the body. It then makes its way into the veins and pores of the flesh and flows by the veins from the circumference on every side to the center, from the lesser to the greater veins, and is by them finally discharged into the vena cava and right auricle of the heart. It flows in such a quantity or such a flux by the arteries, and such a reflux by the veins, that it cannot possibly be supplied by the ingesta. It is also much greater than can be required for mere purposes of nutrition. It is absolutely necessary to conclude that the blood in the animal body is impelled in a circle and is in a state of ceaseless motion. This is the act or function that the heart performs by the pulse, and that it is the sole and only end of the motion and contraction of the heart."[71] Not surprisingly, *De Motu Cordis* elicited controversy and scorn. After its publication, Harvey lamented that "he fell mightily in his Practize and that 'twas believed by the vulgar that he was crack-brained."[72] Although Harvey had a few early supporters, many understood neither his arguments nor their significance.[73] Only by roughly 1650 did most of the resistance dissipate.[74]

How did Harvey unravel the ancient tangle of observations and assumptions regarding the blood's perambulations? What enabled him to learn what so many others had failed to perceive? New technology has many times paved the way for breakthrough scientific discovery: Apparatus for gas collection advanced early chemistry; microscopes and special tissue stains led to cell theory; measurement of blood oxygen levels was needed to unwrap the meaning of cyanosis. Did new technology—perhaps a better way to visualize blood flowing through vessels, or looking inside the beating heart—fuel Harvey's signal breakthrough?

No.

*De Motu Cordis* clearly recounts Harvey's many experiments, and they are the same that Galen, and countless others after him, performed or could have. Harvey removed the chest wall from animals and, using his eyes and fingers, scrutinized motion of the heart and pulsations of the arteries. Finding it near impossible to deduce the mechanical action of a heart beating two or three times a second—his confession above refers to this challenge—he studied cardiac contraction and relaxation using dying (and thus slowly beating) hearts, and "colder" animals, such as frogs, small fish, and snakes, whose cardiac tempo is relatively slow. He even peered

---

[70] Whitteridge (1971), p. 201.

[71] Harvey, *De Motu Cordis* (ed. Carty), p. 76.

[72] Whitteridge (1971), p. 82.

[73] Keynes (1966), pp. 318–319.

[74] Whitteridge (1971), p. 20.

at hearts in small, transparent shrimp, seeing the pulsations "as through a window."[75] Simple experiments revealed elemental facts: The blood ejected from a pierced heart gave unmistakable evidence of its pumping action; pinching the vena cava just below the heart emptied the pump, while compressing the aorta caused the ventricle to distend. Using sight and touch and simple interventions, Harvey came to understand that arteries expand as the heart contracts and ejects blood, as one distends a glove by blowing in it.

He extended his research to the embryo and fetus, and animals with a single ventricle to confirm his impressions. Harvey chipped away the shell from an incubating hen's egg and "[saw] the first rudiments of the chick as a little cloud in the course of the fourth or fifth day of incubation… . In the middle of the cloud there was a bloody point so small that it disappeared during the contraction and escaped from view, but in the relaxation, it reappeared again as a red pinpoint. So between the visible and invisible, between being and not being, it gave the beginning of life by its pulses."[76] He pointed out that the fetal heart has pathways (the foramen ovale and ductus arteriosus) permitting both ventricles to pump venous blood into the aorta and asked: After birth, why should nature close up these open channels and never open any new channels (that is, transit through the lungs) for the passage of blood? Animals with a single ventricle confirmed that the heart transferred blood from veins to arteries.

The clincher and the coup de grâce to Galenic physiology took the form of simple math: Assume that the volume of the cavity of left ventricle is x while dilated, and y while contracted. Subtract y from x, multiply these times the number of heart beats in any given time interval, and you get the amount of blood ejected in that interval. He estimated the left ventricle capacity from cadavers and assumed the percentage of blood ejected with each contraction. Over a wide range of values he found that volume of blood pumped vastly exceeded the amount of food ingested (and the total amount of blood in the body), thus could not have been supplied from chyle moving from the gut to the liver to the heart. The implication was inescapable: The only way the system *could* work, analyzed quantitatively, was for the blood to circulate.[77] Harvey provided yet further confirmation by pointing out that the valves in veins allow venous blood to flow only toward the heart, not peripherally to the tissues. His oft-reproduced diagrams of venous flow in the arm (see Fig. 1.5) make the direction of flow obvious even to the non-physician or anatomist.[78]

---

[75] Harvey, *De Motu Cordis* (ed. Carty), p. 29.

[76] Harvey, *De Motu Cordis* (ed. Carty), p. 29.

[77] Bylebyl (1973). Historian Walter Pagel thinks that Harvey *first* had the quantitative idea that the blood must circulate, followed by accrual of subsequent observational proof (Pagel 1976, pp. 3–5).

[78] Harvey's quantitative thinking may not have been flawless. In Chap. 17 of *De Motu Cordis,* Harvey stated that that the right ventricle "is of greater capacity (than the left ventricle) since it has not only to supply material to the left ventricle, but also to send ailment to the lungs" (Harvey, *De Motu Cordis* [ed. Carty], p. 87). But the only way that the right ventricle could pump more blood than the left (assuming no cardiac defects) would be if the right side were continuously supplied with blood to replace that consumed in the lungs as nutriment; did he have that in mind, or was he

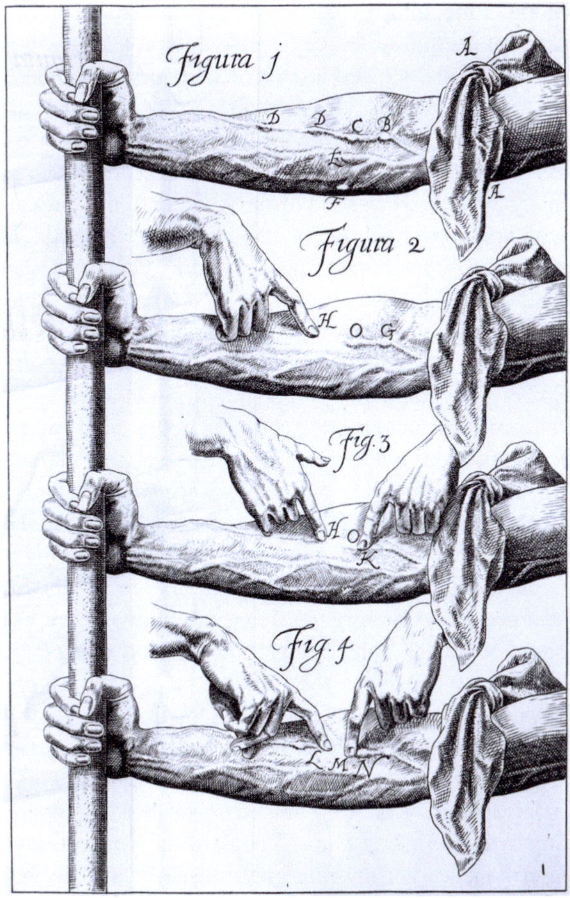


**Fig. 1.5** Diagram illustrating William Harvey's experiments on the valves of the veins; after a drawing by S. Gooden for the Nonesuch edition of De Motu Cordis, London: 1928. (William Harvey, experiments on the valves. From the Wellcome Collection, free to use with attribution)

So: Harvey's technology and experimental models were *the same as those available to Galen and inquiring minds after the Roman physician*; no new physical tools were available or required for Harvey's investigations. His research strategy—experimental study of dead and living animals, and observations in living humans—was anything but new. And Harvey apparently made his observations mostly on his own, so he didn't have an entourage to multiply his efforts.

If Harvey's technological implements were no more advanced than his predecessors, his *intracranial tools* may have been keener and more supple. Finding a rapidly beating heart almost impossible to analyze, he tumbled to the idea—apparently never before employed[79]—of using animals with slower heart rates to get a purchase on the problem. He turned tourniquet-distended arm veins, long used for

unclear on the need for the two ventricles to pump the same volume (neglecting bronchial artery flow)?

[79] Whitteridge (1971), p. 97.

bloodletting, into a window onto the circulation, and easy-to-apprehend evidence in favor of his theory. Harvey's preternatural tenacity in the service of fierce curiosity, not new tools, yielded an unmatched perspective on the puzzle of blood flow: He inspected a long list of mammals, birds, snails, fish, shellfish, reptiles, amphibians, sponges, worms, and even insects in his quest to trace blood flow through the body. Performing countless experiments, he peered at the cardiovascular system from many angles and worried his problem until there wasn't anything left. Not satisfied with discovering the action of the heart and the pulse, and confirming the passage of blood across the lungs, Harvey—unlike Columbo—continued to ponder and probe until he could advance his story to the next level. Intellectual courage and casting aside preconceptions—that is, thinking differently—underlay his discovery. Harvey biographer Gweneth Whitteridge pointed out that one of the tenants of the Royal Society was *nullius in verba* (nothing was to be accepted "on any man's word,"), reflecting this increasingly common notion in the mid-seventeenth century.[80] But all too many of his contemporaries remained under undue influence from ancient sages, and Harvey's intellectual independence was far from standard issue at the time.

*De Motu Cordis* left many questions unanswered. Harvey, to cite only one example of his necessary ignorance, had no understanding of the circulation's most temporally acute function—supplying the materials of respiration[81]; the required advances in respiratory physiology were two centuries distant. But showing that the blood circulates is the Declaration of Independence *and* the Constitution—a thread in the tapestry seems too frail a metaphor here—of cardiovascular and even all physiology. It's hard to exaggerate the importance of Harvey's contribution, which was the necessary prelude of so many more to come.

*De Motu Cordis'* arguments were derived from observable structures and physiological activity, but they hinged on the idea that blood somehow made its way from tiny arteries to tiny veins. Veno-arterial connections (*synanastomoses*) had been inferred since ancient times but had never actually been observed. In fact, Harvey denied their existence and thought that blood extravasated from end arteries into the tissue and was then forced by tissue pressure into the small veins.[82] But some of his peers were unwilling to subscribe to Harvey's physiology absent clear demonstration of some sort of connection.[83] Harvey had hoped to definitively settle this matter,[84] but he lacked the needed technology—a microscope—and the skills to effectively use it. This revolutionary tool, one of the most important in science, had first appeared in about 1600 but was little exploited until the mid-seventeenth century. Robert Hooke's *Micrographia* (1665) is the best known of the earliest books

[80] Whitteridge (1971), p. 126.

[81] Wilson (1960).

[82] Wilson (1960); Whitteridge (1971), pp. 184–186.

[83] Meli, "The New Anatomy of Marcello Malpighi," in Meli (Ed.; 1997), pp. 38–39.

[84] Keynes (1966), p. 183.

devoted to microscopic studies,[85] but our story intersects with Marcello Malpighi, the Bolognese father of histology.

Born just outside Bologna, Malpighi got his degree in medicine and philosophy at its University in 1653 and was recruited to the University of Pisa in 1656.[86] Like Galen and Harvey, he was a highly-regarded practicing physician,[87] but he is best known for mapping large tracts of what had been biological terra incognita, employing special fixation, staining, and other techniques to coax new information from sundry tissues under his lens.[88] His instruments were hopelessly crude by modern standards, but were crafted by Eustachio Divini in Rome and of the highest quality of the times..[89] Malpighi moved back to Bologna in 1659 and had a laboratory in his home as well as his Villa in Ronchi di Corticella, near Bologna.[90]

Malpighi's curiosity ranged widely: lung, brain, nerve, kidney, spleen, blood, gland, tongue, skin, sense organs, insects, silkworms, chicks in eggs, and plants were all examined. Laying first eyes on many microscopic biological structures, his contributions are too many to summarize; suffice it to say that his name lives on in multiple micro-structures, most famously the kidney's Malpighian corpuscles. His studies of the lung, which yielded the first description of the microscopic architecture of any organ, are what interest us.[91]

Finding the frog lung a suitable model ("For in this [frog anatomy] owing to the simplicity of the structure, and the almost complete transparency of the vessels which admits the eye into the interior, things are more clearly shown"), Malpighi "destroyed the whole race of frogs" in his quest to define this organ's micro-architecture.[92] In a letter to his friend Alphonsus Borelli in 1661, Malpighi described his findings, the first account of the fine connections between arteries and veins we call capillaries: "looped vessels…they extend out hither and thither from the vein and artery, that no larger system of vessels will be served, but a network appears, formed from the offshoots of the two.

vessels. This network not only occupies the whole floor (of the air space) but is extended to the walls and adheres to the outgoing vessel" (see Fig. 1.6.)[93] (Anton van Leeuwenhoek, another early microscopist, described capillaries in fish and amphibians 7 years later.)[94] Much too small to spy with the unaided eye, these vessels are at the far end of the vascular continuum: The diameter of the aorta is roughly ten thousand times greater, and its thickness one thousand times that of a capillary.

---

[85] Bardell (2004).

[86] Foster (1970), pp. 86–90.

[87] At the tail end of his career, Malpighi served as chief physician for Pope Innocent XII.

[88] Meli (2011), pp. 12, 19, 42.

[89] Bennett, "Malpighi and the Microscope," in Meli (Ed.; 1997), pp. 66–69.

[90] Meli (2011), p. 7.

[91] Meli (2011), p. 4.

[92] Young (1929).

[93] Wilson (1960).

[94] Foster (1970), p. 98.

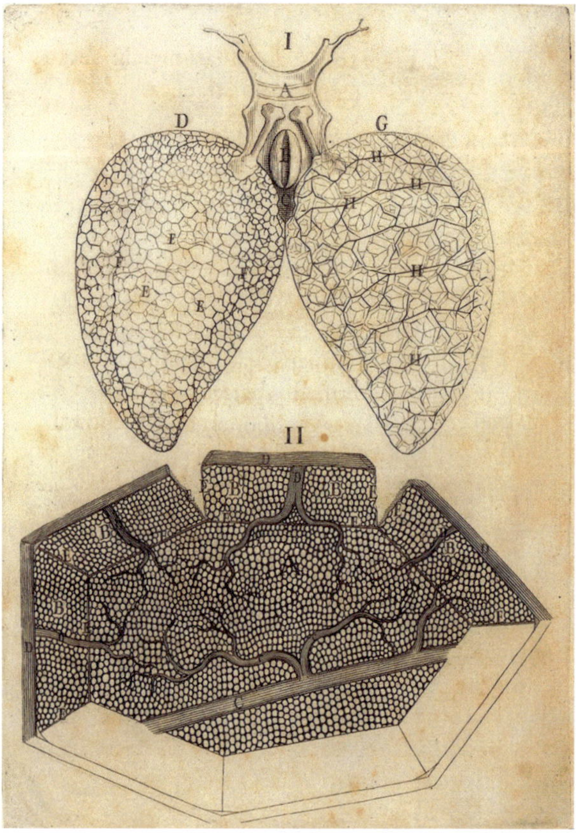


**Fig. 1.6** MALPIGHI, Marcello, (1628–1694). M. Malpighi, De pulmonibus observationes anatomicae. Bononiae: Typis Jo. Baptistae Ferronii, 1661. Engraving: figs. I and II, showing lungs and capillaries. From the Wellcome Collection, free to use with attribution

Malpighi thus closed circulation's loop and demonstrated a micro-architectural characteristic of tissue that would take on meaning only two hundred years later, as people began to understand cellular respiration. Blood—even if confined in a (thin) tube—is in such intimate proximity with the tissue within which it runs that oxygen and other molecules can quickly and efficiently rush from blood to ravenous cells.

> It therefore behooves the historian of science to be very charitable, very forbearing, very humble, in his judgments and presentations of those who have gone before him. He needs to remember that he is dealing with the work of erring and imperfect human beings, each of whom had, like himself, at best a partial view of the truth, but many of whom had a sweep of genius far beyond his own.
>
> – Charles Singer.[95]

Singer was a venerable science historian who had pondered millennia of scientific toil and theories, some stunning, some fatally flawed. Brilliant people with imagination (occasionally too much), alpha dogs in the idea economy of their day, sometimes were—put charitably—inconceivably off base. Why care? Because what we

[95] Singer (1959), p. 2.

learn from past misconceptions and faulty constructs, or ought to, is humility. And perspective. People every bit as capable as us evolved coherent theoretical systems, once widely read as gospel but impossible to square with today's objective reality. What leaves of today's conventional wisdom will someday disintegrate? What assumptions and logical and experiential frameworks *misinform* our everyday practice and efforts at therapy invention today?

Surely, we are much less vulnerable to faulty theories than five hundred years ago. Skeptical of received wisdom, we transmit information faster and further, with tremendous capacity to access accumulated data, and our cannon of physiology is vastly deeper and more solid. The massive accretion of facts and evidence, having stood well the test of time, suggests that we may be over the hump—we've gotten the big stuff right, though many details lag behind.

Maybe. But I'm pretty sure that we have yet to develop immunity to Daniel Kahneman's theory-induced blindness. Perhaps more on a micro than a grand scale, some of today's standard view is bound to eventually be torn from the textbook. Our patients throw us a few too many curveballs, and their phenotypes list off "known" physiology's axis just often enough; we must be missing some important stuff and have even gotten some "facts" wrong. The nearly unrelenting momentum of Galen's theory suggests to me—as many wiser people have opined—that knotty problems should push us outside of ourselves to ask: What other way can I think about this?

Harvey's contribution concerned the relatively large, easily visualized structures involved with energy production. But after the stuff of power generation reaches its destination, it is transformed into the energy-rich molecules which animate nearly all cellular processes. This great English physician and researcher and his peers had no understanding of these energy-related molecules, much less of their transformation inside cells. *Oxygen: What's It Good For?* examines how curious people, bit by bit and step by step, carved out an understanding of how air, and oxygen, are related to life. Compared with modern laboratories stuffed with ever more complex and sophisticated devices, the equipment and experiments used to lay the foundation of respiratory physiology were disarmingly simple, but the investigators were complex and driven. We learn much more about this "vital spirit" in Chap. 2.

## References


Alighieri D (1954) *Comedia* [The divine comedy]. (trans: Ciardi J). New American Library, New York, NY

Bardell D (2004) The invention of the microscope. Bios 75:78–84

Blainton RH (1951) Michael Servetus and the pulmonary transient of the blood. Bull Hist Med 25:1–7

Boylan M (2007) Galen: on blood, the pulse, and the arteries. J Hist Biol 40:207–230

Bylebyl JJ (1973) The growth of Harvey's *De Motu Cordis*. Bull Hist Med 47:427–470

Bylebyl JJ (1977) Nutrition, quantification and circulation. Bull Hist Med 51:369–385

Bylebyl JJ (1978) William Harvey, a conventional medical revolutionary. JAMA 238:1295–1298

Bylebyl JJ, Pagel W (1971) The chequered career of Galen's doctrine on the pulmonary veins. Med Hist 15:211–219
Coppola ED (1957) The discovery of the pulmonary circulation: a new approach. Bull Hist Med 31:44–77
Dobson JF (1927) Erasistratus. Proc Royal Soc Med 20:825–832
Fishman AP, Richards DW (1964) Circulation of the blood. Men and ideas. Oxford University Press, New York, NY
Fleming D (1955a) Galen on the motions of the blood in the heart and lungs. Isis 46:14–21
Fleming D (1955b) William Harvey and the pulmonary circulation. Isis 46:319–327
Foster M (1970) Lectures on the history of physiology. Dover Publications, New York, NY
French RK (1994) William Harvey's Natural Philosophy. Cambridge University Press.
Harris CRS (1973) The heart and the vascular system in ancient Greek medicine. Oxford University Press, Oxford
Harvey W (1628/2016) *Exercitatio anatomica de motu cordis et sanguinis in animalibus* [On the motion of the heart and blood in animals]. Carty JA (ed), (trans: Willis R). Resource Publications, Eugene.
Kahneman D (2011) Thinking, fast and slow. Farrar, Strauss and Giroux, New York, NY
Keynes G (1966) The life of William Harvey. Oxford University Press, Oxford
Meli DB (ed) (1997) Marcello Malpighi, anatomist and physician. Leo S. Olschki, Florence
Meli DB (2011) Mechanism, experiment, disease: Marcello Malpighi and seventeenth century anatomy. Johns Hopkins University Press, Baltimore
Meyerhof M (1935) Ibn A-Nafis (XIIIth cent.) and his theory of the lesser circulation. Isis 23:100–120
Mountcastle VB (ed) (1980) Medical physiology, vol 1, 14th edn. C.V. Mosby Company, St. Louis
Negro GD (ed) (2001–2003) The University of Padua: eight centuries of history. Signum Padova Editrice s.a.s, Padua
Nutton V (1984) Galen in the eyes of his contemporaries. Bull Hist Med 58:315–324
Nutton V (2002) Logic, learning, and experimental medicine. Science 295:800–801
Nye EW. Pounds sterling to dollars: historical conversion of currency. Accessed 31 Jan 2019. http://www.uwyo.edu/numimage/currency.htm
Pagel W (1976) New light on William Harvey. S. Karger, Basel
Poynter FNL, Keele KD (1961) A short history of medicine. Mills & Boon, London
Schultz SG (2002) William Harvey and the circulation of the blood: the birth of a scientific revolution and modern physiology. News Physiol Sci 17:175–180
Shackelford J (2003) William Harvey and the mechanics of the heart. Oxford University Press, Oxford
Singer C (1946) Book review. Bull Hist Med 247:122–124
Singer C (1959) A short history of scientific ideas to 1900. Oxford University Press, London
Singer PN (1997) Galen: selected works. Oxford University Press, Oxford
Temkin O (1940) Was Servetus influenced by Ibn an-Nafis? Bull Hist Med 8:731–734
Temkin O (1973) Galenism: rise and fall of a medical philosophy. Cornell University Press, Ithaca
Toledo-Pereyra LH (1973) Galen's contribution to surgery. J Hist Med All Sci 28:357–375
Whitteridge G (1971) William Harvey and the circulation of the blood. Macdonald, London
Wilson LG (1959) Erasistratus, Galen, and the *Pneuma*. Bull Hist Med 33:293–314
Wilson LG (1960) The transformation of ancient concepts of respiration in the seventeenth century. Isis 51:161–172
Young J (1929) Malpighi's "De Pulmonibus.". Proc Royal Soc Med 23:1–11
Young RA (1940) The pulmonary circulation: before and after Harvey. Part 1. Brit Med J 2:489–485

# Chapter 2
# Oxygen: What Is It Good For?: Respiration

*One thing learned leads to another.*

*–Julia Child*

For the body's various tissues, a continuous and adequate supply of the materials for respiration[1] is mission-critical, and their delivery is job one for the cardiovascular and respiratory systems. The circulation also carries signaling agents (such as hormones) and other non-energy generating molecules, and feeds blood to the filtering kidneys. But without energy generation, all this would be pointless, even were it possible. Since disability from most cardiac defects flows, ultimately, from the fact that they reduce transport of the stuff of respiration to the body's tissues, knowing how the body generates energy was fundamental to advancing therapy.

If you lift a kid on a swing chest-high, or stretch the bands on a slingshot a few inches, turning the potential energy you've generated into useful work is easy: Let go. Using gasoline's chemical energy to power you down the road is more involved because of the machinery required, although the molecular dance of the burning fuel is straightforward. But, unlike auto engines, living organisms are isothermal—that is, their temperature is the same throughout—so they cannot use heat to perform work. For heat to do work, it must flow from an area of greater to lesser heat, or a hot area cooled; the body contains no heat differentials great enough for significant energy generation.[2] Transforming chemical energy into work in biological systems is complicated. As it turns out, Nature has arranged for oxygen to play a key

[1]The word *respiration* can refer to the act of breathing or, more generally, the many metabolic processes (including breathing) involved in generating energy in the tissues; I use the word in the latter sense. The history of respiratory physiology is sprawling and could smother a much longer book than the one in your hands. This review is focused on conveying some sense of how simple equipment and observations led to seminal discoveries, and the importance of certain human qualities in advancing our knowledge. It necessarily leaves multiple important developments out. Proctor (1995), Perkins (1964), and Fishman and Richards (1964) provide more comprehensive accounts, and John B. West (2011) has published many excellent historical reviews.

[2]Lehninger (1971, pp. 23–24).



T. J. Kulik, M. Dick, *Reimagining a Child's Heart*,
https://doi.org/10.1007/978-3-031-88608-9_2

role, at least in most of the animal world. And it is this biological/molecular process which constitutes respiratory physiology (not just the lungs and breathing).

We need molecular oxygen for power generation, but it is not a fuel. Carbohydrates, fats, and amino acids are the fuels that we burn. Organisms have evolved a complex scheme, using enzymes and other molecules, to transform the chemical energy stored in foods into the common currency of biological energy via a molecule called adenosine triphosphate (ATP).[3] In a series of mitochondrial chemical reactions, using substrates or molecular products derived from the metabolism of the three fuels noted above, electrons are transferred from multiple donor molecules to receptor molecules, with energy being released with each transfer; molecular oxygen is the final electron receptor in this chain. (Water and carbon dioxide are waste products.) Oxygen isn't a fuel or a catalyst; rather, evolution has recruited it to complete the biochemical chain of events which most efficiently convert foods into energy in animals. (Other molecules serve as terminal electron acceptors in other forms of life.) We generate a limited amount of energy without using oxygen (via anaerobic [no oxygen], as opposed to aerobic [with oxygen], metabolism), but the anaerobic pathway is too feeble to meet the body's needs.

Oxygen might therefore seem a perfect place to begin exploring how the mystery of respiration was unraveled, but history suggests that we start with *air*. Oxygen, comprising 21% of the gas we breathe, is where the respiratory action is, but people pondered the life-sustaining role of air long before discovering oxygen.[4] We must assume that even pre-historic people connected the act of breathing with life, given that the lack of one invariably implies absence of the other. Ancient Greeks, some of whom you may have heard of—Aristotle, Plato, Hippocrates—and others perhaps not—Anaximenes, Empedocles, Herophilus, Erasistratus—speculated at length on what air brings to life. Air as a coolant, to moderate the innate heat of the heart, was favored by some, a notion which lies quite opposite to that of air as *promoting* energy production. Others thought that air was transformed into a vital spirit (*pneuma*). This concept is, in a very loose way, consistent with its actual function, although the very idea of a vital spirit—somehow existing outside the realm of the observable physical world, is distinctly contrary to the precisely described biochemistry that underlies respiration.[5] As to the mechanistic significance of air sucked into the lungs, much less other facets of respiration, the ancients hadn't a clue.[6]

---

[3] Adenosine triphosphate (ATP) fuels contraction of muscles, powers molecular pumps, is a component of cellular signaling, is required for building molecules, and participates in yet other cellular events. It is continuously cycling: ATP → P + energy + ADP; ADP + energy + P → ATP, where P is phosphate and ADP is adenosine *di*phosphate. Every day, ATP roughly equal to your body weight is turned over in this rapidly churning cycle (Törnroth-Horsefield and Neutze 2008). Paul Boyer, winner of a 1997 Nobel Prize for his work on this molecule, estimated that the net synthesis of ATP is the most prevalent chemical reaction in the human body and, considering the enormous size of the biomass, "that the formation and use of ATP is the principal chemical reaction in the whole world" (Boyer 1997).

[4] Dobbin (1933), citing Rutherford (1772).

[5] Dobson (1927), Wilson (1959), and Fitting (2015).

[6] Proctor (1995, pp. 3–16), citing Rosen (1953).

But how could they? Air reveals its presence in fluttering leaves or as it brushes against your face, but when you and it are at rest, nothing. No color or smell or obvious weight. Its components—mostly nitrogen and oxygen, with a little carbon dioxide and other gases—are so intimately mixed that pulling one from another, and knowing that you have, takes serious ingenuity. Mercury—now that's in your face. And iron and limestone and water and many other materials with properties easily accessible to our senses, yet even they were in many ways inscrutable for thousands of years. Furthermore, the ancient Greek conceptual framework (the four elements—earth, air, fire, and water—along with the associated humors of black bile, yellow bile, blood, and phlegm[7]) throttled new (and true) ways of thinking about physical and biological phenomena until well into the Renaissance.

The first of air's many not-so-obvious properties to be discovered is that it has weight. Galileo knew this, but despite his most excellent grey matter, he could not connect that dot with a question which perplexed the Duke of Florence's pump-makers: Why can't a suction pump raise a column of water up more than about 32 feet? But Galileo's 35-year-old pupil Evangelista Torricelli (1609–1647) could.[8] He reasoned that a vacuum could only lift a column of water that distance because the weight of the atmosphere above it equaled the weight of 32 feet of water; the water's levitation was affected by the atmosphere pushing down on it, not the vacuum attracting the water up. But how to prove it? Well, Torricelli reasoned, if I use the atmosphere to push up a column of a fluid denser than water—he chose mercury, which is 13.5 times as dense as water—then the column should be raised proportionally less high than the maximum height of pumped water (for mercury, about 0.074 × 32 feet = 2.4 feet). He filled a three-foot glass tube, closed at one end, with mercury, used his finger to keep the liquid from escaping and plunged that end into a dish of mercury with the tube held vertical.[9] The mercury in the tube fell to a height consistent with his prediction. This Italian of uncommon insight (with help) thus invented the barometer in 1643, and further work by other scientists confirmed and extended his work (Fig. 2.1).

Robert Boyle (1627–1691), a son of the 1st Earl of Cork, and his then assistant (and later major scientist and polymath) Robert Hooke (1635–1703) improved a recently invented air pump and studied the physical properties of air (1660). They also evacuated air from chambers occupied by a lit candle, and a variety of animals, first demonstrating that combustion and life both demand air.[10] Hooke reckoned that some portion of air was consumed by both combustion and respiration, and both he and Boyle conducted experiments hoping to demonstrate what that portion was. They failed, owing to the fact that oxygen consumed is replaced by carbon dioxide

[7] Porter (1997, pp. 57–59) and McClellan and Dorn (2015, pp. 88–99).

[8] Timbs (1868, pp. 38–42) and Singer (1959, p. 269).

[9] Proctor noted that it was actually Torricelli's young collaborator, Vincenzo Viviani, who first put a finger on the glass tube and constructed the barometer (1995, pp. 83–84).

[10] Singer (1959, p. 271) and Perkins (1964, p. 17).

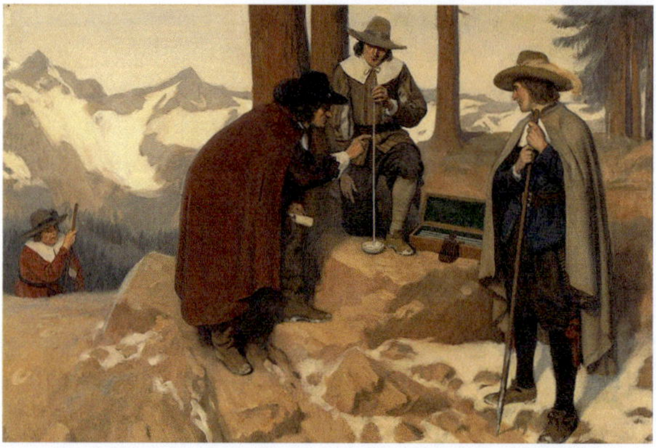

**Fig. 2.1** The discovery of the barometer: Torricelli experimenting in the Alps, 1643. Oil painting by Ernest Board. Wellcome Collection, free to use with attribution. It was actually Florin Perrier, at the behest of Blaise Pascal, who hiked a barometer up the Puy-de-Dôme in 1648 to test the relationship between atmospheric pressure and altitude. (West 2011)

produced, so that the total volume of gas in a chamber with an animal or flame shows little net change.[11]

John Mayow (1641–1710), an English physician and physiologist, following Boyle and Hooke, also believed that some fraction of air is consumed with respiration, but used a different experimental setup: "Thus let a small animal placed on a suitable support be enclosed in an inverted glass, or better, let the animal be put into a suitable cage and suspended in a glass jar. … Then let the inverted glass be sunk a little into the water, so that the water enclosed in the glass may stand at the same level as the water outside… And so, you will soon see the water sensibly rising into the cavity of the glass (Fig. 2.2)."[12]

Mayow was lucky: Because the water absorbed some of the carbon dioxide produced, the breathing animal *did* reduce the volume of gas in the chamber, but the identity of the substance apparently consumed was unknown. Mayow thought that it was a *nitro-aerial spirit*, related to saltpeter, a far cry from the molecule we now know is responsible. His work strikingly anticipated Lavoisier's, 100 years hence, but was soon forgotten, perhaps related to the advent of phlogiston theory.[13]

Richard Lower (1631–1691) was an English physician and scientist, successful enough to have Charles II's life in his hands, but whose lasting fame derives from his skill as a physiologist rather than as a practitioner. For the student of cyanosis, Lower deserves special attention, since it was he who first discovered that contact with air in the lung is what turns blue (venous) into red (arterial) blood. He had alleged in 1664 that pulmonary arterial and pulmonary venous blood were both dark, and that arterial blood must therefore have been reddened in the left ventricle.

[11] Wilson (1960).

[12] Wilson (1960).

[13] Partington (1956), Guerlac (1954), and Proctor (1995, pp. 137–139).

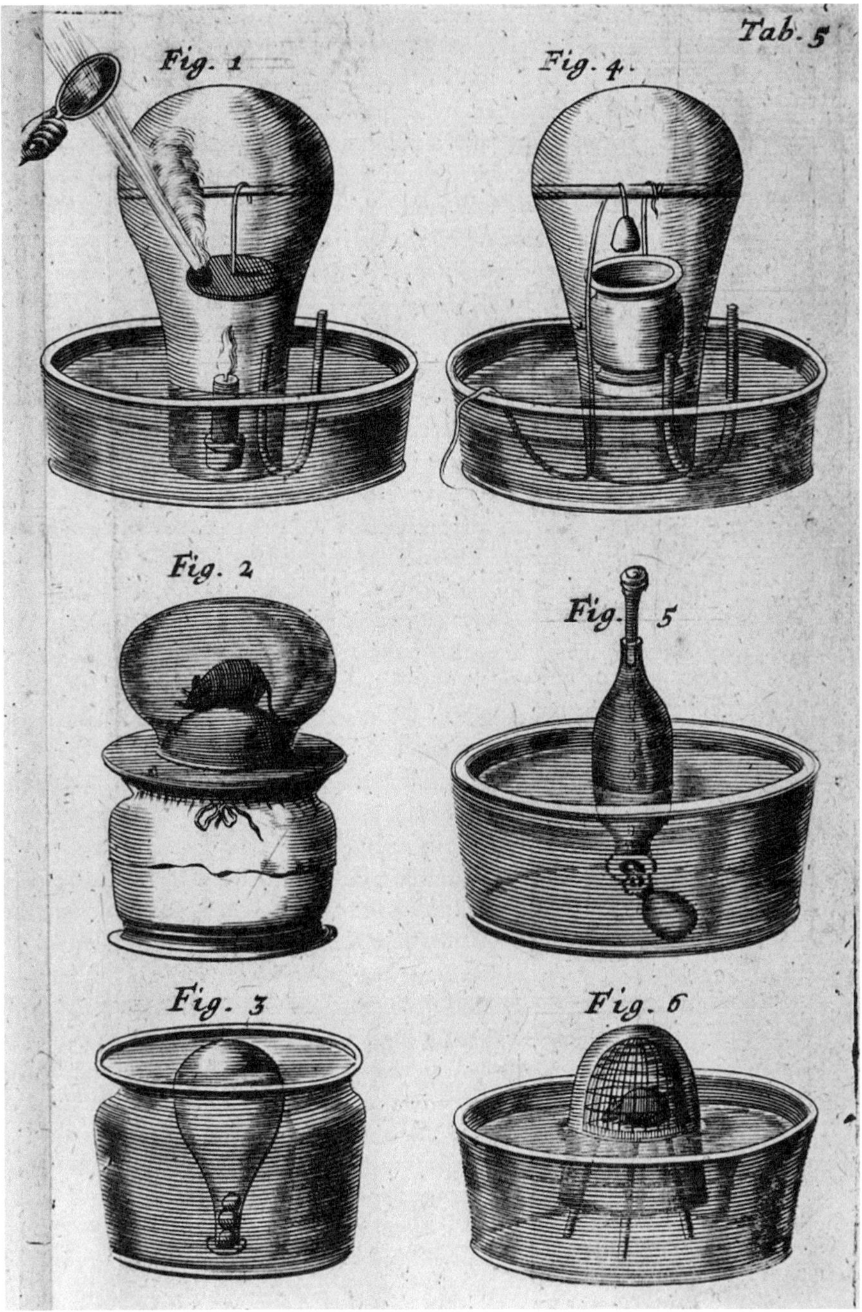


**Fig. 2.2** John Mayow: combustion and respiration. 1674. From the Wellcome Collection, free to use with attribution

But in his classic *De corde* (1669), he admitted that he had "relied more in this matter on the authority and preconceived opinion of his teacher, the learned Dr. Willis, than on my own experience … as, too, the lapse of time has now taught me differently, I shall not be loath to exchange my former view for a better one."

Lower based his argument on several complimentary experimental observations: (1) Venous and pulmonary arterial blood are both dark, while pulmonary venous and arterial blood are red; (2) with occlusion of the trachea, or in a strangled animal, blood in the left ventricle and cervical artery are dark; (3) in what must be the first reported case of something like cardiopulmonary resuscitation, Lower took a dead strangled dog, "forced" vena cava blood through the right ventricle and the (insufflated with air) lungs, and found that the pulmonary venous blood was red; (4) against the notion that the red color is due to heating of the blood in the heart, Lower pointed out that arterial blood, out of the body, does not lose its color when it cools; (5) some thought that blood is "fragmented" in the lungs, imparting the red color, but Lower argued that any such fragmentation would be more likely in the muscles than the lungs; and (6) venous blood in a dish becomes scarlet with exposure to air. With respect to the question of how oxygen made its way from the airways to the blood, he suggested that if cooling particles can penetrate glass or metal into the "drinks of gourmets and … (cool) summer wine," how much easier should the "nitrous spirit of the air" find its way from the lungs into the blood. This argument was based upon the then-current misconception of the nature of heat, but the rest of his case is watertight, even to the modern physiologist.[14] Lower knew what it takes to advance science: open minds and rigorous—usually multiple, complementary—experiments, interpreted with deep insight.

A critical step in opening respiration's kimono was dissecting air into its component gases and uncovering the role that each one plays in energy generation. The book of chemistry was pretty slim until the eighteenth century, when several seminal discoveries, compressed into a few rich decades, added many critical leaves. The Reverend Stephen Hales greatly facilitated the investigation of gases when he invented a "pneumatic trough" (1727); this simple apparatus isolated gases generated by heating substances and stored them over water for examination.[15] Scottish chemist Joseph Black (1728–1799) heated calcium carbonate and generated "fixed air" (carbon dioxide), the first gas distinct from air to be discovered, in 1756.[16] He also showed that this gas was absorbed and precipitated in alkali liquids, making it possible to easily identify and subtract carbon dioxide from mixtures of other gases, and then measure its amount.[17] In the 1770s, oxygen was isolated; air was shown to be mostly composed of two different gases (now known as oxygen and nitrogen);

---

[14] Wilson (1960).

[15] Wilson (1960) and Singer (1959, p. 334).

[16] Singer (1959, pp. 336–337) and Kuhn (1996, p. 70).

[17] Guerlac (1957a, b).

and natural philosophers learned that carbon dioxide and "vitiated air" (nitrogen) did not support combustion or respiration, while "pure air" (oxygen) did.[18]

The physical tools used to acquire this knowledge were simple, but the ingenuity applied was extraordinary. Consider how English scientist Henry Cavendish cleaved oxygen and carbon dioxide from nitrogen in air: He "transferred some common air out of one receiver through burning charcoal into a second receiver by means of a bent pipe, the middle of which was filled with powdered charcoal and heated red hot, both receivers being inverted into vessels of water … so that no air could get into it but what came out of the first receiver and passed through the charcoal." Having removed oxygen using burning charcoal, he used an alkali solution to eliminate the carbon dioxide thus formed and measured the weights of the air he started with and the nitrogen that remained. He found that nitrogen did not support combustion and determined its specific gravity by filling a bag with the gas and weighing it.[19] Another man of the cloth, Joseph Priestley (1733–1804) focused a 12-inch burning lens on mercuric oxide and produced oxygen, distinguishing it from air using the most rudimentary of observations: "[A] candle burned in the (pure) air with a remarkably vigorous flame," and a mouse confined in a chamber lived longer in this gas than in air.[20]

Eighteenth century scientists used simple contraptions to collect, store, and manipulate gases, and elegant and precisely constructed balances to weigh the materials investigated. Using simple assays, they determined fundamental properties of gases: Does it support life or flame (and, if so, how well), or rapidly snuff it out? They climbed the ladder constructed of previous discoveries, such as the fact that "fixed air" precipitated out in alkali solutions, making it possible to remove it from a mixture of gases and measure its amount. Simple tools ingeniously applied were used to mine information buried well below the level that our senses can directly access.

But by the third quarter of the 1700s, these discoveries had yet to congeal into a coherent picture, a big part of the holdup being *phlogiston* theory. According to this theory, combustible materials contain an inflammable principle called phlogiston, and burning the material releases its phlogiston, leaving a residue of ash. Combustion ceases in a closed vessel—so this idea goes—because the air becomes saturated with phlogiston, preventing its escape from the material. Phlogiston also explained the fact that heating metals in air causes formation of a calx (the metallic oxide); the calx is what remains after the phlogiston escapes.[21] Adding charcoal—a phlogiston-rich material—and heating the calx returns the metal because, so goes the theory, the charcoal donates phlogiston back to the metal. One obvious problem with this notion is that metal calx weighs *more* than the un-calcined metal, the opposite of what would be expected if a material substance escaped during calcination. But

[18] Singer (1959, pp. 338–339) and Kuhn (1996, pp. 53–55).

[19] Perkins (1964, pp. 24–25).

[20] McKie (1962, pp. 34–37).

[21] Kuhn (1996, pp. 99–100).

many observations were consistent with this concept, and with imaginative contortions (such as stipulating that phlogiston has negative weight), hands were waved and inconsistencies in the theory were explained away.[22]

Science is as much about interpretation, and construction of testable theories, as making accurate observations. Systematically flawed ways of thinking, such as phlogiston theory, can distort interpretation of experimental observations and lead to blind alleys. Indeed, progress in respiratory physiology was greatly retarded by the perceived need to attach empirical data onto phlogiston's tenuous skeleton. Joseph Priestly thought that "the function of the blood is not to receive the phlogiston of the air, or to meet with the phlogisticated air while it circulates, but to communicate phlogiston to air."[23] Experiments designed to search for a non-existent substance moving in and out of the blood, and experimental results interpreted in this light, slowed rather than accelerated real comprehension.[24] Even though it was at striking odds with what we know to be true today, phlogiston was as tenacious as skunk pee until a French scientist finally scrubbed it from the scaffolding.[25]

> I have had a fairly long life, above all a very happy one, and I think that I shall be remembered with some regrets and perhaps leave some reputation behind me. What more could I ask? The events in which I am involved will probably save me the troubles of old age. I shall die in full possession of my faculties, and that is another advantage that I should count among those that I have enjoyed. If I have any distressing thoughts, it is of not having done more for my family; to be unable to give either to them or to you any token of my affection and my gratitude is to be poor indeed.[26]

Antoine Lavoisier wrote his ultimate letter, to his cousin, 1 day before falling victim to the Terror in revolutionary France. The allegations which authorized his trip to the guillotine were trumped up, and mostly related to his previous work as a Farmer-General. The revolutionaries in charge had no taste for the "bloodsuckers" who were the *Ferme Générale* (Tax Farm)—the organization in pre-revolutionary France that collected taxes for the state—and besides, these charges provided justification for looting the wealth of the Farmers and their families. We don't care about Antione Lavoisier because his blood mingled with the scarlet streams of 1793—he was only one of many. He is woven into our tapestry by virtue of his foundational contributions to respiratory physiology, and because he so splendidly displays one species of human motivation which powers medical innovation. We will start with the first strand.

Using an experimental setup that a precocious grade-schooler could cobble together, Lavoisier was the first to provide real insight into oxygen's action inside the body. Even more, his physiological contributions were only a fragment of a

---

[22] Fishman and Richards (1964, p. 41), citing André Cournand.

[23] See Keilin (1966, pp. 24–27), for a discussion of how phlogiston theory got in the way of Priestley's interpretation of his experimental data.

[24] Kuhn (1996, pp. 70–72).

[25] McKie (1962, p. 287).

[26] Keilin (1966, p. 28).

greater body of work that certifies him as one of the greatest of scientists.[27] In Thomas Kuhn's highly influential *The Structure of Scientific Revolutions*, only four names are highlighted as fomenters of such disruptions: Copernicus, Newton, Lavoisier, and Einstein. Lowering a candle snuffer over the taper of phlogiston theory, Lavoisier showed people a better way to think about the chemical world and, by the lights of many scholars, founded modern chemistry.

Lavoisier was born in 1743 into a well-to-do Parisian family, his father a lawyer.[28] Starting university studies at age 11 at the Collège des Quatre Nations—commonly known as Collège Mazarin—he first concentrated on the humanities, then directed his energies to science. He finished with a degree in law, though he never practiced. We mostly remember Lavoisier for his science, but the sheer volume and variety of his other responsibilities is astonishing. What follows is a grossly deficient accounting of his myriad contributions in the public and political sphere, giving only an inkling of his activities outside the laboratory. Lavoisier was:

An elected member of the Royal Academy of Sciences
A Farmer-General at the *Ferme Générale*
One of four commissioners on the Gunpowder Commission
Secretary of the Committee of Agriculture, the Royal Society of Agriculture, and undertook experimental agricultural studies at his farm at Fréchines.
An elected representative of the Provincial Assembly of Orleanais
President of the Bureau of Consultation of Arts and Crafts
Director of the Discount Bank and Commissioner of the National Treasury
National Commissioner of Weights and Measures
A founder of Lycée des Arts
A contributor in the Constituent Assembly, the Commune of 1789, the Committee on Assignats and Coinage, the Committee on Public Health, and the National Guard at the beginning of the Revolution

These were not honorary positions, and many required huge expenditures of time and work.[29] His wide-ranging intellect and boundless energy intersected with chemistry, geology, meteorology, agronomy, economics, education, public administration, public policy (including public health), philanthropy, and politics. Lavoisier wasn't just a Swiss army knife; he was the machine shop.

But it was his work in his laboratory in his home at the Royal Arsenal that we remember best. To understand Lavoisier's contribution, you need to juxtapose our understanding of gases with that up until the late 1770s. If one says "oxygen" or "nitrogen" today, the mental picture formed is instantaneous: atoms of a specific and uniform type, with well-defined physical properties and known effects on materials and organisms. If you buy a tank of it, you know exactly what you've got. The eighteenth century scientist's perception of gases was much fuzzier. People knew

[27] Kuhn (1996, p. 6).

[28] Weeks (1934).

[29] McKie (1962, pp. 54–55) and French (1941, p. 142).

that an animal or burning candle confined in a closed chamber eventually changed the gas in that space so that it would no longer support life or flame but did not know why. Scottish physician Daniel Rutherford (1749–1819), even before Henry Cavendish, separated nitrogen from oxygen and carbon dioxide in air, but thought that the nitrogen was air saturated with phlogiston.[30] Scientists heated chemicals and generated a gas (oxygen) that supported life better than air—without perceiving the nature of its relationship to air. They could produce "fixed air" (carbon dioxide), which precipitated in alkali solutions, and knew that gas was also generated by animals. Joseph Black demonstrated this in the real world: He dripped limewater over rags in a ceiling air duct of a Glasgow church, exposed it to 15,000 person hours of exhaled breath during the service, producing a significant quantity of crystalline lime.[31] But what fixed air had to do with oxygen or carbon was unknown. And, as we've seen, phlogiston theory hobbled investigators, suggesting, for example, that a candle in a bell jar eventually goes out having saturated the air with phlogiston. (Thus, "dephlogisticated air" was the term Priestly used for oxygen.) The scientist of the day was like a blind pedestrian in a strange neighborhood with a directionally impaired guide dog.

By 1777, Lavoisier, by dint of his own experiments and those of others, realized that "Eminently respirable air (oxygen) that enters the lung, leaves it in the form of chalky aeriform acids (carbon dioxide) … in almost equal volume… Respiration acts only on the portion of pure air which is eminently respirable … the excess, that is the mephitic portion [nitrogen], is a purely passive medium… The respirable portion of air has the property to combine with blood and its combination results in its red color."[32]

He had therefore deduced that there were *two* processes going on in respiration, oxygen uptake and carbon dioxide production, concluding that either oxygen is changed in the lungs into carbon dioxide, or exchanged for carbon dioxide. Very importantly, he found that fixed air is given off with both respiration and when charcoal burns and surmised that heat must be generated by both processes. His quantitative demonstration of the equivalence of burning and respiration is a classic, illustrating how profound insight can be gleaned using only the simplest of tools if one is clever enough.

To define the relationship between the heat generated and the carbon dioxide produced, he needed to measure the amount of heat produced by an animal, and by burning charcoal. To do this, working with Pierre-Simon Laplace in the winter of 1782–1783, Lavoisier employed an ice calorimeter, the idea being that the quantity of ice melted in a period of time is directly related to the amount of heat applied to it. The calorimeter, crafted by tinsmith Pierre Naudin to their specifications,[33] consisted of an inner basket (f), where a guinea pig, or burning coal, resided during the

---

[30] Weeks (1934).

[31] Guerlac (1957a).

[32] West (2011).

[33] Poirier (1996, p. 137).

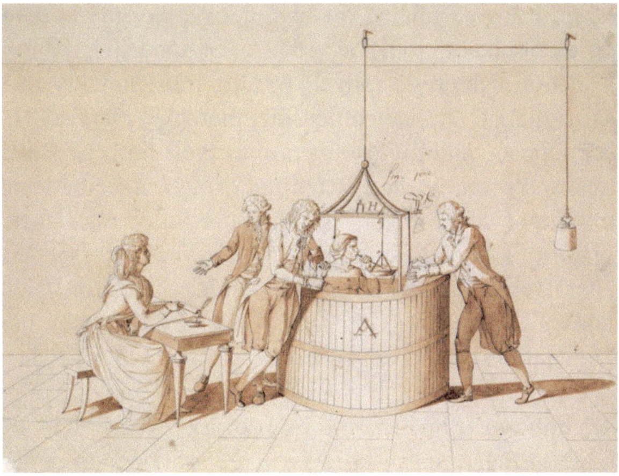


**Fig. 2.3** Pen and ink drawing on Antione Lavoisier performing a respiration experiment while his wife takes notes. Attributed to Marie-Anne-Pierrette Lavoisier, c. 1970. From Wellcome Collection, free to use with attribution

experiment (Fig. 2.3). Outside this basket was a chamber holding ice (b), surrounded by a second chamber (a), also filled with ice. (Basket “a” insulated the inner one from external heat so that any melting in “b” would be due only to the animal or charcoal.) The volume of water from melted ice in “b” was measured and reflected the amount of heat generated. Gas from the chamber was collected, and the quantity of carbon dioxide was determined.

Lavoisier and Laplace found that the ratios of carbon dioxide produced to heat generated were very similar (albeit not identical) with the animal and burning coal, leading Lavoisier to conclude that “Respiration is then a combustion, admittedly very slow, but nevertheless completely analogous to that of charcoal; it takes place in the interior of the lungs.”[34] He was wrong about the site of combustion (which, of course, occurs throughout the body), and knew not what substance(s) combined with air during combustion. There was still a lot to learn, but Lavoisier had provided a glimpse into *how* air works to support life.

I hope that the copperplate engraving of the calorimeter—as sharp and clean as an engineer’s blueprint, but warmly textured—caught your eye. That contrivance was just one of Lavoisier’s many scientific tools rendered onto paper by his wife Marie. Marie-Anne Paulze was just shy of 14 when she married Lavoisier (he, 28), a union that would provoke a gimlet eye in many quarters today. But things were different then, and there were exigent circumstances: Marie’s father, Jacques (who, like Lavoisier, was a Farmer General), was under considerable pressure from Joseph Terray, the Controller-General of Finance, to give her hand to Count d’Amerval, a man of 50 with little money and “whose character … cannot please either my daughter or you or myself, I am, indeed, well assured.” (Marie, with all the tact and subtlety typical of her tender age, said the proposed husband was a “fool, stupid and ill-mannered, a kind of ogre.”) But Paulze was in a tough spot since his position at the Farm depended on Terray. In an effort to slide the proposed arrangement off the

[34] Underwood (1943).

table, Paulze arranged for his junior colleague at the Farm to marry Marie.[35] The union turned out to be, as a master of understatement might declare, fruitful.

Marie's interests ranged widely, most notably in science, art, and politics. A skillful host, she welcomed innumerable scientists (Benjamin Franklin was one), economists, and philosophers into their home.[36] But it was her absorption in her husband's (really, their) scientific work that secured her place in history. A close and important collaborator, starting soon after marriage, Marie displayed a level of maturity and dedication seldom seen, much less in an early teenager. She studied chemistry and learned English (Antione never did), allowing her to read and translate scientific works from English scientists for her husband's personal use.[37] Drawing lessons taken from the well-known artist Jacques Louis David paid dividends in the crisp and precise engravings and drawings she made of her husband's scientific instruments, and even of the experiments themselves. Sitting at a small table in the Arsenal lab, Marie recorded experimental protocols and results, and edited manuscripts reporting the data (Fig. 2.3—[the VO2 experiment]). As her assessment of Count d'Amerval suggests, Marie was a tough cookie,[38] which doubtlessly proved useful in the Lavoisier's' long but ultimately successful campaign to convince skeptical scientists to ditch phlogiston theory for the "new chemistry."[39] We cannot know what fraction of Antione's profound scientific impact flowed from Marie's strenuous efforts, but it seems certain that his scientific oeuvre could have been much smaller without such magnificent support on the home front.

The famous Jacques David painting of M. and Mme. Lavoisier seems to suggest as much (Fig. 2.4). The scene is resplendent, with Antoine and Marie richly dressed, the adjacent desk draped in striking crimson, and several pieces of labware, beautifully crafted in blown glass with turned brass fixtures and containing the ever-present mercury, scattered about. Your eye is drawn most insistently to Marie, not her husband. Her gaze is soft, almost beseeching, but her mouth is firm. One senses a lack of emotional connection with Antoine, an impression strengthened by the knowledge of her current (and long-standing) affair with Pierre Samuel Dupont.[40] Antoine, too, signals little affection, but rather seems to be seeking enlightenment or approval from his wife. The painting's center of gravity may reflect the fact that it was Marie who commissioned the painting,[41] but even if so, Mme. Lavoisier's compelling presence in this eighteenth century scientific tableau squares nicely with what we know of life at the Arsenal lab.

---

[35] McKie (1962, pp. 65–68).

[36] Poirier (1996, pp. 95–96) and West (2013).

[37] Rayner-Canham and Rayner-Canham (2001, p. 18).

[38] Poirier (1996, ch. 20) and McKie (1962, pp. 282, 306).

[39] Guerlac (1975, p. 107) and Keilin (1966, p. 27).

[40] Poirier (1996, pp. 125–126). Dupont was the father of Eleuthère Irénée Dupont, founder of the Delaware gunpowder manufacturing firm which grew into the well-known industrial chemical giant.

[41] Poirier (1996, p. 1).

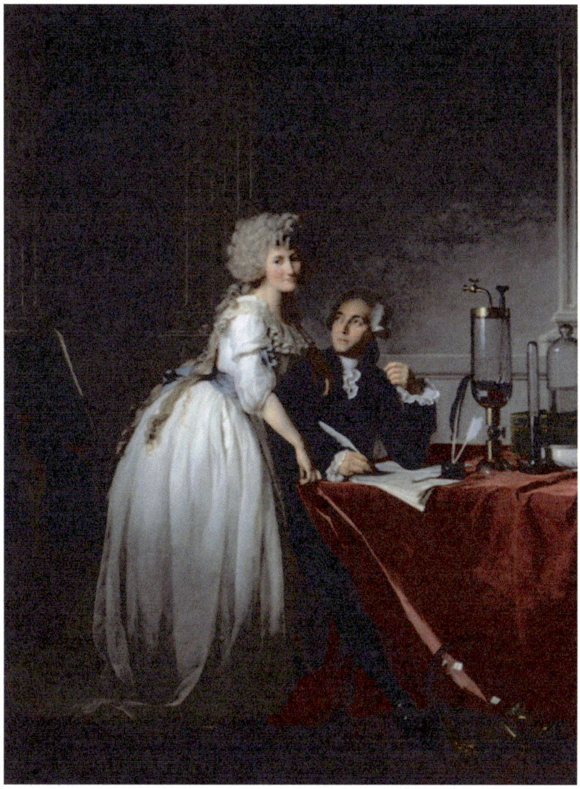

**Fig. 2.4** Jacques Louis David: M. and Mme. Laviosier. (With permission from the Metropolitan Museum of Art, NY, NY)

Rather late in her life, after Antoine was gone, Marie "devoted herself entirely to her friends and the people she entertained with a rather singular mixture of rudeness and courtesy. She was always very good company and showed a great understanding of the world, although her language could be brusque, and she was subject to authoritarian whims."[42] Marie combined sociability and pungent self-confidence, scientific inclination and artistic flare, and loyalty and dedication in stoking the fire under one of the greatest of scientific careers.

It's hard to draw a bead on Lavoisier the man, as information regarding his personal life is regrettably limited.[43] Given his early matriculation at Mazarin, his extraordinary intelligence must have soon been obvious. But Lavoisier's mind was more than formidable, it was *supple*. While other brilliant contributors, such Joseph Priestly and Henry Cavendish, clung tenaciously to the existing paradigm,[44] Lavoisier had the intellectual flexibility—a quality far less abundant than high

[42] Poirier (1996, p. 409).

[43] McKie (1962, p. 179) and Poirier (1996, p. 126).

[44] Perkins (1964, p. 26).

IQ—needed to let go of the jetsam of phlogiston. He was also careful and methodical, which was essential for his laboratory work, which necessitated making innumerable accurate measurements and observations.

It seems that Lavoisier had many friends but, outside his family, few or nonclose.[45] But he deeply cared for people, and his efforts of social reform and public service were legion. He had sympathy for the poor, offering that "If it is allowable to make exceptions in favor of any class, especially with regard to taxes, it can only be in favor of the poor." Generous in his support of younger scientists, peasants working at his farm in Fréchines, and others, he made loans at low or no interest, many never paid off.[46] He was as honest as he was tireless in public service.[47] Lavoisier cannot have had much time for activities outside his public and scientific life, although, like his wife, he enjoyed music.[48]

But he could be prickly, lacked a sense of humor, and was stubborn.[49] One of his biographers observed that "flexibility and diplomacy were not [Lavoisier's] strong points."[50] When Talleyrand asked him to critique—with "great severity"—a report on public education, Lavoisier obliged: "Education, as it exists in almost all of Europe, was set up not to produce citizens, but priests, monks, and theologians. The spirit of the Church has always loathed any innovation, and because the first Christians spoke and prayed in Latin … it was necessary to pray in Latin until the end of time." "This is how everything that might tend to destroy errors and prejudices was kept in the hands of those who had an interest in propagating them."[51]

His ambition was boundless, and one might be tempted to suspect that it was the need for public recognition that drove his laboratory efforts. He took a highly proprietary view of his work and demanded at least a full measure of credit.[52] While many scientist-innovators are eager to demonstrate public generosity—sharing credit with others for advances that they have spearheaded—Lavoisier was not. Commenting in 1792 on the "new chemistry" that he ushered in, he wrote that "This theory is not, as I have heard it said, the theory of French chemists, it is *mine*, and it is a property that I claim before my contemporaries and posterity."[53] Many have accused him of appropriating the observations of Priestly and Cavendish without due credit, although others find these charges to be of little merit.[54]

One biographer observed that "[Benjamin] Franklin, like Lavoisier, was a distinguished scientist and public servant, but unlike Lavoisier, Franklin had won hearts

[45] McKie (1962, p. 13) and French (1941, p. 109).

[46] McKie (1962, p. 184) and French (1941, pp. 141–145).

[47] French (1941, p. 129).

[48] McKie (1962, p. 182).

[49] Poirier (1996, pp. 186, 382) and French (1941, p. 129).

[50] Poirier (1996, p. 289).

[51] Poirier (1996, pp. 337–378).

[52] Poirier (1996, pp. 66, 143) and McKie (1962, p. 186).

[53] Donovan (1993, p. 182).

[54] French (1941, pp. 125, 146–162) and McKie (1962, pp. 186–187).

as well as minds. The French thought of Franklin … as a man of mythical grandeur and avuncular wisdom, attributes of greatness never attributed to Lavoisier."[55] Astringent rather than avuncular, rational rather than warm, Lavoisier never enjoyed the popular veneration we might expect for someone who contributed so generously to the commonweal.

We come now to Lavoisier's paramount quality, and the second reason why this French scientist is woven into our tapestry: *curiosity*. Driven to discover and to understand, he exemplifies the unmatched power of curiosity for rendering the concealed visible. One of his many biographers concluded: "For Lavoisier the most profound pleasures associated with experimental enquiry clearly came, not from dominating the activities of his research associates or commanding the assent of his academic peers, but rather from pursuing truths about how nature operates."[56] A contemporary observed that Lavoisier "spared nothing to discover a truth and counted neither labor nor money when it was a question of advancing a step."[57]

Stronger indication that Lavoisier's impetus was curiosity, not hunger for fame, was furnished by Marie. He devoted 6 hours each day and one whole day a week to experiments: "It was a day for him," she wrote, "a day of happiness; some friends who shared his views and some young men proud to be admitted to the honor of collaborating in his experiments assembled in the morning in the laboratory. There they lunched, there they debated; and it was there that the theory that immortalized its author was created. It was there that you could have heard this man with his precise mind, his clear intelligence, his high genius, the loftiness of his philosophical principles illuminating his conversation."[58] Containing over 13,000 items of chemical apparatus and other specimens and 250 instruments,[59] Lavoisier's lab was state of the art and *très cher*, funded only on his dime. It seems to me that his incalculable investment of resources—temporal, monetary, creative—into science's vineyard can only be traced to a furious need to understand the physical world.

As we have seen in the Introduction, to create therapy for mitral stenosis, Charles Bailey (Chap. 5), willingly put himself at grave professional risk. Was his readiness to imperil his career compelled by the challenge of perfecting his idea, the urge to heal, or a desire for recognition? Probably all three, in variable measure, were in the mix, but shear curiosity wasn't.[60] Taussig and Blalock (Chap. 6), it seems, were motivated mostly by the urge to heal. Maude Abbott's drive, as we will see in Chap. 4, was more complex and unusual. Medical doctors work in the here and now, and even those with an inventive bent generally aim to create near-term practical results.

---

[55] Donovan (1993, p. 183).

[56] Donovan (1993, p. 280).

[57] French (1941, p. 124).

[58] McKie (1962, p. 183).

[59] McKie (1962, p. 185).

[60] Weisse (2002, pp. 79–80). In an oral interview with Allen Weisse, Bailey admitted that there was intense competition between him and Dwight Harken, a second surgeon striving to develop similar therapy (and accrue priority bragging rights), indicating that an unalloyed desire to heal was *not* his sole motive for pursuing his invention.

In contrast, Lavoisier's scientific exertions were not primarily directed at producing useful stuff, but rather reflected a compulsion to know for knowing's sake.

The exquisite force of curiosity is an old and recurring story among scientists, and its footprints are many. My favorite anecdote concerns Isaac Newton, related by Richard Westfall: "[W]hen he was developing a theory of colors [Newton] slipped a bodkin [needle] 'betwixt me eye & y^e^ bone as neare to y^e^ backside of my eye as I could' in order to alter the curvature of the retina and to observe the colored circles that appeared as he pressed. How did he fail to blind himself? In the grip of discovery, Newton did not pause to reckon the cost."[61] But medical innovators mostly aim for the utilitarian (including, at times, fame, and money), which tends to get the most attention. Yet without a thirst for discovery for its own sake, we would pursue only endeavors with a reasonable prospect of delivering practical results in the not-so-distant future; longer-slog quests for deep understanding would be unusual. But these extraordinarily precious threads of fundamental knowledge are what separate our tapestry from burlap.

> A living cell requires energy not only for all its functions, but also for the maintenance of its structure. Without energy life would be extinguished instantaneously, and the cellular fabric would collapse. –Albert Szent-Györgyi, in his 1937 Nobel Prize lecture[62]

Lavoisier's critical insight about combustion was a breakthrough, but it was also misleading. It provoked investigators to focus on *heat*, and where in the body it is produced,[63] while *energy*, in the form of ATP, is actually the point of respiration. Following the French scientists' findings, multiple investigators conducted many experiments, yielding no consensus; the site of heat's generation was held to be the lungs or in the blood, notions which persisted until at least the 1870s.[64] What should have been a widely resonating signal that the locus of combustion lay elsewhere was issued in the late eighteenth century by Lazzaro Spallanzani (1729–1799), an Italian scientist who found that *tissues* from freshly killed animals both consumed oxygen and gave off carbon dioxide. But, like John Mayow, his findings were little appreciated for reasons unclear; the sheer volume of extraneous material one had to plow through to uncover the nuggets in Spallanzani's massive corpus may offer partial explanation.[65]

In fact, even whether air moved from the lungs into the blood was unsettled, despite Lower's work. Only in the 1830s did Gustav Magnus (1802–1870), using a better way of measuring blood gases, demonstrate that oxygen existed in greater quantity in arterial than venous blood, with the reverse being true for carbon dioxide. While this German scientist finally dislodged energy production from the lungs, he mistakenly situated it in the capillaries, rather than the tissues.[66] More evidence

---

[61] Westfall (1980, p. 94).

[62] Szent-Györgyi (1937).

[63] Mendelsohn (1961).

[64] Scheer (1939).

[65] Scheer (1939) and Keilin (1966, p. 36).

[66] Mendelsohn (1961).

of tissue respiration was adduced by Justus Liebig, who, working in Giessen in 1850, showed that isolated frog muscle consumed oxygen and emitted carbon dioxide. Italian Carlo Matteucci confirmed these findings and concluded that "one must admit, as proved by experiments, that the chemical action of muscular respiration during contraction is the cause of the force which is developed in muscles."[67] But not everyone so admitted, even until the late 1870s, although the tide had begun to turn with the influential physiologist Claude Bernard's strong support of tissue respiration in 1876. That the site of respiration is the tissues, rather than the lung or blood, was pretty much settled by the turn of the century.[68]

What was combusting, and how, was learned concurrently. Liebig understood that food and oxygen were utilized by the body for movement. Parsing food into three categories (carbohydrate, protein, and fats), by the mid-nineteenth century he not only showed that they were used for repair and energy, but also how much oxygen was used and the quantity of heat produced.[69] By the *fin de siècle* and early twentieth century, scientists knew that the circulation transported oxygen and food to the tissues, where energy was generated, although they knew very little of the biochemistry of energy production.

The ultimate locus of energy production is the cell and sub-cellular structures, especially the mitochondria. Between the late 1800s and 1925, chemists and biochemists intensively studied hemoglobin, the chemical that gives blood its color and carries almost all of its oxygen. They defined pathways of carbohydrate metabolism, identified relevant enzymes, and discerned the mechanisms underlying biological oxidations.[70] Many of their tools are surprisingly analogous to those of previous generations. Unlike their predecessors, who used animals and candles for assays, biochemists employed chemicals with known characteristics (e.g., methylene blue) to detect certain types of chemical reactions. Naturally-occurring substances—not chalk or mercury, as was the case for earlier scientists, but biological agents, such as milk, yeast, tissue extracts, and red blood cells—were exploited as sources of enzymes and other relevant molecules. Reagents (for example, cyanide and carbon monoxide) known to inhibit certain reactions shed light on the nature of biochemical pathways by altering reactions in a defined way.[71]

Otto H. Warburg (1883–1970), a German physician and physiologist and winner of the 1931 Nobel Prize for Physiology or Medicine, sliced tissues into fragments only a few cells thick, bathed them in solution, and measured the amount of oxygen they consumed under various experimental conditions. He used a "Warburg manometer," whose operating principle was simple: The quantity of oxygen consumption was a function of the change in the height of a column of fluid between the reaction flask and the atmosphere. Anticipating today's high throughput biological screening

---

[67] Scheer (1939).

[68] Scheer (1939).

[69] Rosen (1955) and Perkins (1964, pp. 34–38).

[70] Keilin (1966, pp. 117–139).

[71] Ball (1974).

systems, this meticulous German scientist used multiple manometers to study several samples simultaneously.[72]

Conceptually newer instruments and techniques facilitated more fruitful interrogation of biochemical pathways in tissues and cells. Absorbance spectroscopy, for example, provides a very different type of information than what was available to Lavoisier and colleagues. Pass light, which is composed of a spectrum of wavelengths, through a material, and some wavelengths are absorbed more than others; the pattern of transmitted light is characteristic of the molecules interrogated. This exceedingly useful tool, which identifies chemicals otherwise difficult or impossible to discern, was one that David Keilin—another scientist "stimulated solely by the urge to understand the living world"—put to superb use.[73]

Keilin (Fig. 2.5) was born in Moscow in 1887, but his family soon moved back to Warsaw, where his father was a successful businessman. He took courses at the University of Liège for a year, then moved to Paris in 1905. Jobless, he studied the arts and philosophy until chance intervened: After leaving a Henri Bergson lecture, he took shelter from the rain in a building where Maurice Caullery, a notable French biologist, was lecturing. Keilin wandered into the lecture and found it so interesting that he wound up training under Caullery at the Laboratoire d'Évolution des Êtres Organisés.

Keilin developed into an entomologist and parasitologist, specializing in parasitic insects. Moving to the University of Cambridge in 1915, he was, like Lavoisier and Warburg, meticulous and prolific, publishing 50 original papers by 1920, including important original contributions.[74] From 1919 onward, he was especially interested in how flies respire, especially *Gasterophilus intestinalis*, a horse parasite. In the course of these studies, which were only very tangentially aimed at the biochemistry of respiration (recall that he was not a biochemist), Keilin noticed that, while hemoglobin was present in fly larvae, it disappeared as they matured into adults. Using a spectroscopic microscope, he found that a light passed through an adult fly's wing muscles showed something unexpected: *four distinct absorption bands,* none hemoglobin.]Worried that the bands might only represent a transformation product of hemoglobin, Keilin made many additional observations—in

[72] Warburg knew how to write a grant. In (probably) 1921, he applied to the Emergency Association of German Science for funds: *Dr. Otto Warburg / Application / I require 10,000 (ten thousand) Mark / Otto Warburg*. He was fully funded (Otto 2016; Koppenol et al. 2011).

Biochemist Eric G. Ball recalled that Warburg visited Johns Hopkins in the fall of 1929 and gave a paper bag luncheon. Ball, a postdoctoral fellow at the time, was there: "Here together were two of the most precise and accurate experimenters I have ever known. For this special occasion Bill Clark (a professor of biochemistry at Hopkins) had purchased cigars. After lunch he handed them out, bit off the end of his own cigar, spit it out, and proceeded to light his cigar. Warburg sat watching quizzically, then reached into a pocket, pulled out a penknife, and meticulously cut off the end of his own cigar. This is all I remember now about what was for me at the time a most impressive occasion" (Ball 1974). Science, perhaps *especially* for scientists, is much more than technical developments and exciting discoveries.

[73] Hartree (1973).

[74] Mann (1964) and Hartree (1963).

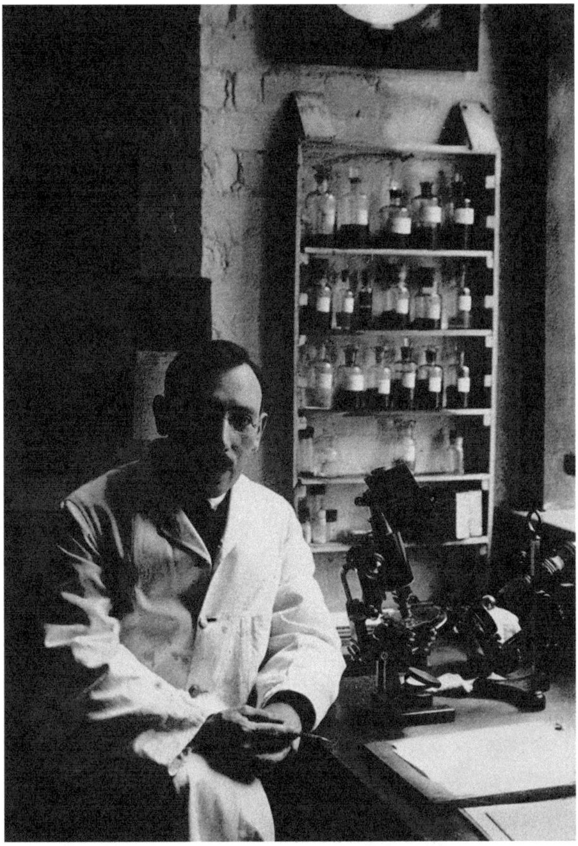

**Fig. 2.5** David Keilin from Welcome Trust, free to use with attribution. Note the simplicity of the lab vs. profundity of discoveries made

blowflies, other insects, and *Bacillus subtilis* (a type of bacteria)—all with similar results. For one last proof that the substance was novel, he put fresh baker's yeast under his microscope and saw the same bands, which "clearly showed that this pigment which gave a four-banded absorption spectrum was completely independent of hemoglobin and its derivatives. At that time, I had no knowledge of the main property of cytochrome, namely its reversible oxidation and reduction."[75]

The biochemical phenomenon of reversible oxidation and reduction was what made Keilin's discovery so important, and it was revealed through serendipity and the other side of that coin, acute observation and interpretation. Keilin had vigorously shaken a bit of yeast in water and placed a drop of the suspension under his microscope. What he observed was totally unexpected: *no* bands at first, but moments later the four bands suddenly appeared. He repeated this experiment "time after time and always with the same result: the absorption bands disappeared on shaking with air and reappeared within a few seconds of standing. I must admit that

[75] Keilin (1966, p. 145).

this first visual perception of an intracellular respiratory process was one of the most impressive spectacles I have witnessed in the course of my work."[76] The four-banded molecules—*cytochromes*—were oxidized when exposed to air during shaking, which changed their absorbance characteristics, causing them to lose the bands. A few seconds later, these proteins were reduced, causing the bands to appear. Keilin, initially curious about the fate of larval hemoglobin, had stumbled onto some seriously important molecules needed for energy production. Cytochromes transfer electrons from hydrogen atoms of intermediary metabolites, and the protons thus created drive ion transport and ATP generation. Keilin's discovery[77] was a landmark in the quest to understand some of the most basic of basic biology.[78]

Much more work on the molecular and atomic mechanisms of respiration remained after Keilin's landmark discovery. ATP was discovered in 1929, but only after another 10 years was its role as the main currency of cellular energy discerned. Other important discoveries and refinements were made yet later,[79] as increasingly powerful probes, such as radioisotopes and genetic modification of proteins, enabled scientists to peer ever deeper into the cell's interior. But Peter Mitchell commenced his 1978 Nobel Prize lecture[80] by looking back five decades, with words of praise for David Keilin as "one of the greatest of biochemists and—to me at least—the kindest of men, whose marvelously simple studies of the cytochrome system … led to the original fundamental idea of aerobic energy metabolism: the concept of the respiratory chain." Keilin is a fine example of curiosity melded with painstaking and precise effort—aided and abetted with good luck—culminating in a major brick in biology's wall.[81]

We've learned how scientists used simple pieces of apparatus to discover why, and how, breathing is critical to life. Having grown up in an era whose laboratories are decorated with complex instruments crammed with electronics and precision optical systems, I was gratified to learn how pieces of blown glass, measuring instruments containing nary an electronic component, and a limited number of reagents were used to make many foundational discoveries. Rudimentary experiments yielded fundamental insights about gases and chemical processes,

[76] Keilin (1966, p. 145).

[77] Keilin (1966, pp. 86–116) and Mann (1964).

[78] Slater (2003), Keilin (1966, pp. 140–165), and Hartree (1963). Keilin was nominated for a Nobel prize many times over a span of nearly 30 years. In a section entitled "David Keilin and the possible disadvantages of competing with a Swedish candidate," Erling Norrby discusses in detail the history of the failed nominations (Norrby 2016, pp. 244–250). Keilin's report of cytochromes was in 1925, and he was not the first to identify these proteins. Very similar observations were described in 1884 by Irish physician Charles A. MacMunn. Keilin acknowledged this and called attention to reasons that MacMunn's work had been neglected (Keilin 1966, pp. 86–116; Mann 1964).

[79] For example, Nobel prizes were awarded in 1953, 1978, and 1997 for work on cellular respiration (Krebs 1953; Mitchell 1978; Boyer 1997; Walker 1997).

[80] Mitchell (1978).

[81] I'm not sure why the "to me at least" is included here; many people who knew Keilin well attested to his kindness, professional generosity, and modesty (Hartree 1963; Slater 2003; Mann 1963, 1964).

and—because one thing learned led to another—a detailed canon evolved. People made painstaking and accurate observations, doggedly following one experiment with another and yet another. Scientists had the flexibility and self-confidence to shatter deeply entrenched (and nearly universally accepted) conceptual traditions. Investigators, burning with curiosity, pursued surprise leads. Good luck also helped. And we also saw how published work can somehow get lost in the shuffle, for reasons not always apparent. In short, advances in respiratory physiology mirrored the scientific enterprise in general.

We've explored, in these first two chapters, the creation of a singularly important installment of respiratory physiology: oxygen's primacy and its delivery. Cardiology's spine. We do not breathe to cool a fiery heart. Quite the contrary: The gas we breathe contains a component—oxygen—that makes blue blood red, which is required for life-sustaining "combustion" in the body's tissues. And it is the heart and blood vessels that distribute oxygen to tissues and cells, feeding molecular engines of energy production. These discoveries were the walking preceding the running needed for a working comprehension of congenital heart disease. We've left many details unexplored—for example, gas exchange in the lung and tissues, and control of the heart and blood vessels—but the human factors are the very same as those underlying other chapters in physiology's corpus.

It's time now to edge closer to single ventricle therapy. The early twentieth century found surgery, so inventive when faced with challenges outside the chest, with little to offer the limping heart. As outlined in the Introduction and Appendix 2, general, orthopedic, ophthalmologic, plastic, otorhinolaryngologic, neurologic, and urologic procedures have (admittedly in a limited way) offered relief for hundreds and even thousands of years, but cardiac surgery is really a child of the mid-twentieth century. But first we will look at the *State of the Art* prior to and in the early twentieth century.

## References

Ball EG (1974) The development of our current concepts of biological oxidations. Mol Cell Biochem 5:35–46

Boyer PD (1997) Energy, life, and ATP. 1997 Nobel Lecture. Accessed 18 Oct 2018. https://www.nobelprize.org/prizes/chemistry/1997/boyer/lecture/

Dobbin L (1933) Daniel Rutherford's inaugural dissertation. J Chem Educ 12(8):370–375

Dobson JF (1927) Erasistratus. Proc R Soc Med 20:825–832

Donovan A (1993) Antoine Lavoisier, science, administration, and revolution. Blackwel Publishers, Oxford

Fishman AP, Richards DW (1964) Circulation of the blood. Men and ideas. Oxford University Press, New York

Fitting J-W (2015) From breathing to respiration. Respiration 89:82–87

French SJ (1941) Torch and crucible. The life and death of Antoine Lavoisier. Princeton University Press, Princeton

Guerlac H (1954) The poet's nitre. Isis 45:243–255

Guerlac H (1957a) Joseph Black and fixed air: a bicentenary retrospective, with some new or little known material. Isis 48:124–151
Guerlac H (1957b) Joseph Black and fixed air: part II. Isis 48:433–456
Guerlac H (1975) Antoine-Laurent Lavoisier: chemist and revolutionary. Charles Scribner's Sons, New York
Hartree EF (1963) Obituary notice: David Keilin (1887–1963). Biochem J 8:1–5
Hartree EF (1973) The discovery of cytochrome. Biochem Educ 1(4):69–71, 74
Keilin D (1966) The history of cell respiration and cytochrome. Cambridge University Press, London
Koppenol WH, Bounds PL, Dang CV (2011) Otto Warburg's contributions to current concepts of cancer metabolism. Nat Rev Cancer 11:325–337
Krebs HA (1953) The citric acid cycle. 1953 Nobel Lecture. Accessed 22 Oct 2018. https://www.nobelprize.org/prizes/medicine/1953/krebs/lecture/
Kuhn T (1996) The structure of scientific revolutions, 3rd edn. University of Chicago Press, Chicago
Lehninger AL (1971) Bioenergetics: the molecular basis of biological energy transduction, 2nd edn. W.A. Benjamin, Menlo Park
Mann T (1963) Obituaries: Prof. David Keilin, F.R.S. Nature 198:736–737
Mann T (1964) David Keilin, 1887–1963. Biogr Mem Fellows R Soc 10:183–205
McClellan JE, Dorn H (2015) Science and technology in world history: an introduction, 3rd edn. Johns Hopkins University Press, Baltimore
McKie D (1962) Antoine Lavoisier: scientist, economist, social reformer. Collier Books, New York
Mendelsohn E (1961) The controversy over the site of heat production in the body. Proc Am Philos Soc 105:412–420
Mitchell P (1978) David Keilin's respiratory chain concept and its chemiosmotic consequences. 1978 Nobel Lecture. Accessed 18 Oct 2018. https://www.nobelprize.org/prizes/chemistry/1978/mitchell/lecture/
Norrby E (2016) Nobel prizes and notable discoveries. World Scientific, Singapore
Otto AM (2016) Warburg effect(s)—a biographical sketch of Otto Warburg and his impacts on tumor metabolism. Cancer Metab 4:5
Partington JR (1956) The life and work of John Mayow (1641–1649), part one. Isis 47:217–230
Perkins JF (1964) Historical development of respiratory physiology. In: Fenn WO, Rahn H (section eds) Handbook of physiology, section 3: respiration, vol I. American Physiological Society, Washington, DC
Poirier J-P (1996) Lavoisier: chemist, biologist, economist. University of Pennsylvania Press, Philadelphia
Porter R (1997) The greatest benefit to mankind: a medical history of humanity. W.W. Norton, New York
Proctor DF (ed) (1995) A history of breathing physiology. Marcel Dekker, New York
Rayner-Canham M, Rayner-Canham G (2001) Women in chemistry: their changing roles from alchemical times to the mid-twentieth century. Chemical Heritage Foundation, Philadelphia
Rosen G (1955) Metabolism: the evolution of a concept. J Am Diet Assoc 31:861–867
Scheer BT (1939) The development of the concept of tissue respiration. Ann Sci 4:295–305
Singer C (1959) A short history of scientific ideas to 1900. Oxford University Press, London
Slater EC (2003) Keilin, cytochrome, and the respiratory chain. J Biol Chem 278:16455–16461
Szent-Györgyi A (1937) Oxidation, energy transfer, and vitamins. 1937 Nobel Lecture. Accessed 19 Oct 2018. https://www.nobelprize.org/prizes/medicine/1937/szent-gyorgyi/lecture/
Timbs J (1868) Wonderful inventions: from the Mariner's compass to the electric telegraph cable. George Routledge and Sons, London
Törnroth-Horsefield S, Neutze R (2008) Opening and closing the metabolite gate. Proc Natl Acad Sci USA 105:19565–19566

Underwood EA (1943) Lavoisier and the history of respiration. Proc R Soc Med 37:247–262
Walker JE (1997) ATP synthesis by rotary catalysis. 1997 Nobel Lecture. Accessed 19 Oct 2018. https://www.nobelprize.org/prizes/chemistry/1997/walker/lecture/
Weeks ME (1934) Daniel Rutherford and the discovery of nitrogen. J Chem Educ 13:101–107
Weisse AB (2002) Heart to heart: the twentieth century battle against cardiac disease—an oral history. Rutgers University Press, New Brunswick
West JB (2011) History of respiratory gas exchange. Compr Physiol 1:1509–1523
West JB (2013) The collaboration of Antoine and Marie-Anne Lavoisier and the first measurements of human oxygen consumption. Am J Physiol Lung Cell Mol Physiol 305:L775–L785
Westfall RS (1980) Never at rest: a biography of Isaac Newton. Cambridge University Press, Cambridge
Wilson LG (1959) Erasistratus, Galen, and the *Pneuma*. Bull Hist Med 33:293–314
Wilson LG (1960) The transformation of ancient concepts of respiration in the seventeenth century. Isis 51:161–172

# Chapter 3
# State of the Art ~1800 to ~1940

Congenital heart disease was a surprisingly hot topic in the 18th and 19th centuries, long before anyone had a clue about any sort of definitive remedy. John Farre, an English physician and a conspicuous early contributor (Fig. 3.1) wrote in 1814 that "the desire to inquire into the vital functions (of the heart and lungs) has been so strongly expressed by philosophers, that even detached facts, and single cases of malformations of the heart, have engaged the attention of some of the most eminent members of the medical profession; and have been deemed worthy of a place in the transactions of the most learned societies of his and other countries."[1] Thomas Peacock (Fig. 3.2) prefaced his 1858 classic *On Malformations, &c., of the Human Heart* with: "There are few subjects which have attracted more attention in the profession than the irregularities in the development of the heart and large vessels" and cited six systematic treatises on the subject published earlier in the nineteenth century, and many other works from as far back as the 1700s.[2] Peacock described many types of defects, including several types of single ventricle, and the signs and symptoms that run with them. A 2009 review cited ten textbooks published between 1814 and 1905 containing variable amounts of material on congenital cardiac defects.[3]

Cardiac malformations have indeed afforded a unique window onto cardiovascular physiology, pathophysiology, and embryology. (And the shear variety of malformations—after over 30 years of practice, I still encounter new variations—holds a certain odd appeal for some of us.) But the first couple of centuries of fascination with congenital heart disease culminated in very little in the way of therapy. Dr. Farre recognized that practitioners could only "sooth and mitigate the evil which nature does not, and art cannot cure." He offered "clothing the skin in flannel," the

[1] Farre (1814, pp. b, 44).

[2] Peacock (1858, p. v); other articles on congenital heart disease are cited throughout the book.

[3] Evans et al. (2009), Keating and Edwards (1888, pp. 44–47), and Campbell (1971).



T. J. Kulik, M. Dick, *Reimagining a Child's Heart*,
https://doi.org/10.1007/978-3-031-88608-9_3

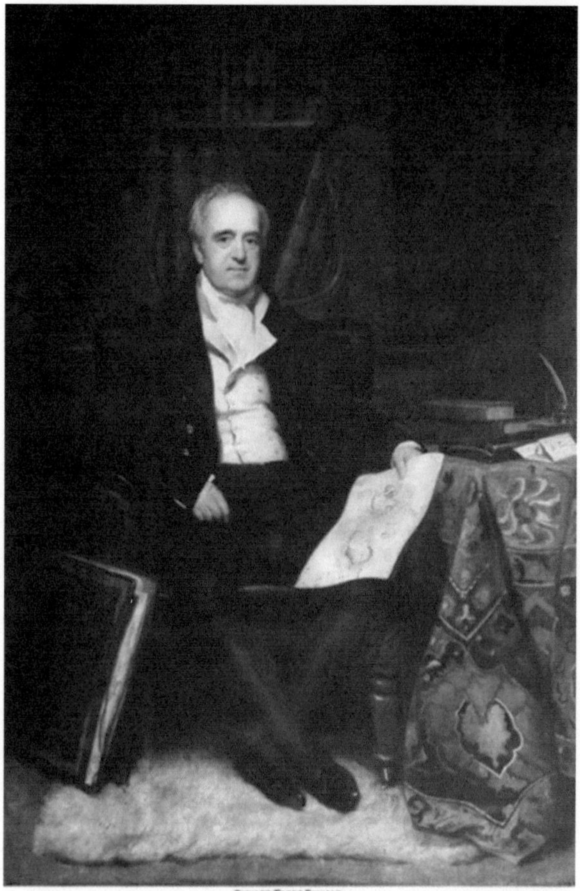

**Fig. 3.1** John Richard Farre (1775–1862), from the Wellcome Collection, free to use with attribution

"soothing medium of warm water," changing the position of the patient, attending to the correct quality and quantity of food, and "regulating any deficiency or excess in the evacuations from the intestines only by the mildest remedies in our possession."[4] All very salutary, no doubt, but pretty paltry palliation.

Forty years later, Thomas Peacock's prescription was much the same. Practicing in London, Peacock was about as close to a cardiologist as you could find in those days. Born in York, England, in 1812 to a Quaker family, he took his medical training from a number of individuals and institutions, eventually receiving his M.D. from the Edinburgh Royal Infirmary. "An ordinary man who put his powers to extraordinary use,"[5] Peacock was both a practitioner and an investigator, and by dint of enthusiasm and hard work made many important contributions. If you spend a couple of minutes with his *On Malformations*, you will find that the good doctor's

[4] Farre (1814, pp. 45–46).

[5] Porter (1962).

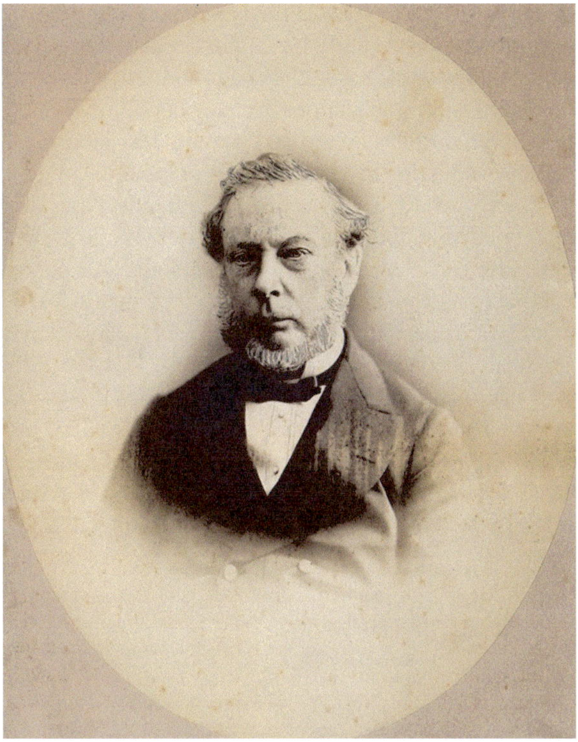

**Fig. 3.2** Thomas Bevill Peacock. From the Wellcome Collection, free to use with attribution

prescriptions differ little in substance from Farre's, although there are a few additions: remedies for gastrointestinal symptoms, pains, and palpitations; a few leeches to the temples for convulsions; and advice (activity restrictions and "over-excitement of the brain should be especially guarded against").[6] Many more treatments were inflicted on cardiac patients (not only those with congenital defects) than offered by Peacock, but he was wise to ignore most. Mercury, in the form of calomel or blue pills, was widely prescribed; bleeding was a mainstay; and a raft of ineffective medications were used for diuresis. Purgatives, emetics, and blistering added to the patients' misery. Rene Laennec, the French physician who invented the stethoscope, treated angina by placing strongly magnetized steel plates over the front and back of the chest. ("It should be remarked that they who witnessed the application of the magnet by Laennec did not, in general, form so favorable an opinion of its utility as the author himself."[7]) A few drugs we still use—digitalis, morphine, salicylates, and nitroglycerine—were in the mix, but the vast majority of the interventions were, at best, palliative rather than definitive, or even perilous.

[6] Peacock (1858, pp. 141–143).

[7] James Hope, quoted in Feil (1960).

Fast-forward to 1940, a few years before the B-T-T shunt. Therapy is still only supportive and strikingly limited in depth and variety; James Brown's textbook[8] on congenital heart disease (1939) devoted fewer than two pages (out of 255) to treatment. His recommendations: treating conditions which really cannot be definitively treated (colds and sore throats), activity restrictions, venesection, possibly immunizations, and a tiny handful of drugs (adrenaline, digitalis, sedatives, cough syrup).[9]

The typical life span for people with most types of single ventricle was at most a few months, with only a few exceptions. While patients with two-ventricle defects generally survived much longer—sometimes a normal life span—even these less complex malformations often subtracted many years.[10] And while alive, their ailments were many. Reduced capacity for physical activity—at its most extreme, utter physical incapacitation—was common, as were difficulty feeding and growing. Some suffered prolonged episodes of unconsciousness, or convulsions. A tendency to develop strokes or brain abscesses, as well as bacterial infection of the heart (endocarditis), round out the many calamities suffered by people with a single ventricle and other malformations. Farre described several miserable patients, including a 15-year-old girl with severe pulmonary valve narrowing:

> She walked slowly, and seemingly with great difficulty, and used to stop a little at every third step; her arms, hands, lips, face, and tunicae conjunctivae, were of a livid colour; she felt a constant pulsation in the left side of her chest, and extreme weakness in all her limbs; she had…a low, faltering voice; an impeded deglutition, so that even thin or liquid aliment could not be swallowed without much difficulty; she had not menstruated, and was generally costive…For three years her complaints gradually became more distressing; and, at the end of that period, in the winter season, when the weather was unusually cold and wet, she began to complain of a pain in her left side, and to discharge, by the mouth, a black grumous blood. Still she continued to place herself in the street as usual, until, on the twenty-fourth day after these last symptoms, she was obliged to be carried home, where she soon died. The first symptoms (by the girl's account) were observed when she was five years old.[11]

Dr. Farre also described a variety of typical symptoms and findings in other patients: being bed-bound, fluid in the abdomen and extremities, emaciation, convulsions, fits, brain abscess, bleeding, and sudden death.

There were, of course, remarkable exceptions. Born in Somerville, Massachusetts in 1868, even as a kid Henry F. Gilbert was blue and frail, with easy shortness of breath and fatigue, dizzy spells, and headaches; he developed black-out spells and transient ischemic attacks as he grew older. But despite his considerable disability, he attended the New England Conservatory, found employment in locations as diverse as Boston, Florida, Chicago, and Paris, and ultimately achieved considerable success as a pioneer of native American music. Once dubbed the Mark Twain of American music, Mr. Gilbert brought his opus

---

[8] James Brown was a largely self-made (he "followed the principle that nothing worth knowing can be taught") English physician who took an interest in congenital heart disease (Bedford and Muir 1959). His *Congenital Heart Disease* (1939) was one of the earliest clinical books on the subject.

[9] Bedford and Muir (1959); Brown, *Congenital Heart Disease* (1939).

[10] Taussig (1947), Appendix.

[11] Farre (1814, pp. 17–18).

to the Continent and Russia in an era when extended travel was stressful even for the robust. In 1927, in preparation for a trip to a music festival in Frankfort, he sought consultation with two prominent Boston physicians, Paul Dudley White and Howard Sprague. The good doctors were amazed—given Gilbert's advanced age—to make the diagnosis of tetralogy of Fallot but offered advice and encouragement for what proved to be a successful journey. He died the following year of a stroke, and a post-mortem exam confirmed their clinical impression of tetralogy.[12] But Gilbert was the rare exception, and the vast majority of people with similar malformations suffered terribly blunted lives.

The tapestry of heart therapy was sparsely yarned during Dr. Farre's tenure, but the early twentieth century saw rapid advances in technology which added color and bulk. New discoveries, such as x-ray technology, were rapidly applied to clinical care. Although at first fickle (one early observer described nascent X-ray equipment as "globes of glass surrounded by zones of profanity"),[13] X-ray imaging was rapidly adopted and improved; Helen Taussig leaned heavily on fluoroscopy (a type of X-ray examination) when diagnosing cardiac malformations.[14] New technology also made possible the *quantitative* studies required to better understand cardiovascular disease. The struggle to understand *cyanosis* illustrates the indispensable role of quantitative data in laying the groundwork for better therapy.

Cyanosis is a bluish discoloration of the skin and mucous membranes, first described in the sixteenth century by Paracelsus, a prominent and prolific Swiss physician and alchemist.[15] The inspiration for a variety of lovely and evocative names—*ictère bleue, ictère violet, mélasictère, maladie bleue, cyanopathie, heliotrope, lilac*, and others[16]—this physical finding occupied some of the best medical minds of the 18th through the twentieth centuries.[17] Cyanosis is the signature sign of tetralogy of Fallot and, in fact, was the manifestation of cardiac malformations (including single ventricle defects) that most consumed the attention of physicians through the early twentieth century.[18] An explanation of cyanosis, even if imperfect,

---

[12] White and Sprague (1929).

[13] Blume, "Medicine, Technology and Industry," in Cooter and Pickstone (2000, pp. 173–174).

[14] Weisse (2002, p. 45).

[15] This historical account of the development of understanding cyanosis is based primarily on Peacock (1858, pp. 121–128), Abbott (1908, pp. 331–335), Lundsgaard and Van Slyke (1923, pp. 64–71), and Brown (1939, pp. 125–126).

[16] Lundsgaard and Van Slyke (1923, pp. 6–7).

[17] Morgagni, de Sénac, Bouillaud, Rokitanski, James Paget, Cruveilhier, Peacock, William Hunter, and many others less illustrious puzzled over the cause of the blue malady, as did Maude Abbott in the century next.

[18] A few of many examples: Farre's book (1814) commences with a discussion of cyanosis and cyanotic defects; Peacock (1858, p. 121) declares that "There are few subjects in the range of medical science which have occasioned more discussion, than the inquiry as to the immediate cause of (cyanosis), which forms so marked a feature in most instances of malformation of the heart"; in Abbott's (1908) authoritative review of congenital cardiac disease, cyanosis is the major item of discussion, outside the anatomy of the defects. Curiously, heart failure, the other common consequence of congenital cardiac defects—and the primary manifestation of some—received much less attention the first half of the twentieth century; see, for example, Abbott (1936), Brown (1939), and Taussig (1947).

was required in advance of inventing effective therapy for people afflicted by many types of cardiac defects.

Early investigators turned to their most powerful investigative strategy, clinicopathological correlation (Chap. 4), as they grappled with cyanosis. The trouble was that the anatomy of dead hearts only inconsistently correlated with the presence of pre-mortem cyanosis. In 1749, on the basis of a cyanotic patient who turned out to have a single ventricle at postmortem, Jean Baptiste de Sénac (Louis XV's future chief physician) concluded that cyanosis is caused by the mixing of (blue) venous blood with (red) oxygenated blood within the heart.[19] But in 1761, Morgagni taught that cyanosis is due to *venous congestion*, not mixing. This maestro of clinicopathological correlation reported a cyanotic patient whose autopsy revealed severe obstruction of the outlet of the right ventricle and concluded that the (presumed) resulting backup of venous blood accounted for the patient's blue coloration. In fact, the patient whom Morgagni interpreted as having cyanosis due to venous congestion probably was blue due to intracardiac shunting. The heart had severe pulmonary stenosis, right ventricular hypertrophy, and a fairly large patent foramen ovale; right-to-left shunting across the foramen ovale under these circumstances is typical.[20]

Observations from other investigators multiplied the confusion. There were hearts with severe right ventricular obstruction, retrieved from people with *no* history of cyanosis, and hearts where venous and arterial blood had surely mixed, but without the patient having been blue. Additional factors were adduced to explain the blue malady, including too much carbon dioxide in the blood, the exuberant growth of capillaries, and an abnormally high hematocrit (red blood cell count), but by the first decade of the twentieth century, the admixture and venous congestion theories were the prime contenders to explain cyanosis.

We know today that cyanosis is due to the fact that deoxygenated (also termed reduced, or unsaturated) hemoglobin is dark blue, in contrast to the bright red of the fully oxygenated (fully saturated) hemoglobin. When blood in the capillaries contains a sufficient *quantity* (not percentage) of unsaturated hemoglobin (about 5 g/100 mL of blood), tissues take on a bluish tinge. Capillary blood may contain enough reduced hemoglobin to cause cyanosis for one, or both, of two reasons: (1) *Insufficiently oxygenated arterial blood*, almost always due to a congenital cardiac defect or abnormal lung function (or both). When unoxygenated venous blood makes its way to the arterial side, either because it mixes with fully oxygenated blood in the heart, or because it passes through the lungs without being fully oxygenated, arterial blood contains less oxygen than normal. (2) *Reduced blood flow through the capillaries of the skin*. When cutaneous (skin) perfusion is reduced, more oxygen is extracted from the blood than normal, increasing the amount of reduced hemoglobin in the capillaries and small veins. This

[19]This was published in his *Traite de la Structure du Coeur, de Son Action, et De Ses Maladies* (1749), the first comprehensive synthesis of the structure, function, and diseases of the heart. Some consider this work to mark the beginning of cardiology as a specialty (Bowman 1987).

[20]Peacock (1858, pp. 81–82, 121).

*acro*cyanosis, especially evident in the tips of the fingers and toes and around the mouth, can be caused by reduced cardiac output. (Acrocyanosis can also occur in healthy people when exposure to cold constricts small arteries leading to the skin's capillaries.)

So, there's more to cyanosis than meets the eye. While at its core it boils down to a single variable (the quantity of reduced hemoglobin in the capillaries), two distinctly different mechanisms can cause low capillary blood saturation. What's more, several other factors impact the color perceived. Since the quantity of unsaturated hemoglobin is a function of the *total amount* of hemoglobin in the blood, with anemia the amount of unsaturated hemoglobin may be so reduced that cyanosis is not present even though the capillary oxygen is low. Conversely, with increased blood hemoglobin, cyanosis is intensified; indeed, babies born with a very high hemoglobin level may be blue despite having a normal arterial oxygen level. The number of capillaries in the skin, and whether they are engorged because of high venous pressure, also impacts how blue the skin appears.

It's not surprising that early observers had a hard time wrapping their minds around cyanosis. A major part of their problem was that *quantitative* information was largely lacking. The variable most germane to understanding the problem—blood oxygen saturation—was not readily measured until the twentieth century. Previous investigators had *qualitative* information (e.g., the color of venous blood is different from arterial, and some cyanotic patients had malformations that presumably permit mixing of venous and arterial blood), but quantitative data required new technology.

The clinical studies which yielded a definitive understanding of cyanosis weren't terribly sophisticated, but they exploited new technology for measuring the blood's oxygen saturation and content. Investigators measured oxygen saturation in the venous blood of both cyanotic and acyanotic patients using a technology (1917) developed by Van Slyke[21] (Fig. 3.3); they found that the amount of unsaturated hemoglobin in the blood correlated best with the degree of cyanosis.[22] These studies culminated in 1923 in Christen Lundsgaard and Donald Van Slyke's *Cyanosis*, the classic monograph which finally delivered a coherent, quantitative understanding of this ancient sign.[23] These Rockefeller Institute for Medical Research investigators lucidly laid out the physiology of cyanosis (and modifying factors) and put numbers on the key variables involved. They explained the confusing observation that some patients with intracardiac mixing of red and blue blood weren't blue, using an equation showing that a fairly large quantity of blue blood shunted into the arterial

---

[21] Van Slyke (1918).

[22] Lundsgaard (1919a, b).

[23] Lundsgaard and Van Slyke (1923). Maude Abbott (Chap. 6) declared this monograph to be "epoch-making," and that the "scope and value of the knowledge both of the circulation and the respiration that has become available to us through the Van Slyke technique, we stand as it were before an open door through which a stream of light radiates into the very heart of cardiac pathology" (Abbott 1923).

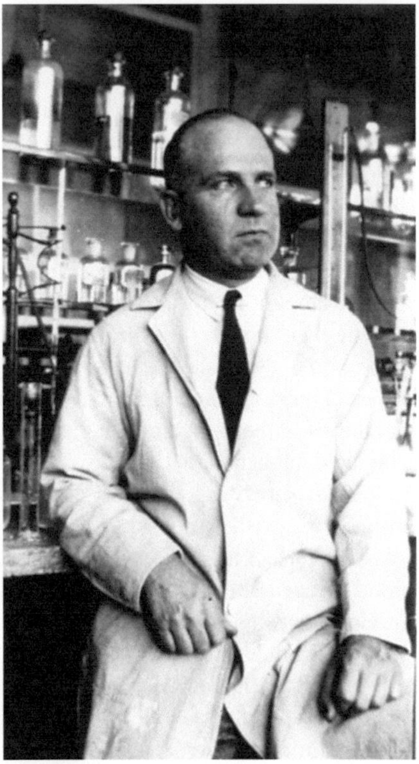

**Fig. 3.3** Donald Van Slyke- source record at Images from the History of Medicine (NLM)- NLM believes this item to be in the public domain

circulation is needed to produce cyanosis.[24] The ability to think about cyanosis quantitatively was therefore key, and understanding this venerable problem had to wait for the necessary information and concepts.[25]

It's just conceivable that the B-T-T (Blalock-Tausig-Thomas) shunt could have been invented without understanding cyanosis. As will be discussed in Chap. 6, Helen Taussig's appreciating that closure of the ductus arteriosus in tetralogy of Fallot coincided with worsening cyanosis was the single most important observation that led to the idea that a surgically contrived duct could be effective therapy. That solo insight, even lacking a deep understanding of cyanosis, might possibly have impelled a bold innovator to invent a substitute duct for therapy. But Blalock

[24] It is actually more complicated than that. A patient with a single ventricle (where all the blue blood mixes with all the red blood from the lungs) may be acyanotic if the ratio of red blood to the lungs to blue blood from the body is high.

[25] The same year the *Cyanosis* monograph was published, Campbell and co-workers (1923) reported studies relating to, among other things, cyanosis with congenital heart disease. They concluded that arterial desaturation, not venous congestion, was the most important factor accounting for cyanosis, and implied that intracardiac mixing predominantly accounted for the desaturation. Their paper, while useful, lacked the quantitative, sweeping analysis of cyanosis provided by Lundsgaard and Van Slyke.

and Taussig kicked off their seminal shunt paper with a detailed and extended exposition of the nature of cyanosis, explicitly based on the *Cyanosis* monograph, as they laid out the rationale for their therapeutic innovation.[26] It's hard to think that these or other pioneers would have undertaken the risks and time investment needed to invent their artifact without a clear biological rationale for its possible utility, a rationale which required a fine understanding the physiology of *maladie bleue*. Resolving the puzzle of cyanosis was a necessary first step along the winding path to single ventricle palliation.

Innumerable bits and bodies of knowledge, and technical developments, were required to realize the B-T-T shunt and other therapies needed for single ventricle palliation. Learning how the body adjusts the heart's force of contraction, and blood flows and pressures to various organs, enabled physicians to treat critically ill patients more effectively. Modern pharmacology added to the clinician's toolbox by providing new and potent drugs. Devices to monitor vital signs (blood pressure, heart rate, and the like), and instruments to quickly measure various chemicals and gases in the blood were invaluable for adjusting these critical variables after surgery. As we've noted, the lack of suitable anesthesia was a major barrier to advancing surgery, especially in the chest; learning to anesthetize patients deeply yet safely, while maintaining respiration with an open chest, was necessary for safe and effective cardiac surgery. Etc., etc., etc. It would be easy to get lost in this forest, but let's don't. Over the six Chaps. 6, 7, 8, 9, 10, and 11, we will admire but a handful of threads of *knowledge*, *technique*, and special *human qualities* that licensed its development. Others could have been chosen, but these are exceptional pieces of our story, and they apply to many other medical innovations as well.

In Aesop's telling, the fox chided a lion for giving birth to only one cub. That's right, retorted the lion, only one…but it's a lion. I don't know if that is actually part of Aesop's oeuvre, but it does convey the root significance of our first two and thickest threads: the hard-won discoveries of how the energy needed for vital cellular processes is both generated and delivered. Animal life quickly vanishes without energy continuously produced, making the conversion of oxygen and food into energy—biology at its most salient. Knowing that blood and oxygen circulate through the arteries, then veins, and back to the heart was an essential prelude to discovering the meaning of blue lips and fingers. Circulation: *Transport and Distribution* (Chap. 1) traced the astoundingly long road to concluding that the heart is a pump—not a furnace—dedicated to propelling blood in a continuous loop around the body. William Harvey uncovered the function of the cardiovascular system in the seventeenth century, but yet more time and toil followed before people learned the *significance* of pumped blood. Respiration: *Oxygen: What's It Good For?* (Chap. 2) described how people came to appreciate why and how breathing separates the quick from the dead and the nature of human cellular

[26] Blalock and Taussig (1945).

energy generation. We have now seen how the seminal sign of many forms of congenital heart disease, especially single ventricle malformations—cyanosis—was explained.

We will now meet Maude Abbott, whose "Collection of Hearts" created the "Periodic Table of Congenital Heart Disease" as I call her magnum opus—a very influential comprehensive compendium of congenital heart disease.

## References


Abbott ME (1908) Congenital cardiac disease. In: Osler W (ed) Modern medicine: its theory and practice, vol IV, ch. IX. Lea Brothers & Co., Philadelphia, pp 323–425

Abbott ME (1923) Cyanosis, Lundsgaard C, Van Slyke, D. Medicine, 1923, vol. II, pp. 1–76 [Review of a monograph]. Can Med Assoc J 13:601–604

Abbott ME (1936/2006) Atlas of congenital cardiac disease. McGill-Queen's University Press, Montreal

Bedford DE, Muir DC (1959) James William Brown. Br Heart J 21:284–288

Blalock A, Taussig HB (1945) The surgical treatment of malformations of the heart. JAMA 128:189–202

Bowman IA (1987) Jean-Baptiste Sénac and his treatise on the heart. Tex Heart Inst J 14:5–11

Brown JW (1939) Congenital heart disease. Staples Press, London

Campbell M (1971) Early anatomical knowledge of cardiac malformation. Br Heart J 33:169–172

Campbell JMH, Hunt GH, Poulton EP (1923) An examination of the blood gases and respiration in disease, with reference to the cause of breathlessness and cyanosis. J Path Bacter xxvi:234–282

Cooter R, Pickstone J (eds) (2000) Medicine in the 20th century. Harwood Academic Publishers, Amsterdam

Evans WN, Acherman RJ, Anderson RH (2009) One hundred years of texts describing congenitally malformed hearts from 1814 to 1914. Cardiol Young 19:12–29

Farre JR (1814) On malformations of the human heart. Longman, Hurst, Rees, Orme, and Brown, Paternoster-Row, London

Feil H (1960) History of the treatment of heart disease in the nineteenth century. Bull Hist Med 34:19–28

Keating JM, Edwards WA (1888) Diseases of the heart and circulation in infancy and adolescence. P. Blakiston, Son & Co., Philadelphia

Lundsgaard C (1919a) Studies on cyanosis, part I: primary causes of cyanosis. J Exp Med 30:259–269

Lundsgaard C (1919b) Studies on cyanosis, part II: secondary causes of cyanosis. J Exp Med 30:271–293

Lundsgaard C, Van Slyke DD (1923) Cyanosis. Medicine monographs. Williams and Wilkins, Baltimore

Peacock TB (1858) On malformations, &c., of the human heart. John Churchill, London. Reprinted in The Classics of Medicine Library. Birmingham, AL: Gryphon Editions, Ltd.; 1981

Porter IH (1962) The nineteenth-century physician and cardiologist Thomas Bevill Peacock (1812–1882). Med Hist 6:240–254

Taussig HB (1947) Congenital malformations of the heart. The Commonwealth Fund, New York

Van Slyke DD (1918) Gasometric determination of the oxygen and hemoglobin of blood. J Biol Chem 33:127–132

Weisse AB (2002) Heart to heart: the twentieth century battle against cardiac disease—an oral history. Rutgers University Press, New Brunswick

White PD, Sprague HB (1929) The tetralogy of Fallot: report of a case in a noted musician, who lived to his sixtieth year. JAMA 92:787–791

# Part II
# A New Dawn

# Chapter 4
# Mens et Manus—Alex Carrel and Robert E. Gross

*Gold is where you find it.*

The seal of the Massachusetts Institute of Technology displays a craftsman poised at an anvil and a scholar absorbed in his book. *Mens et Manus*—mind and hand—is engraved on a ribbon below these, in case you didn't get the point: Inventing stuff requires more than just "scientific" knowledge. Techniques and methods, derived mostly from experience and trial and labor, are what transform a blueprint into an invention, a design into a tapestry. Our first three chapters traced the spinning of the earliest fibers of cardiovascular physiology; while this sort of knowing is vital for invention, including effective therapies, without the ability to effect physical transformations, knowledge is like a page from a Paganini caprice thrust in front of a student after her first violin lesson. Methods for effectively and safely manipulating the body and its tissues are some of the most indispensable implements in the surgeon's toolbox. Although these techniques may seem self-evident today, their invention was purchased with ingenuity and practical experience.[1]

Technique, *per se*, tends to get short shrift in discussions about medical advances. We will shortly meet a Nobel Prize winner honored largely for solving a technical surgical problem, but I can find only a handful of similar examples.[2] This most prestigious of all medical prizes is almost always awarded for basic biological discoveries or therapeutic breakthroughs, implying that for the Nobel Prize Committee (at least for physiology or medicine), technical inventions are the poor cousins.

[1] Technique is required not only for activities like surgery, but also for endeavors whose output is pure knowledge. Lavoisier and other proto-chemists employed simple apparatus and manipulation of materials in their quest to discover matter's hidden nature, and William Harvey did much the same, albeit working with living organisms.

[2] Since the first Nobel Prize in 1901, besides Carrel's, seven prizes in Physiology or Medicine have been awarded primarily for invention of new technology: hybridoma technique for producing polymerase chain reaction; monoclonal antibodies, in vitro fertilization, computer-assisted tomography, radioimmunoassay of peptides, cardiac catheterization, and production of mutations using radiation.



T. J. Kulik, M. Dick, *Reimagining a Child's Heart*,
https://doi.org/10.1007/978-3-031-88608-9_4

But seemingly modest advances in the way tissues are cut or moved and how stiches are driven have animated surgical breakthroughs and hugely improved results. Neonatal and infant cardiac surgery was on the steep part of its learning curve early in my career, and over the last 40 years I've seen and—via my patients' outcomes—benefited tremendously from striking improvements in cardiac surgery's technical puissance. Consider one of many examples: Repair of a complete atrioventricular septal defect (a relatively complex cardiac malformation) was dicey in the 1970s; the Mayo Clinic's operative mortality rate for this operation from 1970 to 1980 was 21%.[3] But by 2002–2005, only one out of 111 patients operated upon for this defect in the state of New York died after surgery.[4] There are many reasons for this decline in operative mortality. Pathologists such as Jesse Edwards, Robert Anderson, and Richard Van Praagh (Chap. 8) parsed the subtly complex anatomy of malformed hearts and taught surgeons and cardiologists what they learned. Better imaging of the heart before and after surgery, micro-surgical technics, more sophisticated post-operative care, and operations undertaken before complications set in—these are only a few of the elements contributing to better results. But I have no doubt that a major factor was cardiac surgeons' greatly improved ability to coax flimsy tissue into complex three-dimensional reconstructions. Not all species of medical innovation have so heavily relied upon technical developments, but for single ventricle palliation (and indeed all of surgery), *manus*' role was indispensable.

So, we turn now to the genesis of the craft of cardiac surgery. While *surgery* dates back to prehistoric times and was surprisingly advanced by the late nineteenth century, *cardiac* surgery is almost strictly a twentieth century invention. The very earliest surgery of the heart was, quite literally, superficial: suturing inflicted wounds and stripping away scar tissue from around the organ. Attempts at surgical remedy for a common, acquired problem—mitral stenosis (narrowing of the mitral valve)—followed, but with little early success. As we saw in Chap. 3, people didn't know enough about congenital defects in the early twentieth century to usefully engage them, but by the late 1930s, creative and doughty souls, flush with recently acquired practical knowledge, had tiptoed onto the congenital landscape. Technical advances, ranging from carefully orchestrated laboratory studies to early experience garnered deep inside the chest of seriously wounded WWII combatants, primed the post-war explosion of cardiac surgery.

Woven into this section of our tapestry are other finely intersecting threads. As you may recall or learn later from *Inventing Interface* (Appendix 4), a paucity of suitable models of disease has long hampered medical invention. As we will see, the absence and, conversely, the availability of animal models both constrained and fueled the early evolution of cardiac surgery. And selecting the *right problem* to tackle can be a challenge for the medical innovator; the correct choice can make the difference between invention and frustration. The first successful operation to

[3] Feldt et al., in Moller and Neal (1990, pp. 428–430).

[4] New York State Department of Health (2007).

correct a congenital cardiac defect is typically—and correctly—recounted as a story of courage and determination. But it also reflects one surgeon's canny choice of a problem, animated by his deeper-than-typical understanding of the natural history of one type of congenital defect entwined with his insight that its correction was a readily solvable technical problem (more later). Finally, like many new things, cardiac surgery aborning encountered the momentum-sapping friction of skepticism and negative biases. The grease that the relieved the resistance came in the form of strong and courageous personalities who could deliver the goods, and then crow about it.

The first third of the twentieth century found cardiac surgery, if not dead in the water, not exactly advancing at flank speed. A major barrier to progress was breeched in 1897 when Professor Dr. Ludwig Rehn, in Frankfurt on Main, successfully sutured the heart of a 22-year-old florist who had been knifed in the left chest.[5] Other surgeons followed suit, and relief of another condition—constrictive pericarditis—was also realized, but more ambitious cardiac operations were seldom ventured. In 1929, then-Cleveland (later Harvard) surgeon Elliott Cutler searched the literature for all previous operations to remedy defective heart valves and could dig up only 12.[6] A few attempts at increasing blood flow to the heart muscle were made in the mid-1930s, but these efforts came to little,[7] and surgeons had yet to hazard repair of a congenital defect. Even as far back as the late 1800s, surgeons had used animal models to explore the physiology of leaky and narrowed cardiac valves. Using mostly dogs, valves were sliced using knives introduced into the heart, and sutures used to narrow the pulmonary artery and aorta just above the valve or restrict the mitral valve ring. Cannulas were introduced from the left atrium through the mitral valve to cause leakage and narrowing.[8] But these models were crude and imparted little forward motion to the infant field.

Concurrent with these little-appreciated exertions, a Lyonnais surgeon with a mind like a kaleidoscope yoked to a perpetual motion machine and phenomenally deft fingers was inventing foundational vascular-surgical techniques. Alexis Carrel (Fig. 4.1) was one of the earliest surgeons to develop techniques to access the living heart's interior in the animal laboratory and was awarded a Nobel prize for learning how to splice together blood vessels (and applying this technical advance toward organ transplantation). His subsequent work in tissue culture commanded international attention. In the 1930s, his fame rivaled Einstein's.[9] Many French streets were renamed in his honor, but in the 1990s, "rue Carrel" was shorn from those very same

[5] Actually, there were two closely preceding instances of successful suturing of the heart, but both patients died of post-operative complications (Elsberg 1899).

[6] Cutler and Beck (1929).

[7] Shumacker Jr. (1992, ch. 1–3).

[8] Jarcho (1974a, b, 1975) and Cushing and Branch (1908).

[9] *The Independent* considered Carrel the sixth most useful man in America in 1912 (Hamilton 2017, p. 154). Using Google Ngram as an index of celebrity, David Hamilton found Carrel and Einstein were on a rough par in France in 1930 (Hamilton 2017, p. 337).

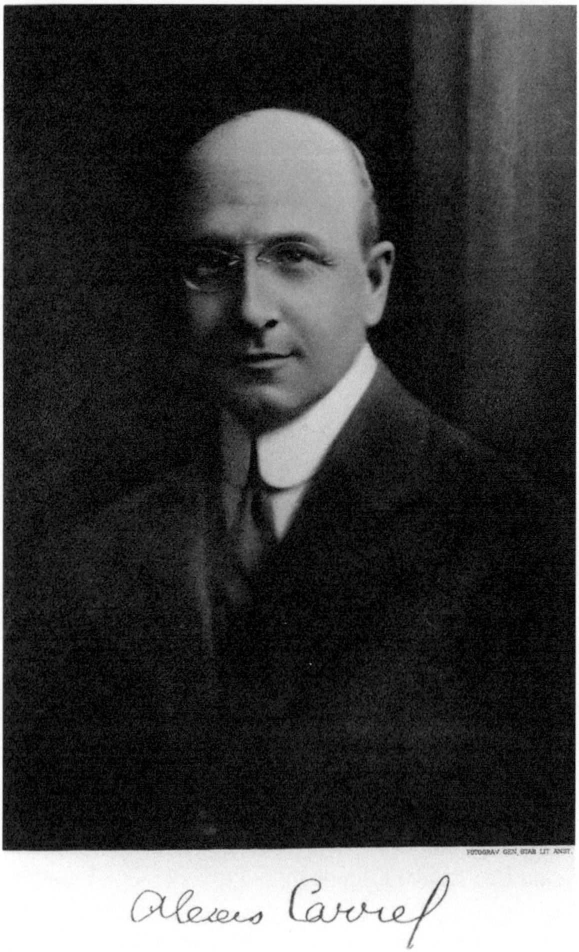

**Fig. 4.1** From the Wellcome Collection, free to use with attribution

streets,[10] as rapt admiration yielded to a more equivocal summing up of this intensely creative but disturbing French innovator.

> Endurance and strength generally develop in the mountains, in the countries where seasons are extreme… Florida and the French Rivera are suitable for weaklings, invalids, and old people, or normal individuals in need of a short rest. –Alexis Carrel, *Man the Unknown*[11]

Born 1873 in Sainte-Foy-des Lyons to a well-to-do family, Marie Joseph Auguste Carrel Billiard (later contracted to Alexis Carrel) enrolled in medical school at the University of Lyon in 1891 after an unexceptional childhood.[12] His student-self

[10] Weksler (2004) and Reggiani (2002).

[11] Carrel (1935, p. 303).

[12] The sources for Carrel's background are primarily Hamilton (2017), Edwards and Edwards (1974), and Stephenson and Kimpton (2001); specific references are given where it seems appropriate.

presaged some of his later characteristics: "*politesse stricte, réserve distante, and un peu d'égoïsme.*"[13] Carrel lacked interest in '*l'alcohol, le tabac, l'amour,*'[14] and his male friends were few. He joined a conservative discussion group, named after monarchist Joseph de Maistre; once a band of Carrel and friends, clubs in hand, tried to disrupt a local meeting, possibly of a human rights group.[15] His medical training was finished by 1899, and 3 years later, Carrel commenced the work on vascular anastomosis (stitching blood vessels together) that lit the fuse on his sky-rocket career.[16] He had been mulling over the problem of vascular repair since 1894, when French President Sadi Carnot died of an assassin's knife; the post-mortem showed a lacerated portal vein, the repair of such being an unsolved problem at the time. Perhaps Carrel had manipulating delicate vascular structures in mind when, as an intern, his hands acquired swift precision thanks to embroidery tutorials from one Mme. Leroudier.[17] His famous 1902 paper described the "triangulation" technique for positioning the ends of two blood vessels to be joined, though he still had much to learn to reliably make satisfactory connections (Fig. 4.2).

Carrel's precocious research program hit heavy air soon after taking off. Something of a mystic, fascinated by telepathy and clairvoyance and keen to study

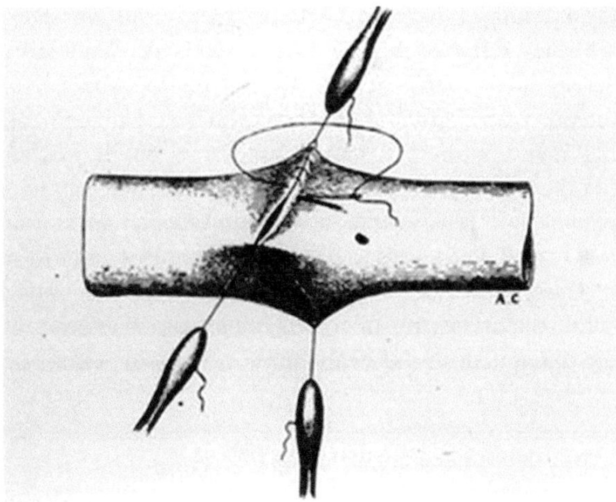


**Fig. 4.2** 1902- plate showing Carrel's technique for vascular anastomosis. From the National Library of Medicine, in the public domain

[13] Descriptions of Carrel's complex personality run the gamut from good and sweet to aloof and haughty; he was certainly hard-working, highly ambitious, unconventional, and a maestro of self-promotion. Carrel took Richard Bing briefly under his wing, who described Carrel as generous, kind, understanding, and humane (Stephenson and Kimpton 2001, pp. 7, 12–21; Hamilton 2017, p. 9, 12; Bing 1983).

[14] Hamilton (2017, p. 31).

[15] Hamilton (2017, pp. 9–11).

[16] Carrel (1912).

[17] Edwards and Edwards (1974, p. 16).

miracle cures, he journeyed to Lourdes with a group of pilgrims in May of 1902; as it happened, he observed a stunningly rapid and unexplainable recovery in a terminally ill young woman. Carrel made pronouncements, and the Lyon *Nouvelliste* quoted him as declaring that he had observed a supernatural event. This he denied, claiming that he had only offered that the recovery could not be explained by any known mechanism, but the resulting controversy tarnished his local reputation and throttled any chance for promotion. Fed up, he left Lyon for Paris in 1903, where he attended lectures at the Sorbonne and the College de France and cast about for his next steps. Carrel steamed out of Bordeaux to Montreal in May, with a career in cattle ranching in mind,[18] but with a quick change in plans he soon made his way to Chicago, landing in George N. Stewart's laboratory at the University of Chicago in mid-1905. Charles C. Guthrie, a 25-year-old surgeon already working in Stewart's lab, was pursuing unrelated projects but soon joined Carrel in studying vascular anastomotic techniques and organ transplantation.

Narrowing at the vascular connection, bleeding, thrombosis, and avoiding infection—these were the major challenges Carrel and Guthrie faced as they labored in the laboratory, using dogs and cats, to perfect a method for sewing blood vessels together. Inventing anastomotic technique was partly a problem of learning how the vessels to be connected should be lined up with each other, and the configuration of the stitching. Finding the necessary materials was also key, and these items emphasize the craft-like nature of their endeavor: They sought neither arcane biological agents nor sophisticated analytical devices, but slender needles and smooth silk thread, snarl and tangle resistant.[19] These Chicago collaborators were far from the first investigators to work this problem,[20] but they extended and perfected the efforts of others and quickly applied their new technology to canine and feline organ transplantation.[21] It was for their work on vascular anastomosis and organ transplantation that Carrel was awarded the 1912 Nobel Prize in Physiology or Medicine.

Carrel also published a few papers between 1910 and 1914 describing cardiac surgical experiments in dogs. Though aimed at describing techniques and strategies for manipulating the heart, these reports also confirm Carrel's legendary manual

[18] Edwards and Edwards (1974, p. 21).

[19] Hamilton (2017, p. 44) and Stephenson and Kimpton (2001, pp. 80–81, 83).

[20] Watts (1907), Wangensteen and Wangensteen (1978, pp. 264–265).

[21] They found that the best needles were round, very fine, and sharp; coating suture material with Vaseline prevented blood contacting the suture and wounded vessel. Avoiding damage was paramount: only smooth-jawed clamps, gingerly applied, were used to occlude vessels for temporary hemostasis; forceps were applied only on the adventitia (external sheath) of the vessel. Vessels need to be kept moist using Ringer's solution or Vaseline. Adventitia must be removed from the edges of vessels, lest it attract clot-stimulating fibrin, and coagulated blood and tissue juices are rinsed off the vessel with Ringer's. To avoid narrowing of the connection, stitches should be applied to the vessel under tension and the surfaces precisely approximated. Complete hemostasis must be obtained before closing the wound, and strict asepsis is "absolutely essential." Ultimately, these collaborators perfected techniques for end-to-end, side-to-side, and end-to-side connections; when a small vessel is taken off a larger one, a patch of the larger vessel remains attached to the one removed to facilitate sewing it to the recipient vessel (Carrel and Guthrie 1906; Carrel 1912).

dexterity[22]: Anticipating a surgical approach applied in humans only several decades later, he described interrupting blood flow into the heart, incising the pulmonary artery, manipulating the pulmonary valve, and finally suture-closing the artery, all inside 3 minutes. Seven out of ten dogs survived this virtuoso procedure.[23]

What techniques did Carrel contrive to make this cardiac incursion successful? He learned how to stop the beating heart, trying various approaches before finding that gently clamping the blood vessels as they join the organ, using a special clamp with rubber sheathed jaws, worked best. He found that the heart should be filled with well-oxygenated blood before clamping, and that the clamp could be applied for as long as about two and a half minutes for spontaneous return of function after removal. Carrel discovered where and how (using sharp scissors) to enter the pulmonary artery without damaging the valve (one can cut between the valve cusps into the right ventricle without danger). He determined the optimal suture (coated with "vaselin"), the correct needles, and the most useful (quickest) sewing technique (continuous through and through stitches). Speed being of the essence, Carrel fixed a tiny piece of muscle on the end of the China silk No. 1 suture so that no time was spent making a knot after the first stich. Experience showed that closing the pericardium (the sack around the heart) before bleeding was completely staunched was a bad idea. Seemingly mundane details, all. But taken in aggregate and meshed with other species of knowledge, these sorts of manual maneuvers constitute the métier of a craftsperson—and the surgeon.

Exactly what, if any, influence this French surgeon's experimental cardiac work had on the progression of heart surgery is unclear,[24] although we do know that Carrel and Guthrie's work on vessel splicing was studied by Vivien Thomas and Alfred Blalock (see Chap. 6) as they first forayed into experimental vascular surgery.[25]

Classical surgical experiments, directed at moving tissues about, mark only the inception of Carrel's variegated career. Having moved to the newly formed Rockefeller Institute (now University) in 1906, over the next 25 years he inscribed an investigative portfolio of prodigious variety. While his professional activities were numerous and mostly of little interest for us,[26] Carrel's tissue culture work was a window onto his science and his style.

---

[22] Edwards and Edwards (1974, p. 13).

[23] Carrel (1914).

[24] For example, Russell Brock, the first surgeon to have real success relieving pulmonary valve stenosis, used a different technique than that described by Carrel (1914) and did not refer to Carrel's work as a possible approach when describing his own operation (Brock 1948). Carrel's technique (inflow occlusion) was actually a viable way to treat pulmonary stenosis, and for a time was used by subsequent surgeons.

[25] Thomas (1985, pp. 34–37) and Levy and Blalock (1939).

[26] Two of Carrel's other activities are of special note. In WWI shrapnel-riddled France, Carrel, collaborating with the American chemist Henry Dakin, developed a new way of treating war wounds (irrigation with Dakin's antiseptic solution). And in 1929, he initiated studies of whole organ perfusion, aiming to keep organs viable for prolonged periods in blown glass chambers. Aviator Charles Lindbergh injected formidable energy and imagination into this project as an

Carrel's transplantation experiments stalled in 1909–1910, perhaps because rejection severely limited organ viability. At the same time, he became interested in nerve growth when his limb transplantation experiments proved unsatisfactory, owing to slow and incomplete reinnervation of reattached limbs. Aware of Ross Harrison's pioneering work at Yale suggesting that tissue culture might prove useful for studying nerve growth, Carrel arranged for Montrose T. Burrows, a researcher at the Rockefeller, to visit the Harrison laboratory. After returning to New York, Burrows made important contributions of his own in Carrel's lab,[27] but Carrel soon became sole proprietor of tissue culture at the Rockefeller when Burrows moved to Cornell. The most famous of Carrel's many experiments commenced when he dropped a fragment of embryonal chick heart into culture medium and observed these cells, rudely ripped from their natural environment, still beating away weeks later. This demonstration garnered massive publicity, partly because he repeatedly asserted that these and other kinds of cells could live indefinitely in culture.[28] This claim commanded serious attention: If cells are immortal, so too might people be, if only the life-limiting factors in the intact organism could be discovered and neutralized.

But the rigor of Carrel's science sometimes lagged its press. As one expert observed, "reports of [Carrel's] experiments [have] become much more dramatic and are couched in such a way as to attract the maximum attention… [I]n Carrel's case the drama is associated with a great deal of over-optimistic inaccuracy."[29] His claim that the cultured chick cells were immortal is a prime case in point: His embryonic cells[30] appeared to survive for years, then decades, far longer than other experience would indicate possible. The explanation? Some (non-conclusive) evidence suggests that the culture may have been periodically refreshed by the addition of new cells. (Although, if true, it is unknown whether Carrel himself was aware of this).[31] There are multiple other instances when his claims were ultimately proven inaccurate.[32]

Carrel's optimistic exaggeration can be explained, at least in part, by his ravenous need for public recognition. It is perhaps not surprising that this man who employed a press cutting agency to collect newspaper stories about him[33] neither denied nor discouraged over-the-top newspaper accounts of his work. Early in their Chicago days, word of Carrel and Guthrie's work showed up in the newspapers, prompting Carrel to complain to Guthrie that "Our experiments are infinitely too

unpaid volunteer in Carrel's lab, but they could never get the system to work as hoped (Edwards and Edwards 1974, pp. 89–96).

[27] Harris (1995, pp. 31–35).

[28] Landecker (2007, ch. 2).

[29] Harris (1995, p. 35).

[30] Fibroblasts, another type of cell found in the heart and elsewhere, which do not contract, eventually replaced the cardiocytes (Landecker 2007, p. 99).

[31] Witkowski (1980).

[32] Hamilton (2017, p. 547).

[33] Hamilton (2017, p. 113).

much known, for they are in the preliminary stage" and speculate that their lab personnel had leaked the information,[34] but it seems far more likely that it was Carrel who did the leaking.[35] Shouldering others out of the limelight—at least by the lights of his critics—was also a recurring theme. Carrel was the sole author for an early Chicago paper with Guthrie, even though his collaborator participated in the experiments and even writing the paper.[36] A more serious breech occurred in April 1906 when Carrel presented their results at a Johns Hopkins conference densely populated with prominent surgeons and physiologists; Guthrie went unmentioned and was barely acknowledged in the written reports.[37] (Some Guthrie supporters are critical of the fact that Carrel's Nobel prize was not awarded to both surgeons, even though multiple Nobel awardees were not allowed at the time.)[38] Carrel's tissue culture activities were resonant: Contemporaries alleged that Carrel and the Rockefeller were claiming credit for discoveries better attributed to Harrison (although others strenuously denied this).[39]

By the early 1930s, Carrel's cell culture work was running on fumes, and he was as much preoccupied with philosophy and social engineering as biology. At a friend's urging, he wrote *Man the Unknown* (MTU, 1935), a 300-page declinist rant on man's degradation by the modern industrial environment. The book was a best-seller[40] and received multiple (though not uniformly) favorable reviews.[41]

*MTU* is in part astute and informative, especially its biologically and medically related material. Some if it is surprisingly in tune with modern sensibilities (for example, advice to eat whole grain rather than white bread! [p. 25]). A few passages approach eloquence: "Moral beauty … gives to those who possess its divine gifts, a strange, an inexplicable power. It increases the strength of intellect. It establishes peace among men. Much more than science, art, and religious rites, moral beauty is the basis of civilization" (pp. 103–131). But much of the text is diffuse, open to wide interpretation, or self-contradictory. Some is just goofy. Consider Carrel's take on Florida and the Rivera (above), or: "Men of genius are not tall. Mussolini is of medium size, and Napoleon was short" (p. 62). This, from a self-proclaimed "man of science" (p. ix) and son of the nation of Lavoisier, Pascal, and Laplace? And there are bigger flies in this porridge.

It is Carrel's authoritarian, eugenic, and racial views which grate most painfully. Mussolini and Napoleon, of all the leaders that history has hosted, are singled out for encomium. Coming directly to the point: "Another error … is democratic

[34] Stephenson and Kimpton (2001, p. 48).

[35] Hamilton (2017, pp. 52–54).

[36] Hamilton (2017, pp. 41–42).

[37] Stephenson and Kimpton (2001, pp. 105–111).

[38] Stephenson and Kimpton (2001).

[39] Hamilton (2017, pp. 134–138).

[40] *Man the Unknown* sold 900,000 copies in 19 different languages (Edwards and Edwards 1974, p. 97).

[41] Reggiani (2002).

equality… Indeed, human beings are equal. But individuals are not. The equality of their rights is an illusion. The feeble-minded and the man of genius should not be equal before the law" (p. 271). How to deal with crime? "The conditioning of petty criminals with the whip, or some more scientific procedure, followed by a short stay in the hospital, would probably suffice to insure order. Those who have murdered, robbed while armed with automatic pistol or machine gun, kidnapped children, despoiled the poor of their savings, misled the public in important matters, should be humanely and economically disposed of in small euthanasic [sic] institutions supplied with proper gases." Similar treatment was prescribed for the criminally insane (pp. 318–319). Carrel advocated for "voluntary" eugenics aimed creating an "inherited biological aristocracy" (p. 303). He acknowledged that "the reproduction of human beings cannot be regulated as animals," but insisted that "[t]he propagation of the insane and feeble-minded must be prevented" (p. 300). Have a family history of feeble-mindedness, insanity, or cancer: no marriage for you (pp. 299–301). He complained about the "newcomers, peasants, and proletarians from primitive European countries, who beget large families. But their offspring are far from having the value of those who came from the first settlers of North America" (p. 299).

As if *MTU* wasn't enough, Carrel's reputation has also been battered after leaving the U.S. near the end of his career.[42] Forced to retire from the Rockefeller in July 1939, he returned to occupied France in early 1941. Working closely with the Vichy government, Carrel created, and was appointed regent of, the Foundation Française pour I'Etude des Problèms Humains. His involvement with the Institute was only indirect and his other activities were constrained by illness starting in 1943; Carrel died in Paris on November 5, 1944.[43]

Charges of Nazi collaboration flew at Carrel, and while frank collaboration is unproven, he did not resist the regime in any obvious way and likely provided some forms of support.[44] While *MTU* and his life in Vichy were for a time mostly overlooked after WWII, they ultimately provoked scraping Carrel's name from the medical school in Lyon, as well as over 20 streets in France, and Montreal and Gatineau in Canada.[45] Carrel perhaps suffers the disadvantage of living in our temporal backyard, his sharp edges closer to our nerves than, say, Galen's.[46] Some leeway is perhaps due him since eugenics was regarded as a legitimate subject for discussion by serious thinkers at the time, and something like his brand of authoritarianism has always attracted considerable subscription. Still, his reputation—rising and falling over the years, like a prow in choppy seas—seems unlikely to be headed for lasting redemption any time soon.

[42] Reggiani (2002) and Harrison (pp. 521–560).

[43] Reggiani (2002).

[44] Harrison (pp. 479–526).

[45] Weksler (2004), Montreal Gazette and Canadian Press (2017), and Canadian Broadcasting Corporation (2015).

[46] Reggiani (2002, p. 356).

Summing up the scientist, Carrel's work on transplantation and cell culture helped set the table for subsequent fundamental discovery, though his experiments rarely scratched deeply into basic biology. Certainly for us, Carrel's contribution to the single ventricle story was *practical* and *technical*—inventing a way of joining blood vessels that enabled certain types of congenital heart surgery, including the indispensable Blalock-Taussig-Thomas shunt. As for the bigger picture, where do we situate Carrel relative to our other pioneers? Galen, despite his hypercritical, acerbic, abrading self, has firmly settled into the pantheon of medical giants. Lavoisier, accolade-needy like Carrel but with vastly more agreeable political inclinations, is inextricably embedded in the pantheon of super-elite scientists. William Harvey, with little appetite for plaudits,[47] or political baggage, is perhaps better situated in a Parthenon than a pantheon—his massive contribution and sympathetic history make him, for me at least, close to (if not quite) uniquely revered as a foundational figure. Carrel's contributions, while not nearly clearing the bar of the other three, surely command grateful acknowledgement. But it's hard to see Carrel the man being situated even as close as arm's length to the other trailblazers we've encountered so far.

Some modern observers have attributed early twentieth century cardiac surgery's lobster's pace, at least in part, to what might be termed *non-progressive attitudes* among contemporary surgeons. Two declarations from influential surgeons, famously lacking in prescience, are often adduced to convey the temper of the times. Steven Paget, author of a then-standard textbook of thoracic surgery, averred in that 1896 volume that "Surgery of the heart has probably reached the limits set by Nature to all surgery: no new method, and no new discovery, can overcome the natural difficulties that attend a wound of the heart. It is true that 'heart suture' has been vaguely proposed as a possible procedure, and had been done on animals: but I cannot find that it has ever been attempted in practice."[48] Theodor Billroth, a highly accomplished and influential surgeon, has often been fingered for writing something to the effect that "a surgeon who would attempt such an operation (cardiac suture) should lose the respect of his colleagues."[49] Conventional wisdom insisted that the heart was "very sensitive to the smallest mechanical insult or injury", subject to stopping with "smallest mechanical insult"; nor would stitches hold in this incessantly twisting muscle. But animal experiments and Ludwig Rehn's repair showed that the heart could take a thread like any other organ, and cardiac surgery set sail as general surgery had thousands of years before: fixing wounds.[50]

---

[47] Keynes (1966, pp. 425–426).

[48] Paget (1896, p. 121).

[49] Clowes Jr. (1960) and Litwak (1971). For the notion that the early development of cardiac surgery was retarded by the (ancient and unproven) bias that the heart simply was not amenable to surgical intervention, see Shumacker Jr. (1992, ch. 1), Clowes Jr. (1960), Sellors (1967), and Swan in Snellen et al. (1981, pp. 139–141).

[50] Elsberg (1899), Cushing and Branch (1908), and Clowes Jr. (1960).

Billroth was probably given a bum rap—there is actually little to suggest that he tried to discourage surgeons from performing cardiac procedures[51]—and besides, the nascent century saw plenty of imaginative and influential practitioners interested in attempting more complex cardiac surgical procedures. It is widely appreciated that Scottish physician Lauder Brunton advocated operation for mitral stenosis in 1902, and in 1907, John Munro, surgeon-in chief at Carney Hospital in Boston, proposed ligation of the patent ductus arteriosus.[52] In 1929, Elliott Cutler and Claude Beck discussed the work of nine surgeons who actually attempted repair of valve lesions in humans,[53] and there were undoubtedly others who were more than receptive to the idea of novel cardiac operations.

On the other hand, the attitudes and inclinations of medical doctors—the primary source of patients referred for operation—served as a millstone around innovation's neck. Contemporary papers and personal reminiscences vividly document surgeons' frustration with medical colleagues who refused to submit patients for novel cardiac operations.[54] This disinclination to refer patients for surgery doubtlessly had multiple roots. Charles Bailey, one of three surgeons who first established effective surgical treatment for mitral stenosis,[55] felt that the medical man simply didn't properly appreciate the severity of the illness. He commenced his seminal 1949 paper on the subject by scolding the should-be referring doc for "a general lack of appreciation of the extreme seriousness of (mitral stenosis). Many internists, among whom are cardiologists, feel that with proper medical management and limited activity these patients may live a normal span of life … and know a case or two … which has survived to an advanced age. Unfortunately, these men do not have any roughly accurate idea of the much larger number of cases which have died at an early age. It is also notable that these same older patients will admit that they have not especially enjoyed their prolonged life of limited activity."[56] Robert Gross (of more anon), though less lecturing in tone, was also mindful of the need to lay out the case for the perniciousness of the patent ductus in his first paper describing his operation to eliminate the same.[57]

Many others have written about lack-of-faith-based delays in the introduction of new cardiac surgery, none being more annoyed with troglodyte attitudes than Harris Shumacker, Jr. A cardiac surgeon who had written extensively about the history of his field, Shumacker bemoaned the reticence of referring doctors to submit their patients to novel surgery, greatly delaying progress, including a *cri de coeur*: "How often has the introduction of a new concept of study or management been

---

[51] Absolom (1983) and Weisse (2002, p. 389).

[52] Brunton (1902) and Munro (1907).

[53] Cutler and Beck (1929).

[54] Shumacker Jr. (1968, 1992, pp. 33, 39–40), Brock in Snellen et al. (1981, pp. 165–172), Harken (1989), Johnson (1970, p. 91), and Brock (1951).

[55] Clowes Jr. (1960).

[56] Bailey (1949).

[57] Gross and Hubbard (1939).

frustratingly delayed because no one in authority recognized its worth, spoke out for it, and influenced his confreres to provide the needed patients!"[58] Henry Swan, a member of the crop of pioneer open-heart surgeons, acknowledged the crucial importance of the courage factor when he generously gave "primary credit" for the first operation to correct a congenital cardiac defect (discussed later) not to the surgeon, but to the pediatrician who referred the patient![59] Even closer to the subject of this book, a breakthrough treatment for babies with a certain type of single ventricle—the Norwood palliation—was rejected by many practitioners for years, as we will see in Chap. 11.

One factor which mitigated against surgical referrals was the fact that many physicians, including such influential practitioners as Sir Thomas Lewis and Sir James Mackenzie, mistakenly thought that it was weakness of the heart muscle, rather than the narrowed valve, that led to symptoms in patients with mitral stenosis, making repair of the valve seem irrelevant.[60] There were doubtless other reasons why so few medical people referred patients for mitral operations, but the bottom line for surgeon Tom Treasure and cardiologist Arthur Hollman is that "What held up progress (with surgery for mitral stenosis) was clearly a solid wall of opposition to the notion that a surgical approach to the valve was the right way to treat the illness. It seems likely that the arguments, rather then being re-examined, were marshaled ever more strongly, so as to halt what was seen to be surgical recklessness."[61]

But what is often left out of cogitations about why cardiac surgery was slow to pick up steam is the pesky fact that anything much more complex than suturing a lacerated heart *simply didn't work very well* until Robert Gross' ductal ligation in 1939. The aforementioned report by Cutler and Beck revealed the sorry state of valve surgery: 12 operations were attempted with only three survivors, and it was unclear how much any of them had actually benefited from operation. Since the doctor's primary responsibility is to provide optimal care for a given patient, not to advance the field by supplying experimental subjects, referring a live and (at least somewhat) functional patient for a procedure with a high *a priori* risk of mortality is a tough proposition for most. If nothing succeeds like success, then the converse is also true—it's difficult to recommend an innovative procedure if pioneer subjects run a high risk of harm.

Multiple reasons account for the discouraging surgical results, which are all too apparent in the Cutler and Beck paper. One patient had an inaccurate diagnosis, and another apparently died of anesthetic complications. Several succumbed to postoperative complications, including pneumonia, cardiac tamponade, and the then-limited means of treating low cardiac output and other hemodynamic disturbances. While it was then possible—in theory—to put a patient asleep, perform a fairly

---

[58] Shumacker Jr. (1968, 1992, ch. 6–7), Snellen et al. (1981, pp. 165–168), and Bing (1999, p. 93).

[59] Swan in Snellen et al. (1981, p. 141).

[60] Hollman (1997, pp. 172–174), Lewis (1942, pp. 147–148), Mackenzie (1918, pp. 329–330), and Shaw (1902).

[61] Treasure and Hollman (1995).

complex cardiac operation, and get the patient to recover, it was actually a dicey proposition, with success seeming to hinge upon proper alignment of several celestial bodies. People knew little about anesthesia for open chest operations, how to access the heart without provoking abnormal rhythms or other problems, managing abnormal heart rhythms and blood pressure, and the many other details needed to negotiate the cardiac minefield.[62] Furthermore, for nearly all of the cases, the surgeon lacked the technical wherewithal to physically improve the valve as needed, because he didn't have a clear idea of how to relieve the stenosis without causing lots of leakage.

You may recall (or may learn in the future) from Appendix 3 (*Inventing Therapy*) that the medical innovator is often severely hemmed in by testing limitations, and this was plainly true for those struggling to develop a remedy for mitral stenosis. Imagine that Cutler and colleagues had had dogs whose mitral valves were deformed in the same way as diseased human valves, and whose physiology was altered similarly. Assume that these dogs would have symptoms like humans, that with relief of the stenosis the symptoms would abate, and that the canine's response to anesthesia and other medical interventions would be very similar to that of people. Not only would this model have made it easier for the innovators to tumble to solutions to the technical problems involved with the operation, but with it they could have *demonstrated* their therapy's efficacy and safety to the community at large. Proof of principle using animal models has long been an important early step in introducing novel therapy to humans. Surgeon Harvey Cushing was interested in developing surgery for mitral stenosis, but he felt that an experimental model of this disease, with relief of symptoms by surgery, was necessary "before attempting, by a similar procedure, to relieve the corresponding pathological lesion in man,"[63] well-reflecting the typical sequence for inventing new therapies.

But early surgeon-innovators utilized experimental models of mitral stenosis, using mostly dogs and the occasional cat, that were crude, and none accurately replicated the human situation. The valves—mostly normal canine mitral valves—bore little resemblance to human rheumatic valves, and other characteristics of these models were unlike the human equivalent. To be sure, the information garnered from these experiments was invaluable for the ultimate creation of the artifact: Surgeons learned how to best gain access to the heart, how to cut and sew the organ, and how it responded to manipulation. Inserting their index finger into the left atrium and palpating the mitral valve in the beating heart, they gained a better appreciation of how the valve functions. They found that if the mitral valve was made grossly insufficient (leaky) while trying to relieve stenosis, death followed. Surgeons learned all this and more from their animal models, but these surrogates weren't sufficient for either perfecting the therapy or convincing skeptics that the time for mitral valve surgery had come.[64]

---

[62] Brock (1965), Harken (1989), Johnson (1970, pp. 98–99), and Litwak (1971).

[63] Cushing and Branch (1908).

[64] Ravitch (1966, p. 26).

In fact, I can't help wondering whether the heavy emphasis on lab investigation, while crucial for developing cardiac surgery, didn't also *impede* invention of successful mitral valve surgery. Cutler and Beck doggedly pursued the chimera of creating mitral stenosis for 7 years, without success.[65] It was only after other surgeons focused on, and better, understood normal and diseased *human* mitral valves that effective surgery was created. Careful and analytic observation of stenotic valves post-mortem, not experiments, supplied the missing piece of the puzzle. Cutler and Beck may have been as much trapped (or perhaps distracted) by their search for an experimental model as aided by it.

In 1925, Henry Souttar, working at London Hospital, relieved mitral stenosis in a single brave soul. Lily Hines, 19 years old, was incapacitated by a right ventricle weakened by high pressure caused by the narrowing. Souttar used his finger, gaining entry into the left atrium via the left atrial appendage, to split open the scarred-together leaflets of the valve at their commissures—an operation later dubbed a commissurotomy (or valvuloplasty). Lily recovered well and lived "in very fair health" for another 5 years. But "At the time however, it was an article of faith with physicians that the valves were of no importance and the only thing that mattered was the condition of the cardiac muscle" wrote Souttar to Brian Blades, another prominent and uncannily-named heart surgeon. "In that atmosphere I was naturally unable to obtain another case, in spite of this one complete success. It was a pity, but easy to understand."[66] Commissurotomy was frozen out for another 20 years.

Widespread application of mitral valve surgery hung fire until the late 1940s and early 1950s, when Charles Bailey, Dwight Harken, and Russell (later, Lord) Brock posted consistently good results, convincing the medical community of this operation's merit. Positive words and acceptance spread in many ways, but one story is of note, if only because of its resonance with Blalock and Taussig's promotion of their shunt (Chap. 6). In late June 1948, 10 days after his first successful commissurotomy, Bailey spoke about his procedure at the American College of Chest Physicians in Chicago. He had asked the 24-year-old woman upon whom he had operated to attend the meeting, and she was pleased to attest to how much better she felt after operation. Apparently, that wasn't proof enough, and a stethoscope was scrounged from the hotel physician. Hearing no mitral murmur, the influential Evarts Graham and other thoracic surgery muckety-mucks in the crowd confirmed the success of the procedure. Congratulatory words from Graham directly followed, words that Bailey believed did much to convince others of the operation's merit.[67]

As previously noted, excepting Souttar's, prior efforts were mostly aimed at cutting or excising a piece of the valve, relieving stenosis at the expense of making the valve leak, which was poorly tolerated.[68] Commissurotomy actually *worked*, and worked reliably. Multiple developments contributed to the creation of this

[65] Cutler and Beck (1929).

[66] Souttar (1925) and Johnson (1970, pp. 90–91).

[67] Johnson (1970, pp. 96–98).

[68] Bailey (1949), Baker et al. (1950), Harken et al. (1951), and Snellen et al. (1981, p. 171).

operation, including several not specific to the problem at hand (for example, improvements in anesthesia),[69] but when Bailey was asked how he finally solved the problem of mitral stenosis his reasons were three: his facility for operating where he could not see, using his sense of touch; his deep understanding of the anatomy of the normal and diseased mitral valve; and previous experience "[selling] ladies' underwear… [I] was early on impressed by the similarity of the mitral valve structure to the old-fashioned feminine girdle. Perhaps this is what suggested mitral commissurotomy to me."[70] Indeed, Bailey had looked long and hard at the anatomy and function of the normal, and stenotic, human mitral valves and came to understand that repair of narrowed valves was best effected by splitting their fused commissures (often using only the tip of the finger). Cutler and Beck had misunderstood the nature of the problem, being convinced that the rheumatic mitral valve is so thickened and tough that only a powerful cutting instrument, perhaps excising a bit of the valve, could relieve stenosis.[71]

Bailey also used the animal lab to invent solutions to his technical problems. Using roughly 60 dogs, he learned how to access the valve without causing arrhythmia or unmanageable bleeding, that producing mitral regurgitation was not tolerated, and that one has to touch the valve to accurately position a cutting instrument.[72] But these experiments would have come to nothing without his acute inspection of gnarly human valves, and the practical insights which flowed from these observations. Mitral pioneers Dwight Harken and Russell Brock also emphasized the need for a clear understanding of subtleties of the anatomy of the deformed valve for successful intervention.[73]

But new technical tricks were not enough; technique had to be complemented by persistent and iron-willed personalities to push this controversial innovation over the hump. Charles Bailey's story is that of a single-minded zealot. A surgeon on a mission, he pushed past failure and grave professional risk in his quest to develop a new therapy. The first three patients he operated upon for mitral stenosis died, culminating in his loss of operating privileges at three of the five Philadelphia hospitals at which he had practiced. Undeterred by these setbacks, Bailey scheduled patients numbers four and five for operation on the same day, but at different hospitals, so that should the first operation fail (it did), he could hustle across town to operate upon the other patient (who survived) before the news caught up with him.[74] In an interview with cardiologist-historian Allen Weisse in 1979, he talked about how he was able to operate on patient number five, after the first four had died: "Obviously, I felt there were irrelevant reasons for the loss of the first four patients and that the principle was entirely sound and could be developed but just needed further effort…

[69] Baker et al. (1950), Brock (1965), and Litwak (1971).

[70] Weisse (2002, p. 76).

[71] Cutler et al. (1924) and Cutler and Beck (1929).

[72] Bailey (1949).

[73] Harken et al. (1951) and Brock (1952).

[74] Johnson (1970, pp. 94–98) and Weisse (2002, pp. 77–78).

Finally, however, you have to face the 'moment of truth,' and the poignancy is so great that I can't really express it. You know that almost all the world is against it; you know that you have a great personal stake and might even lose your medical license, or at least your hospital privileges if you persist. In fact, the thought crosses your mind that maybe you really *are* crazy. And yet you feel that it has to be done and it must be right. At the time I did the last of those five operations, the successful one, I was sure that I was, at the least, in danger of losing all my hospital operating privileges."[75]

Dwight Harken's saga is resonant, although this time with the twist that it was a *medical man* who helped stiffen his resolve to persevere until he perfected his mitral valve operation: "[S]ix of my first 10 patients died. This was so devastating that with the tenth patient and the sixth death, I left the operating theater, insisting that I would never do another heart operation. I went home to bed. The late Dr. Laurence Brewster Ellis, my wonderful cardiologist friend and collaborator, drove to my house and asked Anne Harken if it were true that I said that I would never do another heart operation. She confirmed this, and he asked if he could see me. She urged him to wait until the next day. The next day I again insisted that I intended to do no more heart surgery. He said, 'I think that would be very irresponsible of you.' I replied, 'What in the world is irresponsible about that? I refuse to kill any more people.' He said, 'You have never killed anybody. I have never sent you a patient who wasn't dying.' I replied that 'I would not expect any responsible physician to send me another patient.' He replied, 'I am president of the Heart Association and generally regarded as responsible. I would certainly send you patients and I would criticize you if you did not operate. You must have learned something from those six disasters.' I went back to work, and we lost only one of the next 15 patients."[76] Innovating was almost as hard on the innovators as it was on the innovatees!

Harken had served as a lieutenant colonel in the U.S. Army Medical Corps at the 160th General Hospital in England, where he pioneered techniques required for extraction of foreign objects in soldier's hearts and blood vessels. He learned optimal approaches to open the chest—from the front, back, or sides, left or right—depending upon the location of the foreign body. He found that lifting the heart out of its pericardial sac reduced its output and provoked arrhythmias, so he left the heart in place during missile extraction; techniques for entering the heart to remove fragments and for securely suturing the incised myocardium were evolved.[77] Yet more invention was needed to fracture open a stenotic mitral valve,[78] but practical experience in war's operating theater helped Harken—and via his publications, other surgeons—get their bearings for tangling with the heart.[79]

---

[75] Weisse (2002, p. 77) and Goor (2007, pp. 143–164).

[76] Harken (1989).

[77] Harken (1946), Harken and Williams (1946), and Harken and Zoll (1946).

[78] Harken et al. (1951).

[79] Harken and Williams (1946).

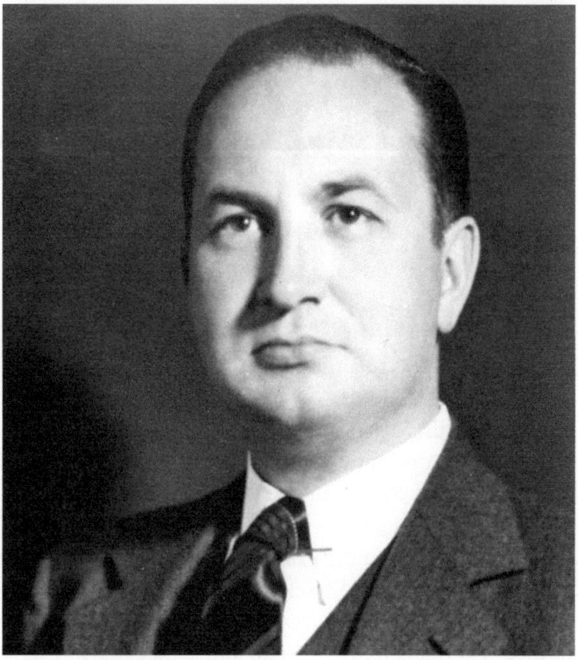

**Fig. 4.3** Robert E Gross MD. **Boston Children's Hospital Archives, Boston, MA**

We got a little ahead of ourselves with the mitral valve story. This cardiac ship of state actually set sail in 1938, 10 years before mitral commissurotomy, when Robert Gross (Fig. 4.3) at Boston Children's Hospital first successfully ligated a patent ductus arteriosus.[80] Gross's operation for the patent ductus "changed everything dramatically … [and] set into motion a chain of achievements. One success led to another, then a host of others, and suddenly an entirely new age in cardiac surgery was born." Many agree Gross' achievement launched modern cardiac surgery[81] and a career heavily decorated with encomiums. Among many medals, honorary degrees, and awards, including election to the National Academy of Sciences, Gross twice won the highly prestigious Albert Lasker Award for Clinical Medical Research

[80]The ductus almost always closes within the first few days of life. But, depending upon its diameter, if may persist and cause problems (congestive heart failure, bacterial endocarditis, damage to lung blood vessels, rupture).

[81]Gross was not the first attempt to close a patent ductus. Boston surgeon John Streider had previously attempted ligation of an infected ductus, but the vessel could only be partly closed, and the patient died 4 days postoperatively (Graybiel et al. 1938). There have been claims of other unsuccessful or successful ductal ligation attempts, but these lack documentation (Alexi-Meskishvili and Bottcher 2010). Not everyone singles out ductal ligation as a singular turning point in cardiac surgery (e.g., Clowes Jr. 1960; Meade 1961), and one observer acknowledges the tendency to afford Gross' operation special historical significance without exactly understanding why (Richardson 1970, p. 106).

(in 1954, with Blalock and Taussig, for distinguished contributions to cardiovascular surgery and knowledge, and again in 1959, for ductal ligation).[82]

The story of the first ligation of a patent ductus recalls that of mitral commissurotomy. Ductal closure was first proposed in 1907 by John Munro, a Harvard surgeon,[83] but the operation remained theoretical for the next three decades. Most of the factors which impeded the development of mitral interventions were operative here, with the challenge of making an accurate diagnosis especially germane. It was known that a patent ductus can serve as a compensatory structure in the presence of other cardiac anomalies (in which case ligation would prove disastrous), but the crude diagnostic tools of the day made confident exclusion of these anomalies problematic. The fact that some lucky people lived indefinitely with a ductus with few symptoms also dampened enthusiasm. Resistance from the medical community didn't help. Russell Brock related how another great surgeon, Evarts Graham, was road-blocked from attempting ductal closure by a professor of pediatrics at St. Louis Children's Hospital, and there are other examples of such friction.[84]

Baltimore-born in 1905, Robert Gross' father was manager of the Stieff Piano Company. Like Alexis Carrel (who had one blue and one brown eye), Gross had an ocular anomaly, but one rather more significant. Robert had a congenital cataract and therefore monocular vision, not a propitious characteristic for someone whose craft would demand sub-millimeter three-dimensional hand-eye coordination. In hopes of improving Robert's depth perception, his father had Robert disassemble, then reassemble smaller and smaller clocks. (The cataract was removed only after Gross' retirement.) He graduated from Carleton College, followed by Harvard Medical School, graduating in 1931. Staying in the Harvard system, Gross studied pathology for 2 years, followed by surgical training at the Peter Bent Brigham Hospital under Elliott Cutler (1933). Gross' landmark operation was performed while he was chief resident under William Ladd at Boston Children's Hospital.[85] Gross, knowing that Ladd would nix the surgery, performed the ligation while his chief was on vacation. When the two happened to run into each other at a sporting event, Ladd asked Gross how things were back at the hospital: "The laconic answer of Dr. Gross was that nothing unusual had happened."[86] Although he had considerable cover—the acting chief of the surgical service, Dr. Thomas Lanman, had given Gross the go-ahead, and consultation with highly influential cardiologist Paul Dudley White at the Massachusetts General Hospital also netted a thumbs up[87]—Gross' surgical foray took serious courage; had the operation failed, the repercussions for Gross could have been devastating.

---

[82] Shumacker Jr. (1992, p. 41), Sellors (1967), Castañeda (1980), Swann in Snellen et al. (1981), Naef (1990, p. 82), Hurt (1996, p. 425), and Moore and Folkman (1995).

[83] Munro (1907).

[84] Brock (1965) and Alexi-Meskishvili and Bottcher (2010).

[85] Moore and Folkman (1995), Hendren and Folkman (n.d.), and Murray et al. (2013).

[86] Castañeda (1980), Ravitch (1981, p. 814), Harken (1989), and Bing (1999, p. 94).

[87] Moore and Folkman (1995) and Warren (1984).

Gross' first patient was well-chosen. Lorraine Sweeney was a frail seven and a half year-old in well-compensated heart failure. As she related during a touching 2012 interview, "I just was very, very weak" and had to watch other kids doing hopscotch and jumping rope from her window.[88] She was at risk for long-term complications of the ductus and was significantly symptomatic; the ligation was therefore not only prophylactic but aimed at debilitating symptoms, providing additional justification for a subjecting her to a new, possibly hazardous procedure. Lorraine was referred by John P. Hubbard, a physician at Boston Children's. Far more than simply a "referring doc," Hubbard collaborated with Gross in the preliminary studies needed for the first operation, and was first author of a lead *New England Journal of Medicine* article thoughtfully outlining indications for ductal ligation.[89] Friday, August 26, 1938, must have been a day of living anxiously for the referring and operating doctors, to say nothing of Lorraine and her mother, but one can imagine the admixture of relief and elation felt by Gross and colleagues as Loraine emerged from anesthesia after a successful operation, and their delight in giving the good news to her family.[90] Up and walking within 3 days, she was "detained" in the hospital for another ten because of "interest in the case."[91] She survived for many years (Fig. 4.4)

Gross, as it turns out, was lucky. His twelfth patient, a 14 year old girl, collapsed dead 2 weeks after the ligation; the suture had worked its way through the ductus,

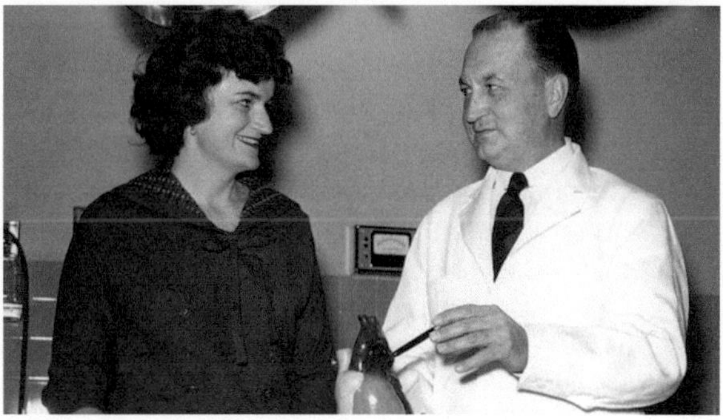

**Fig. 4.4** Robert E. Gross MD with his patient, Mr. Sweeney, first patient with patent ductal arteriosus ligation. Circa 1963. **Boston Children's Hospital Archives, Boston, MA**

[88] Nicoli (2012) and Murray et al. (2013).

[89] Gross and Hubbard (1939).

[90] Robert L. Replogle and Judson G. Randolph claimed that Gross, à la Charles Bailey a decade later, had scheduled two ductal ligations for the same day, ensuring another crack at the procedure should the first fail; neither could have had firsthand knowledge of this, since their association with Gross commenced much later (1956 and 1960, respectively; Replogle 2003; Ferguson 2016; Stoney 2008, pp. 197–198). More credibly, Richard Warren (1984)—based upon written communication from Gross—wrote that a second patient had been scheduled for the *next* day, in case of failure. Gross's second ductal ligation took place on September 12, 1938 (Alexi-Meskishvili and Bottcher 2010).

[91] Gross and Hubbard (1939).

and massive hemorrhage ensued.[92] There is a fix for this, dividing and sewing the ends of the ductus closed instead of simple ligation, which Gross subsequently employed. But had his very first patient suffered such a catastrophic demise, it seems likely that further referrals—and institutional forbearance for the procedure—would have been seriously compromised for some time to come.

Besides chutzpah, there are a couple of notable reasons why Gross was able to create his therapeutic artifact. First, the rationale for ductal ligation (and its justification) was strongly endorsed by Maude Abbott's (see Chap. 4) beautifully systematized observations of congenital heart lesions and the patients wrapped around them. Her work provided statistical evidence that the patent ductus was, much more than generally appreciated, a pernicious, life-shortening lesion, supplying Gross a powerful rationale for eliminating this fetal remnant. In papers reporting his ductal ligations, Gross quoted Abbott's findings: Of 92 patients autopsied with a patent duct, 74% died of a cardiac cause at an average age of 24 years. Abbott's data also indicated that patients with ductal-dependent heart defects usually die very young, implying that one could close the ductus in an older patient with little risk of inadvertently eliminating a life-sustaining compensatory structure. In pursuing this novel intervention, Gross was paddling upstream of prevailing opinion, and he used Abbott's data as an oar.[93]

Just as important, Gross chose his problem wisely. Ligation of the (extracardiac) ductus was fairly straightforward. That's not to say that ductal ligation was without technical challenge. Before touching a scalpel to his first patient, Gross undertook a meticulous program of studies, first utilizing human cadavers, then dogs in the laboratory, and finally finishing up using human autopsy material again to identify the optimal approach to gaining access to the ductus. He wasn't so much worried about what to do when he got to the ductus, but more about the best way to get there. The innards of our chests are not arranged with the convenience of the surgeon in mind; how to get to and isolate the ductus without bleeding, nerve damage, and other trauma is what Gross needed to know before he could transform a simple idea into a safe operation.[94] But the key technology of the innovation (i.e., closing off a blood vessel using suture) was old stuff, unlike the problem of improving a stenotic valve situated deep within the heart. The relatively modest conceptual and technical leap this innovation required made it easier for Gross and Hubbard to justify attempting their first attempt than if a chancier technical exercise was required. The situation with early mitral valve surgery (and the first Blalock-Taussig shunts, and many other new surgical procedures) was quite different; since the surgery was perceived as being risky, justifying the operation was difficult except in very symptomatic patients. The catch-22 is that these highly symptomatic patients are often very fragile, increasing the risk of operation and reducing the likelihood of a good result. In retrospect, surgeons who went after the more interesting problems of intracardiac

---

[92] Moore and Folkman (1995).

[93] Gross (1939b).

[94] Gross (1939a, b).

pathology in the 1920s and early 1930s had bitten off more than they could chew, while Gross had the insight to tap the thin edge of the wedge into the problem of structural heart disease.

But now a case of perhaps not enough imagination; we come to with what must be the most storied refusal in all of cardiology. Shortly after Gross' duct ligation, Helen Taussig journeyed from Baltimore to Boston, asking him to build an artificial ductus for her tetralogy patients. He famously sent her packing, declaring in effect that he was a destroyer, not a builder, of ducts. Gross' refusal to provide a ductus for Taussig is perplexing. If this was a technical challenge that he had no time to tackle—in other words, his priorities lay elsewhere—well OK, busy people have to make choices. But he reported creating in dogs what could have been known for the ages as the Gross-Taussig shunt (left subclavian artery to pulmonary artery connection) in 1941,[95] and apparently had created these shunts by the time of Taussig's visit.[96] The development work was therefore mostly done. Taussig recalled that Gross had said that "as he was in the full glory of the successful ligation of a patent ductus arteriosus, to build a ductus seemed foolish,"[97] but one wonders what this offhand explanation leaves unsaid. At the time, people struggled with the physiology of cyanotic defects, as we discuss in Chap. 3; in fact, Russell Brock, an innovative and perceptive contemporary surgeon, had reservations about the conceptual basis of the B-T shunt for tetralogy even after its utility had been clearly demonstrated.[98] Did Gross fail to apprehend that a shunt would be helpful? Or perhaps he imagined that deeply cyanotic patients were at too high a risk for operation? Maybe Gross wasn't comfortable with Taussig as a collaborator on a perilous venture. John Hubbard was a physician of unusual presence—he served as the Chief of Public Health for the military mission in Denmark during WWII and ultimately wound up as chief executive officer of the National board of Medical Examiners[99]; Taussig may not have been as compelling a potential collaborator. Possibly she made only a weak case for her artificial ductus. But whatever the proximate reason, Gross's refusal ultimately must come down to a failure of imagination: He was ambitious and surely would have craved the fame attached to solving the problem of severe cyanosis. Had he envisioned the success that Blalock would soon enjoy, he surely would have thrown in with Taussig—or sought collaboration closer to home—rather than brusquely turning his back on this idea.

As one might surmise from his defying Ladd to hazard a new and potentially catastrophic procedure, Gross's self-confidence and ambition registered many standard deviations above the mean. So did his need for recognition. Trainees flocked to train with him, but many of the best were driven away at the end of their residency, so jealous was he of the limelight. More interesting and peculiar were his

[95] Eppinger et al. (1941).

[96] Taussig (1979).

[97] Taussig (1981)

[98] Snellen et al. (1981, p. 168).

[99] Piemme et al. (2012).

psychological quirks. He would, for example, famously disappear for days at a time after the death of a patient. One trainee recounted an incident during his training suggesting something exceeding mere eccentricity: One day, Gross was operating while the small observational gallery above the operating table was packed with famous surgeons; one of them dropped a newspaper on the floor, and Gross abruptly demanded that all the surgeons immediately vacate the gallery, or so the story goes. While some found Gross easy to work with, and a warm and sympathetic man if you could penetrate below his surface, many were put off by his aloofness. Others felt that Gross was more shy than aloof and point to his generosity with his trainees and the tight bond he formed with his patients. Gross had exceptional technical skills, but the progress in open-heart surgery in the 1960s saw his preeminence fade as surgeons with greater facility inside the heart strode onto the scene. In fact, late in his career, cardiologists at Boston Children's quietly transferred babies with transposition of the great arteries to another hospital with better surgical results for this malformation. Gross retired at age 66, moving to Vermont, where he died in October 1988.[100]

If gold is where you find it, so too are the pathways to medical innovation. A trailhead might appear through the lens of a microscope, or in the breath of a hamster in an ice calorimeter. Many are grounded in canny clinical observations made of one's patients, as is displayed in the next few chapters. Many lie in advancing the *craft* of therapy, especially in the case of surgical procedures. We've seen that cardiac surgery's venues of technical invention have ranged from the academic environment of the animal laboratory to the somber undertone of the morgue, to the often highly-charged atmosphere of the surgical theater. Models—almost always animal—were critically useful, but never as good, and never as useful, as innovators would like. And staring perceptively at a piece of tissue can yield more crucial information than many an elaborately planned and executed experiment.

Ancient preconceptions of impeccable provenance, and newer but just as flawed ideas, have resisted the Lavoisiers and Harveys in the scientific domain; cardiac surgery's fledgling history demonstrates much the same. Strong—or at least persistent—and confident personalities provided the energy of activation to push a novel therapy over the hump, never better exemplified than by the surgeon-innovators we've met. And the challenge of selecting the *right problem*—the important *and* likely soluble problem—is limned by the Robert Gross story. This Boston surgeon chose well when he decided to attack the patent ductus, but he missed a much bigger opportunity when he sent Taussig back to Hopkins empty handed. And luck. Gross' ductal ligation, while not exactly contingent on good fortune, could have been roadblocked for months or years had his twelfth patient been his first.

We've come to the end of our brief excursion into cardiac surgery's "ancient" past, and to the threshold of the first effective therapy for cyanotic heart disease. The Blalock-Taussig-Thomas shunt was more exciting and more palpably impactful than ductal ligation, its story more richly textured, and this invention is still indispensable in single ventricle therapy.

[100] Cooper (2010, pp. 9–25).

## References


Absolom KB (1983) Theodor Billroth and cardiac surgery. J Thorac Cardiovasc Surg 86:451–452

Alexi-Meskishvili VV, Bottcher W (2010) The first closure of the persistent ductus arteriosus. Ann Thorac Surg 90:349–356

Bailey CP (1949) The surgical treatment of mitral stenosis (mitral commissurotomy). Dis Chest 15:377–397

Baker C, Brock RC, Campbell M (1950) Valvulotomy for mitral stenosis: report of six successful cases. Br Med J 1(4465):1283–1293

Bing RJ (1983) Carrel. A personal reminiscence. JAMA 250:3297–3298

Bing RJ (ed) (1999) Cardiology: the evolution of the science and the art, 2nd edn. Rutgers University Press, New Brunswick

Brock RC (1948) Pulmonary valvulotomy for the relief of congenital pulmonary stenosis: report of three cases. Br Med J 1:1121–1126

Brock RC (1951) Discussion on the surgery of the heart and great vessels. Proc R Soc Med 44:995–1003

Brock RC (1952) The surgical and pathological anatomy of the mitral valve. Br Heart J 14:489–513

Brock RC (1965) The development of heart surgery in children. Arch Dis Child 40:123–127

Brunton L (1902) Preliminary note on the possibility of treating mitral stenosis by surgical methods. Lancet 1:352

Canadian Broadcasting Corporation (2015) Gatineau renames two city streets after complaints over Nazi links. Accessed 13 Aug 2024. https://ca.news.yahoo.com/gatineau-renames-two-city-streets-124410805.html

Carrel A (1912) Nobel Lecture. Accessed 7 Aug 2018. https://www.nobelprize.org/prizes/medicine/1912/carrel/facts/

Carrel A (1914) Experimental operations on the sigmoid valves of the pulmonary artery. J Exp Med 20:9–18

Carrel A (1935) Man the unknown. Harper & Brothers Publishers, New York

Carrel A, Guthrie CC (1906) Anastomosis of blood vessels by the patching method and transplantation of the kidney. JAMA 47:1648–1651

Castañeda AR (1980) Patent ductus arteriosus: a commentary. Ann Thorac Surg 31:92–96

Clowes GHA Jr (1960) The historical development of the surgical treatment of heart disease. Bull Hist Med 34:29–51

Cooper DKC (2010) Open heart: the radical surgeons who revolutionized medicine. Kaplan Publishing, New York

Cushing H, Branch JRB (1908) Experimental and clinical notes on chronic valvular lesions in the dog and their possible relation to further research of the cardiac valves. J Med Res 17:471–486

Cutler EC, Beck C (1929) The present status of the surgical procedures in chronic valvular disease of the heart. Final report of all surgical cases. Arch Surg 18:403–416

Cutler EC, Levine SA, Beck CS (1924) The surgical treatment of mitral stenosis, experimental and clinical studies. Arch Surg 9:689–821

Edwards WS, Edwards PD (1974) Alexis Carrel: visionary surgeon. Charles C. Thomas, Springfield

Elsberg CA (1899) An experimental investigation of the treatment of wounds of the heart by means of suture of the heart muscle. J Exp Med 4:479–520

Eppinger EC, Burwell CS, Gross RE (1941) The effects of the patent ductus arteriosus on the circulation. J Clin Invest 20:127–143

Ferguson MK (2016) Robert Lee Replogle, September 30, 1931-May 9, 2016. Ann Thorac Surg 102:1406–1408

Goor DA (2007) The genius of C. Walton Lilllehei and the true history of open heart surgery. Vantage Press, New York

Graybiel A, Strieder JW, Boyer NH (1938) An attempt to obliterate the patent ductus arteriosus in a patient with subacute bacterial endarteritis. Am Heart J 15:621–624

Gross RE (1939a) A surgical approach for ligation of a patent ductus arteriosus. N Engl J Med 220:510–514
Gross RE (1939b) Surgical management of the patent arteriosus. Ann Surg 110:321–351
Gross RE, Hubbard JP (1939) Surgical ligation of a patent ductus arteriosus. JAMA 112:729–731
Hamilton D (2017) The first transplant surgeon: the flawed genius of nobel prize winner Alexis Carrel. World Scientific, Singapore
Harken DE (1946) Foreign bodies in, and in relation to, the thoracic blood vessels and heart, I: techniques for approaching and removing foreign bodies from the chambers of the heart. Surg Gynecol Obstet 83:117–125
Harken DE (1989) The emergence of cardiac surgery, I: personal recollections of the 1940s and 1950s. J Thorac Cardiovasc Surg 98:805–813
Harken DE, Williams AC (1946) Foreign bodies in and in relation to the thoracic blood vessels and the heart. Am J Surg 72:80–90
Harken DE, Zoll PM (1946) Foreign bodies in and relation to the thoracic blood vessels and the heart. Am Heart J 32:1–19
Harken DE, Dexter L, Ellis LB, Farrand RE, Dickson JF (1951) The surgery of mitral stenosis. III. Finger-fracture valvuloplasty. Ann Surg 134:722–742
Harris H (1995) The cells of the body: a history of somatic cell genetics. Cold Spring Harbor Press, Plainview
Hendren H, Folkman J (n.d.) Harvard Medical School faculty memorial minute, Robert E. Gross. [Undated article]. Accessed 20 Apr 2019. https://fa.hms.harvard.edu/files/memorialminute_gross_robert_e.pdf
Hollman A (1997) Sir Thomas Lewis: pioneer cardiologist and clinical scientist. Springer, London
Hurt R (1996) The history of cardiothoracic surgery from early times. Parthenon, New York
Jarcho S (1974a) Experimental mitral insufficiency. Am J Cardiol 33:904–907
Jarcho S (1974b) Experimental production of cardiac murmurs (Thayer and MacCallum, 1907). Am J Cardiol 34:834–837
Jarcho S (1975) Experiments on heart valves (1908) by Harvey Cushing and J.R.B. Branch. Am J Cardiol 36:506–508
Johnson SL (1970) The history of cardiac surgery, 1896–1955. The Johns Hopkins Press, Baltimore
Keynes G (1966) The life of William Harvey. Oxford University Press, Oxford
Landecker H (2007) Culturing life: how cells became technologies. Harvard University Press, Cambridge
Levy SE, Blalock A (1939) Experimental observations on the effects of connecting by suture the left main pulmonary artery to the systemic circulation. J Thorac Surg 8:525–530
Lewis T (1942) Diseases of the heart: described for practitioners and students, 3rd edn. Macmillan and Co., Ltd., London
Litwak RS (1971) The growth of cardiac surgery: historical notes. Cardiovasc Clin 3:6–49
Mackenzie J (1918) Diseases of the heart, 3rd imp edn. Henry Frowde and Hodder & Stoughton, Oxford University Press, London
Meade RH (1961) A history of thoracic surgery. Charles C. Thomas, Springfield
Moller JH, Neal WA (eds) (1990) Fetal, neonatal, and infant cardiac disease. Appleton & Lange, Norwalk
Montreal Gazette, Canadian Press (2017) Montreal moves to rechristen street named after Nazi sympathizer. Accessed 8 Apr 2019. https://montrealgazette.com/news/local-news/montreal-moves-to-rechristen-street-named-after-nazi-sympathizer
Moore FD, Folkman J (1995) Robert Gross, 1905–1988. National Academy of Science. Accessed 11 Apr 2019. https://nap.nationalacademies.org/read/4961/chapter/8
Munro JC (1907) Ligation of the ductus arteriosus. Ann Surg 46:335–338
Murray L, Hendren WH, Mayer JE, Rockoff MA (2013) "A thrill of extreme magnety": Robert E. Gross and the beginnings of cardiac surgery. J Pediatr Surg 48:1822–1825
Naef AP (1990) The story of thoracic surgery: milestones and pioneers. Hogrefe & Huber Publishers, Toronto

New York State Department of Health (2007) Pediatric congenital cardiac surgery in New York State, 2002–2005. Accessed 1 May 2019. https://www.health.ny.gov/statistics/diseases/cardiovascular/heart_disease/docs/2002-2005_pediatric_congenital_cardiac_surgery.pdf

Nicoli LS (2012) Oral history interview. Boston Children's Hospital Archives. Accessed 13 Aug 2024. http://www.youtube.com/watch?v=JOq_-L24WBs

Paget S (1896) The surgery of the chest. John Wright & Co., Bristol

Piemme TE, John T, Hubbard MD (2012) Physician Assistant History Society. Accessed 13 Aug 2024. https://pahx.org/bios/hubbard-john-p/

Ravitch MM (ed) (1966) The papers of Alfred Blalock, vol I and II. The Johns Hopkins Press, Baltimore

Ravitch MM (1981) A century of surgery. The history of the American Surgical Association. J.B. Lippincott Co. Philadelphia, vol. 1

Reggiani AH (2002) Alexis Carrel, the unknown eugenics and population research under Vichy. Fr Hist Stud 25:332–356

Replogle RL (2003) Cardiac surgery in the age of the dinosaurs. Perfusion 18:171–177

Richardson RG (1970) The scalpel and the heart. Charles Scribner's Sons, New York

Sellors TH (1967) The genesis of heart surgery. Br Med J 1:385–393

Shaw LE (1902) Surgical operations for mitral stenosis. Lancet 1:619

Shumacker HB Jr (1968) Authority, research, and publication: reflections based upon some historical aspects of vascular surgery. Ann Surg 168:169–182

Shumacker HB Jr (1992) The evolution of cardiac surgery. Indiana University Press, Bloomington

Snellen HA, Dunning AJ, Arntzenius AC (eds) (1981) History and perspectives of cardiology: catheterization, angiography, surgery and concepts of circular control. Leiden University Press, The Hague

Souttar HS (1925) Surgical treatment of mitral stenosis. Br Med J 2:603–606

Stephenson HE, Kimpton RS (2001) America's first nobel prize in medicine or physiology: the story of Guthrie and Carrel. Midwestern Vascular Surgery Society and Hugh E. Stephenson, Boston

Stoney WS (2008) Pioneers of cardiac surgery. Vanderbilt University Press, Nashville

Taussig HB (1979) Difficulties, disappointments, and delights in medicine. Pharos 42:6–8

Taussig HB (1981) Little choice and a stimulating environment. J Am Med Womens Assoc 36:43–44

Thomas VT (1985) Pioneering research in surgical shock and cardiovascular surgery: Vivien Thomas and his work with Alfred Blalock. University of Pennsylvania Press, Philadelphia

Treasure T, Hollman A (1995) The surgery of mitral stenosis 1898–1948: why did it take 50 years to establish mitral valvotomy? Ann R Coll Surg Engl 77:145–151

Wangensteen OH, Wangensteen SD (1978) The rise of surgery: from empiric craft to scientific discipline. University of Minnesota Press, Minneapolis

Warren R (1984) Patent ductus arteriosus. JAMA 251:1203–1207

Watts SH (1907) The suture of blood vessels: implantation and transplantation of vessels and organs: an historical and experimental study. Ann Surg 46:373–404

Weisse AB (2002) Heart to heart: the twentieth century battle against cardiac disease—an oral history. Rutgers University Press, New Brunswick

Weksler M (2004) Naming streets for physicians: "L'affaire Carrel". Perspect Biol Med 47:67–73

Witkowski JA (1980) Dr. Carrel's immortal cells. Med Hist 24:129–142

# Chapter 5
# Collector of Hearts—Maude Abbott

> Abbott was almost obsessed by her interest in congenital malformations of the heart and would talk all day, and with an occasional catnap, would continue all night on the subject.
> – Helen Taussig.[1]

Big Data is currently all the rage. Twenty years from now, it may be something else, but as this is being written (2019), mining, smelting, and refining innumerable bites of patient-related information animates some of the smartest people in healthcare. The Data in Big Data can be clinical information (lab test, X-rays, doctor's notes, and the like) or biological data (for example, genes or proteins and small molecules). By capturing massive amounts of information from many people (millions in some cases), and applying sophisticated analysis, so the notion goes, diagnosis, disease mechanisms, prognosis, treatment, and other valuable information will ensue. Loaded with promise, Big Data may prove revolutionary, the day eventually arriving when we can't imagine how medicine ever advanced this far without it.

But all congenital heart cognoscenti had before the dawn of the modern (that is, surgical) era was Tiny Data. As Chap. 3 noted, the 18th and 19th centuries welcomed many papers and even textbooks describing cardiac malformations, Thomas Peacock's *Malformation and Conditions of the Human Heart* (1858) with original cases being the classic example. Although Peacock presented only nine cases of his own, he described roughly another 60 hearts from the literature, along with analysis and commentary. In most cases, symptoms and age at death (and occasionally physical findings) connected with a heart were included, and Peacock grouped the cases by their anatomy (for example, the number of cardiac chambers), imparting rudimentary organization to this chaotic subject. A treasure trove, *Malformations*' usefulness far exceeded reports with only one or a few cases. But its utility was limited partly by its presentation—narrative text—which demands the reader's time and concentration to organize and condense it into a big picture. And the number of patients was tiny, especially considering the bewildering variety in anatomy and outcomes. To have an even rough idea of length of survival, for example, you need many more of observations than Peacock's. Keating and Edwards's *Diseases of the*

[1] Taussig (1965).



T. J. Kulik, M. Dick, *Reimagining a Child's Heart*,
https://doi.org/10.1007/978-3-031-88608-9_5

*Heart and Circulation in Infancy and Adolescence* (1888) is heftier than Peacock's book, but it adds little new relative to congenital malformations and seems to have barely hit practitioners' radar screens.

In 1905, William Osler (ultimately Sir William) fired up a human bulldozer who would provide quantum enhancement and expansion of the corpus of congenital cardiology (Fig. 5.1). One of the great physicians of his or any era,[2] Osler had started his career at McGill University, subsequently advancing to the University of Pennsylvania before being recruited to Johns Hopkins Hospital as one of the legendary four founding professors. Although he couldn't have known this when he approached the young Maude Abbott to contribute a section on congenital heart disease for the *System of Modern Medicine*, this task proved to be of extraordinary yield, culminating in a groundbreaking chapter in Osler's book[3] and kindling a passionate interest in cardiac malformations in this unique Canadian physician. Maude had precious few credentials for this assignment—only a monograph on heart murmurs and one relevant case report. But her energy and capacity for hard work were huge, surfacing repeatedly in her associates' reminiscence. W.W. Francis distilled

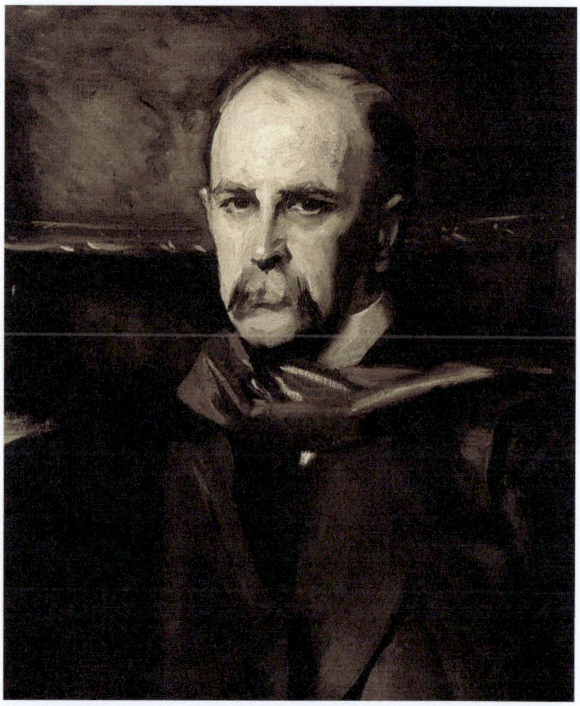

**Fig. 5.1** John Singer Sargent's impression of Sir William Osler. From the Wellcome collection, free to use without restriction

[2]Possibly the single best indicator of Osler's towering reputation and substance is the fact that Harvey Cushing—a surgeon of legendary stature—devoted the time and labor to write a massive, Pulitzer Prize winning biography of Osler.

[3]Abbott (1908).

her essence as well as any: "Kindness of heart, exuberant enthusiasm, colossal industry, and sheer grit, she had no equal among us. Illnesses and accidents, many of which would have killed a less sturdy mortal, were the only rest she got."[4] Her inexhaustible zeal impaled her friends as well, as Mrs. Blanche Yates recollected: "Maude's energy was appalling, and we were all wrecks when she got through with us."[5] Substituting exuberance for experience, Abbott discharged Osler's assignment brilliantly, then devoted another 30 years laying the groundwork for the explosion in pediatric cardiology and cardiac surgery which followed in her wake.

Evidence of Abbott's profound impact on congenital cardiology is scattered throughout its early history. If her work provided warrant for Robert Gross' breakthrough ductal ligations, as I suggest in Chap. 4, that alone secures her place as a founding figure. Maude's infiltration of the contemporary literature signals her broader influence: Her name in the text or her publications as references appear in roughly 40% of all papers on congenital heart disease published between 1930 and 1949.[6] But lavish endorsements from other creators of pediatric cardiology provide the most compelling arguments of all. Helen Taussig, celebrating a few select pioneers in a major speech for the American Heart Association, recollected that Abbott "above all, truly aroused interest in the malformations of the heart," and that "her contribution was so great it is fitting to review her life."[7] Alfred Blalock, in his 1945 Harvey Lecture, referred to Abbott's work several times, and cited her as one of a handful of people responsible for the then-recent interest in congenital heart disease.[8] John Brown singled out Maude—and her alone—for inciting interest in this domain in his 1939 textbook on the subject, insisting that "she alone has done more than any other person to raise the field of the general heart disease to the plane on which it now stands and dispel much of the obscurity surrounding these cases."[9] Richard Bing and Alexander Nadas (the latter was one of the mainsprings of

[4] Francis (1941).

[5] MacDermot (1941), p. 221. Perhaps the most plangent indicator of Abbott's vital reserves was her dedication to sister Alice (Brooks, 2011; MacDermot, 1941, pp. 210–212). Two years older than Maude and severely afflicted with bipolar disease, Alice had her first breakdown while traveling with Maude in Europe in the fall of 1895. She required hospitalization in Glasgow's Gartnavel Royal Asylum in January 1897, and following her September discharge, Maude transferred her to the family home, Elmbank, on St. Andrews East. Alice was never able to live independently from then on, but rather than institutionalize her, Maude retained attendants to care for her at Elmbank. Living in a rented room in Montreal, Maude was ever ready to rush to Elmbank as the need arose. Never giving up on "Allie," Maude persisted in hoping for her recovery until Alice died in her arms in October 1934. The unremitting drain of time, worry, and money would do many of us in, but not Maude; some of her most productive years ran concurrently with her sister's illness.

[6] I searched PubMed (June 4, 2019), using the key words "congenital heart" ("congenital cardiac" yielded almost identical results) for publications from 1930–1949. All publications available online were inspected (30); for 1940–1949 (553 papers), 10% were randomly inspected.

[7] Taussig (1965).

[8] Blalock (1946).

[9] Brown (1939), pp. vii, 1.

fledgling pediatric cardiology) ventured that "The advances in cardiac surgery and pediatric cardiology would have been impossible without her contribution."[10]

Maude transformed congenital cardiology (my amalgamation of pediatric cardiology and pediatric cardiovascular surgery) from Tiny Data to, well, Small Data, fanning her smoldering field into flames along the way. How did she do it? It turns out that collecting hearts, using a strategy that presaged Big Data nearly 100 years later, was key—if not the only key—to her success.

> January 23rd, 1908, 13 N Gardens, Oxford
> Dear Doctor Abbott
> I knew you would write a good article but I did not expect one of such extraordinary merit. It is far and away the best thing ever written on the subject in English—possibly in any language.... For years it will be the standard work on the subject and it is articles of this sort—and there are not many of them—that make a System of Medicine.
> William Osler.[11]

In December of 1898, a 29-year-old nobody of a woman physician, bedeviled with lifelong insecurities but having enough gumption to venture to meet one of the medical titans of her day, was thrilled to be rounding with William Osler.[12] Traveling from Montreal to Washington, D.C. on business, Maude Abbott had indulged in a quick excursion to Baltimore to introduce herself to the Physician-in-Chief at Johns Hopkins Hospital, a personage she found especially interesting given his previous history at McGill. Osler's invitation to join his rounding entourage must have delighted Maude, but the tail-end of her day abruptly turned painful: with her "hand on the lentil of the half-closed door, someone swung the other heavy half door to, crushing her finger and nearly extracting the nail. Doctor Osler's concern took the form of an invitation to dinner that evening."[13] Her mangled digit—one of many injuries this accident-prone lady suffered over the years—turned out to be the price of admission for a watershed evening for Maude. After dinner, discussions at Osler's house got her "heart beating at the wonderful new world that had opened unexpectedly before [her]."[14] When Osler urged Abbott to throw herself into her new job at the medical museum, she did exactly that. She also stayed in close contact with Osler, who remained Maude's major professional influence—and object of her hero worship—until his death in 1919. While Abbott's energy and drive would surely have culminated in important contributions even *sans* the Osler connection, I believe

---

[10] Nadas & Bing, "Congenital Heart Disease," in Bing (1999). There are many other similar encomiums, such as: Perry (1937); Marquis (1987); R.M. Freedom, "Historical overview: A brief narrative of the modern era of congenital heart disease," in Freedom et al. (2004), p. 1; Alfred E. Cohn, in MacDermot (1941), p. 241.

[11] Abbott (1959).

[12] Biographical material for Abbott is from MacDermot (1941); Segall, in MacDermot (1941); Waugh (1992); Taussig (1965); Paul and Ina White, in Waugh (1992); Martin (1941); Francis (1941); and other specific citations.

[13] MacDermot (1941), pp. 72–73.

[14] Abbott (1959).

it likely—for reasons soon apparent—that her passion would have carried her to places unrelated to malformed hearts absent that carelessly swung door.

Maude Babin saw first light in 1869 in St. Andrews East, Quebec, a small village planted on the Ottawa river's North Shore. Her parents were French Canadian—the Reverend Jeremiah Babin and Elizabeth Abbott. Jeremiah fell into serious trouble—he was tried (but acquitted) for the murder of his pathetically crippled sister—and abandoned his family hard on Maude's birth.

Only 7 months old when tuberculosis carried off Elizabeth, Maude and her older sister Alice were entrusted to the care of their 62-year-old grandmother. Caring for nine children and her husband,[15] Mrs. William Abbott endured the life of Job but remained tough and resourceful. Perhaps reacting to the scandal surrounding Maude's father, she arranged for the sisters' last name to be refashioned to Abbott via an act of Parliament. Grandma was reasonably prosperous, judging from 11-year-old Maude's Christmas haul: a gold cross, two yards of wide ribbon and one of a narrow, black-handled penknife, a silver thimble, a black handled toothbrush, half a dozen handkerchiefs, $0.50, a pencil case, some frilling, fruit, nuts and candies, a pair of seed bracelets, and a coral necklace.[16]

Maude burned with curiosity, manifest early on by an intense desire for schooling. A home governess provided her early book learning, but she was desperate for more. A diary entry at age 15 reveals her desperate yearning: "My wish! Oh, if I were to get it: if that were to come true.... but if I were to go to school, if it were only for one term, how happy I would be. I don't think it is the other girl's society I want or anything of that sort, but the good education I would love—how I long for one."[17] Two weeks later, she declared the same—that she couldn't help thinking about going to school next winter, couldn't help building castles in the air, that she could "scarcely help improving the shining hour (of school) while it lasted"; she would "not care for the competition, but for *the real study and the benefit I would arrive from it*."[18] By December 1885, her air castle had materialized in the guise of Miss Symmers and Smith School in Montreal, but "We are never satisfied. My wish is to go to college and now I am wishing for that almost as ardently as I did last winter for my present good fortune."[19] Securing a scholarship from McGill University, she crossed "the gates of Paradise"[20] a year later. Maude was "literally in love with McGill, or so the girls said,"[21] and her university years presaged her sharply honed social-organizational nature. Elected president of her class, Maude was also a founder of the Delta Sigma Debating Society, the religious society, and a future McGill Alumnae Society. The *McGill Fortnightly* saw fit to appoint her its

[15] MacDermot (1941) says nine children; Waugh (1992), says eight.

[16] MacDermot (1941), p. 6.

[17] MacDermot (1941), p. 10.

[18] MacDermot (1941), p. 11; emphasis mine.

[19] MacDermot (1941), p. 13.

[20] Abbott (1959).

[21] Abbott (1959).

editor, and (just after graduating) Maude organized a soup kitchen. None of these got in the way of her graduating with high honors and as Class Valedictorian in 1890.

The McGill medical school admitted no women, but Maude adored the university and itched to stay for medical training. When her appeal to the Dean and Faculty of Medicine for admission was rejected, her friends congealed into the Association for the Professional Education of Women (A.P.E.W.), petitioned the faculty to reconsider, and vowed to raise the necessary funds. The answer still being no, Abbott organized and agitated, the newspapers got involved, and the controversy evolved into a wrestling match between the A.P.E.W. and the medical faculty. While many of the faculty had no objection to mixed sex classes, others did "for the reasons that must occur to everyone … it is unnecessary to find them, especially for a public newspaper."[22] One Dr. F.W. Campbell considered that McGill might endow a separate college for women to be trained in a few areas (but not surgery, for which "women would not have the nerve"), but he had serious reservations: "And can you think of a patient in a critical case, waiting for half an hour while the medical lady fixes her bonded or her bustle?"[23] Ultimately, the irresistible force of Maude Abbott proved too little to budge the immovable object of hide-bound McGill, obliging her to search elsewhere.[24]

Maude wound up matriculating with the first cohort of women students at Bishop's College of Medicine in Montreal. She found the going tough. Suffering from "rough" students with "lower standards" than she was used to, Abbott was lonely, mostly from feeling out of place in an almost entirely male class. Her assertiveness must have rubbed people the wrong way, but Maude had no choice—she was still plowing upstream. Hands-on patient contact is indispensable for medical students, but Montreal General Hospital had never before accommodated a woman for clinical training; Maude had to pester and agitate to become the first.[25] Despite these distractions, she gathered up the Senior Anatomy and Chancellor prizes—pretty galling, one imagines, for some of her male littermates—before graduating in 1894. After 3 years of travel and medical training in Europe, Abbott returned to Montreal in 1897, hanging her shingle at 156 Mansfield St. But her heart wasn't in private practice, and she soon stumbled into a most unusual job, especially for an ambitious young physician—Assistant Curator of the medical museum at McGill (1898), advancing to Curator the following year. This seemingly milquetoast posting proved a surprisingly potent—if also exasperating—perch for Maude's entire career, excepting a 2-year interlude (1923–1925) as the Chair of Pathology at the Women's College of Medicine in Philadelphia, PA.

---

[22] MacDermot (1941), p. 40.

[23] MacDermot (1941), pp. 41–42.

[24] I include this episode not to preach, from the superior perspective of the twenty-first century, on the medical profession's antediluvian attitudes in Abbott's day (and beyond, for that matter), but rather to give one of many examples of this young woman's force of personality and determination.

[25] Abbott (1959).

The Museum had accreted a profusion of medical specimens over decades—tissues and organs preserved in formaldehyde; bones, many traumatically shattered; wax models of embryos at various stages of gestation; and assorted medical instruments. Situated in hopeless disarray, these sundry items were therefore eventually unusable for those seeking to study human pathology firsthand and close-up. Formulating a scheme to catalog this stuff of unrealized potential was Maude's first challenge, and she hoped to get her bearings by visiting other medical museums, including the Army Medical Museum in Washington, D.C. It was on this trip that she first met Osler.

Maude's passion for congenital heart malformations took fire in 1900 when her eye was arrested by a heart in decades-long repose in a formalin-filled glass jar, a rare type of single ventricle defect known as "Holmes Heart." As far as I know, Abbott never shared *why* she found this heart—hardly a hunk of handsome muscle—so intriguing. (Fig. 5.2) Perhaps it was the utter strangeness of the organ that riveted her: It had only a single pumping chamber, with a pulmonary artery coming off a useless chamber of its own. Osler instantly recalled this specimen when Abbott sent him an inquiry: Doctor Andrew Holmes, the first Dean of the faculty at the McGill medical school had looked after one Isaac N, who died blue at age 21 years of age. Holmes conducted the autopsy and described N's heart in the *Transactions of the Medico-Chirurgical Society of Edinburgh* (1824). Maude was so taken with this specimen that she republished Holmes's paper with commentary of her own in 1901. It was on the strength of this effort that Osler asked her to write a section on congenital heart disease for his and Thomas MacRae's textbook, the *System of*

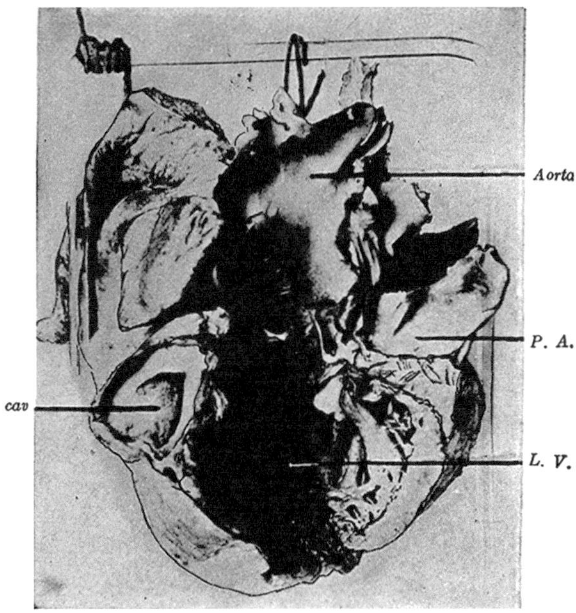


**Fig. 5.2** The heart that launched a thousand clinico-pathological correlations. The 'Holmes heart' at the McGill medical museum. Also in Abbott (1936) p. 51

*Modern Medicine*.[26] Osler, now Regius Chair of Medicine at Oxford, was delighted with her contribution to the *System* (see quoted letter from Osler). His fulsome praise was perhaps to be expected, given that her chapter resided in *his* book, which is only as good as its individual contributions. But there may have been more to Osler's extravagant assessment. Doubtlessly aware of Maude's hero worship, he would have been keenly aware how much she craved his words of praise. Indeed, tucked safely in her handbag, Osler's letter traveled with Maude wherever she went.[27]

Maude's chapter in Osler's *System* was anchored by observations of congenital cardiac defects and the 412 patients wrapped around them. She scrutinized hearts in her museum and linked the cardiac morphology with the clinical history, and also gathered similar information from the literature and hearts via extensive correspondence with other doctors worldwide.[28] The age at death, degree of cyanosis, one symptom (attacks of difficult breathing), and typical murmurs were included. Organized into a table—which I think of as a sort of Periodic Table of Congenital Cardiology—the malformations were split and lumped into 23 categories. Maude discussed the embryology of normal and malformed hearts, and her review of cyanosis, an unsolved puzzle in 1908 (discussed in Chaps. 3 and 6), is interesting reading even today. She concludes with a few discouraging paragraphs on treatment: "a careful hygiene and expectant and preventive treatment may be summed up as the only available assistance that can be given."[29] Like Mendeleev's periodic table of the elements, this was a new way to think about the subject, by virtue of the sheer volume of material, organized in a way that facilitated drawing general conclusions.

Abbott continued to collect cases and refine her thinking as her career blossomed. She was up to 631 by 1915 for the second edition of the *System*, and up to 850 by 1927 for the third edition. By 1932, her table had mushroomed to 1000 cases in *Nelson's Loose-Leaf Medicine*. It was natural for Maude—this most social of creatures—to extend her passion beyond the inscribed page into the flesh and blood world of other enthusiasts (and those who would come, thanks to her). She threw together "a jumble of specimens, photos and diagrams"—pared down and organized thanks to Dr. Lewis Gross—and hauled this exhibit to the New York Academy of Medicine's graduate Fortnight in Cardiology in 1931.[30] Her display was expanded and shipped to the Centenary Meeting of the British Medical Association in London the next year. The 32-foot-long exhibit showcased 50 anatomical specimens, X-rays, various drawings, figures, and the 1000-case table. Attracting the attention of the *British Medical Journal* (it "told a coherent story in which were made apparent the etiological basis of congenital heart disease"), the three-day exhibit was well attended, including by many leading cardiologists.[31] Too successful to consign to

[26] MacDermot (1941), p. 76; Dobell & Van Praagh (1996).

[27] Brooks (2011).

[28] Abbott (1936), pp. vii–viii; MacDermot (1941), p.184.

[29] Abbott (1908), p. 425.

[30] MacDermot (1941), pp. 179–180.

[31] MacDermot (1941), p. 181.

history at meeting's end, Abbott transformed much of the London display into her slim but soon-classic 1936 monograph, *Atlas of Congenital Heart Disease*. She had now constructed 3 broad categories of congenital heart disease—cyanotic, initially acyanotic but with transient or late cyanosis, and acyanotic—with 24 subcategories. The table also displayed more clinical information and the cause of death.[32] Even more than her 1908 initial foray, this grand synthesis enabled physicians to wrap their minds around this arcane and convoluted subject, to perceive the link between defects and symptoms, and to estimate what the clinical consequences of a malformation might be.

Maude also included diagrams indicating the (abnormal) path of blood flow in these malformed hearts, *extrapolating anatomy and physiology*. This was new and important: While Peacock, pondering the nature of cyanosis, speculated about "intermixture of the currents of blood" and the direction of intracardiac blood flow, he supplied no such diagrams with only fragmentary discussion of physiology.[33] Although the heart's architecture influences its function, what matters ultimately is where and how much oxygen is delivered, at rest and with stress, and at what physiologic cost. Boiled down to its essence, classical cardiovascular physiology is largely defined by considering blood oxygen content, and blood flow and pressures in the heart and blood vessels outside of the heart, and the many factors influencing these variables. Abbott's effort to instruct physicians on this crucially important aspect of cardiovascular malformations was a significant contribution considered on its own, although she could only scratch the physiology's surface given the technological limitations of her day.

By the end of the nineteenth century, measuring physiological variables in normal animals was old stuff. The Reverend Stephen Hales, as he reported in *Statistical Essays: volume 2. Containing a Haemastaticks*[34] in 1733, "caused a mare to be tied down on her back… 14 hands high, and about 14 years of age" and measured her arterial pressure by observing how high blood from her leg artery rose in a glass tube; jugular vein pressure was also measured. Pulmonary arterial and right and left ventricular pressures had been registered by the mid-1800s, and cardiac output was quantified a few decades later. Extensive hemodynamic investigations had been accomplished in animals before the twentieth century but not in people, blood pressure measurement being the exception.[35] Heart catheterization, where blood pressure, flows, and oxygen content are measured by using intracardiac catheters, made hemodynamic studies practical in humans and was of such significance that it netted a 1956 Nobel Prize for its earliest pioneers.[36] But cardiac "cath" made its first

[32] Abbott (1936/2006), p 60–61.

[33] Peacock (1858), pp. 121–128.

[34] Hales (1733)

[35] Using a mercury manometer, in 1856 Faivre measured arterial blood pressure in a human during limb amputation (!), although the modern era of BP measurement lagged 40 years behind. See three articles by Cournand, Hamilton & Richards, and Pickering, all in Fishman (1964).

[36] André F. Cournand, Werner Forssmann, and Dickinson W. Richards.

appearance only in 1941, and application to patients with congenital heart disease tarried until about 1947.[37]

The core of Abbott's work derived from *clinicopathologic correlation*—correlating pre-mortem clinical findings with anatomic findings made at autopsy. As we saw in Chap. 3, this is one of the earliest strategies for learning about the pathology of human disease. But this approach is inherently *static*, while physiology is *dynamic*. No blood flowed, nor was pressure generated inside Maude's collection of hearts. Her cardiac physiology was therefore *inferential*. For example, assuming pressures in the aorta and ventricles, Abbott could often—though not always[38]—correctly infer the direction of blood through a hole in a malformed heart. But while her diagram showed what directional effects abnormal intracardiac blood flows might have on blood oxygen levels and other variables, she could not quantify them. Yet quantification is key: the difference between life-limiting cyanosis or heart failure, and few if any symptoms, is as much a function of the *amount* as the *direction* of blood flow in a malformed heart. The virtue of Abbott's physiology is that it imparted a more vivid and complete picture of the clinical relevance of a malformation than anatomic description alone could provide; its vice was that it presented at best a blurred, sometimes even misleading, picture of how a defect actually affects the patient's life.

If Maude's physiology was, understandably, wafer thin and a little unreliable, her *Atlas* was lacking in yet other ways, suffering from limitations obvious even in her day. For a start, its "case ascertainment" was heavily biased. The cases she collected were not representative of the universe of people with a given defect, but rather only patients of doctors inclined to procure postmortem hearts. People with, say, a patent ductus arteriosus who lived long and died a natural death were less likely to figure into her analysis than patients who died younger, of a heart malformation, in the hands of a curious physician. Indeed, Maude found that the mean age of death with a patent ductus was 24 years, but analyzing data from hundreds of patients under observation (not autopsy specimens), cardiologist Maurice Campbell later established that nearly 60% of such patients would live 45 years, and that by age 60 survival was still 40%.[39] And flawed information about the youngest (as well as the oldest) patron skews our perception of consequences of a defect, a fact well demonstrated by Maude's collection of cases. Babies with a large ventricular septal defect usually develop heart failure, but Abbott's table suggests that these patients seldom succumb to this. It turns out that she included very few such patients in the first few months of life, explaining why "cardiac insufficiency" appears to be a minor problem with this defect. Abbott also can be confusing. In 1908, for example, she states that isolated coarctation is of little significance in the infant, yet the five such infants

[37] Baim & Bing in Bing (1999); Bing (1988).

[38] For example, she incorrectly indicated only systemic-to-pulmonary shunting through the ductus arteriosus and atrial septal defect in transposition of the great vessels (Abbott [1936], p. 13, 3c).

[39] Campbell (1968).

in her table died between birth and 5 years of age.[40] And Maude's biggest idea—her three-category classification scheme (see above)—was of little clinical utility, as Helen Taussig observed in her foundational 1947 textbook.[41] Published only 3 years after the Maude's *Atlas*, John Brown's *Congenital Heart Disease* was loaded with vastly more and better clinical information than found in Maude's book.

If Maude's opus was flawed, so was Giorgio Vasari's *Life of the Most Excellent Painters, Sculptors, and Architects Prentice* (first published in 1550). Vasari was a sixteenth century painter, architect and art historian—in fact, arguably the very first of that breed of historians. As is richly described in Ingrid Rowland and Noah Charney's the *Collector of Lives, Giorgio Vasari and the Invention of Art* (2017), *Lives* was anything but objective or even reliably factual history. It promoted his city (Florence) and its artists, especially Michelangelo. Roland and Charney offered that the "the modern conception of art… owes its popularization, if not its origin to Giorgio Vasari."[42] Vasari demonstrated a different and compelling way to think about artists, which overshadowed factual deficiencies in his book. Five hundred years later, *Lives* still thrives despite its many imperfections, serving as required reading for countless students and a subject of serious contemplation by scholars such as Rowland and Charney.[43]

Abbott collected not the lives of artists but malformed hearts, or written accounts of them. Her work, while limited in scope and depth and sometimes even incorrect, did for congenital cardiology something like what Vasari had done for art history. For any discipline to advance, a critical mass of intellectual and social activity must gel. Maude helped many people wrap their minds around this curiously Byzantine, arcane subject by taking a disparate, even bizarre, collection of malformations and demonstrating certain similarities (and differences) in morphology and symptoms. Her table imparted a sense of order, previously unappreciated. She showed how a defect alters the blood path, rather than merely sketching the anomaly. Maude's oeuvre thus precipitated a heightened appreciation and interest in congenital heart disease. By showing her colleagues how to think differently about the malformed hearts, she injected "oomph" into this unformed discipline. Maude's contribution was only secondarily about the actual data that she mined and presented—her impact derived from her opening her obsession to a much wider audience. And what was the deep source of Maude's influence? Abbott's impact turned on the spindle of her *social ability and need to connect* with other people, which was as integral to her contributions as Lavoisier's laboratory apparatus was to his. A generous, warm-hearted, and convivial soul,[44] she had widely scattered colleagues and talked shop at the many parties and dinners that she loved to organize and attend. Carrying on an

[40] Abbott (1908), p. 413.

[41] Taussig (1947), pp. xxxi–xxxii.

[42] Rowland & Charney (2017), p. 15.

[43] Rowland & Charney (2017), p. 347.

[44] Signs of Maude's generosity and humanity range from her innumerable small gifts for friends, to expending precious time assisting a former St. Andrews acquaintance in his efforts to avoid jail time, then sending him gifts in prison when she failed (MacDermot, 1941, p. 86). The ultimate

extensive international correspondence with other enthusiasts, she eagerly shared information, reinforcing her colleagues' interest in congenital heart disease. Since many of her one thousand cardiac cases[45] were contributed from far-flung practitioners, the magnitude of her contribution hinged greatly upon her networking skills. Abbott put ink onto paper—the academic coin of the realm—but she also infused excitement via her lectures and exhibits in New York and London.

Thus, it was the zeal infused, thanks to an enormous need and talent for connecting with other people, that mostly accounts for Maude's edifice in congenital heart disease. At least that was how Dr. Paul Dudley White, one of the era's most influential cardiologists (and famous for having treated President Eisenhower) figured the essence of Maude's seminal contributions: "[W]hen we review Maude Abbott's influence in the field of cardiovascular disease, we find that far more important than any of her written works was her vital stimulus to other workers. Her spirit was indefatigable. She inspired innumerable other workers throughout the world and was always very willing, in fact eager, to place at the disposal of anyone who sought it, her own vast experience… she was an inspiration to us all, pathologists and clinicians alike… her presence act as a ferment, and yet the most pleasant sort of ferment."[46] White was Maude's good friend, and these sentiments need to be interpreted accordingly, but other biographical recollections, as we saw earlier in this chapter, are suffused with similar sentiment.

Maude was cut to the quick in 1936 when she was forced to retire, on account of her age, from McGill. She fought this as she had other battles, with little success,[47] but her energetic engagement of the cardiac community continued unabated even after her connection with McGill was severed. She gave talks on the U.S. Pacific Coast, consulted, and enlivened professional meetings. Maude planned on writing a large textbook, a grand summary of what she had gleaned of congenital heart disease, and even envisioned laboratory and multi-institutional clinical studies.[48] It is a great pity that she had too little time left for these projects, suffering a stroke in July 1940 and finally succumbing on September 2nd of that year at the age of 71.

Antoine Lavoisier lost his life in the Terror when zealots took him too seriously as an agent of economic repression. Abbott had quite the opposite problem at McGill: many of her colleagues didn't take her seriously enough. In fact, she was treated miserably in Montreal, at least by the lights of several of her contemporaries. Harold Segall, a museum assistant and friend, admitted that "in certain circles it was acceptable to regard Dr. Abbott as an inferior character, someone to be tolerated and humored—a 'hen medic.'"[49] She was promoted at a glacial pace, advancing only to

expression of her munificence and profound compassion was her unsparing support of her sister Alice (See footnote 5).

[45] Bauer & Astbury (1944) provide a bibliography for one thousand hearts in Abbott's table.

[46] White (1940).

[47] Waugh (1992), pp. 116–117.

[48] Evans (2008).

[49] Waugh (1992), p. 40.

assistant professor, a ludicrous under-appointment, give her productivity and international renown. Despite her many entreaties, her salary advancement was also slow. Maude did have a few strong supporters, notably Charles Martin (Dean of the faculty), F.J. Shepherd (surgeon par excellence), and J. George Adami (McGill's professor of pathology). and the University made some recompense in 1936 when it awarded Abbott an LL.D. *honoris causa*, its highest honor, although this seems paltry compensation for decades of disregard. Her second-class status is especially striking when one considers her almost Lavoisier-like vitae. In addition to running the Museum and her marathon exertions in the cardiac domain, a few high points include:

- A highly regarded teacher, Maude devoted countless hours to one-on-one sessions with medical students early in her career.
- An amateur historian, Abbot lectured and published on Florence Nightingale, nursing history, the McGill medical faculty, and the history of Quebec medicine.
- In 1906, she, with two other physicians, organized the International Association of Medical Museums (its name later changed to the International Academy of Pathology) and worked tirelessly to foster it.
- Abbott put in a stint as acting director at the Canadian Army Medical Museum and helped organize the Argenteuil Museum at Carillon. Maude served for a time as the editor of the *Canadian Medical Journal* and, as managing editor, took on the 600-page Osler Memorial Volume for the Museums Association, a 6-year labor of love.

McGill's seemingly unaccountable disregard could be easily enough chalked up to sexism. Maude's previous unavailing struggle for acceptance into the medical school, and her need to fight for clinical rotation certainly suggests as much. Segall's "hen medic" indictment shouts out the same. While male chauvinism was likely a culprit, other factors may have resonated with the widespread predisposition to discount a woman physician. Maude presented something of a bumbling visage, lacking the gravitas many associate with her profession. Ambling preoccupied down the street, her skirt sometimes worn backward, sometimes trailing dropped items, Abbott was an absent-minded professor straight out of Hollywood casting. Friends often remarked on her absent-mindedness, and Maude's many accidents suggested she rambled about with a perilous lack of awareness. These mishaps range from the amusing—pitching off a donkey crossing a stream in Greece—to three considerably more consequential encounters with moving vehicles while a pedestrian. Abbott herself injured a pedestrian while driving, bringing her driving to a screeching (and expensive) halt.

H.E. MacDermott, one of Abbott's colleagues and (sympathetic) chief biographer, observes that "her energy sometimes lacked method and concentration," and that her "benevolence was apt to be swayed by impulse alone."[50] One forms the impression that Maude was

[50] MacDermot (1941), p. v.

> surrounded by zone of faint chaos and was perhaps too pungently and relentlessly animated to be enjoyed except in measured doses (as one biography has pointed out, Abbott had no constant intimates[51] which is consistent with this idea). Casual acquaintances, especially those unaware of her many accomplishments and international reputation (Maude shied away from blowing her own horn), may have found her too scattered, too awkward to take seriously.

Whatever the reasons for her sometimes-uncomfortable fit at McGill, those who appreciated and loved her laughed last. How many of those who condescended to this larger-than-life person ever graced a Canadian postal stamp?[52] Or were honored by an anonymous donor, establishing a scholarship in their name? Or had an elegant academic portrait painted in her honor (Fig. 5.3) Or had the artist Diego Rivera paint their likeness onto a panel depicting the greatest cardiac pioneers from Galen on? (Maude is the only woman, and the sole Canadian, gracing these panels in the National Institute of Cardiology in Mexico City.)[53] History has treated Dr. Maude Elizabeth Seymour Abbott well, as well it should.

William Harvey fused acute observations with a gift for thinking differently to radically alter our understanding of how blood courses through the body. Lavoisier

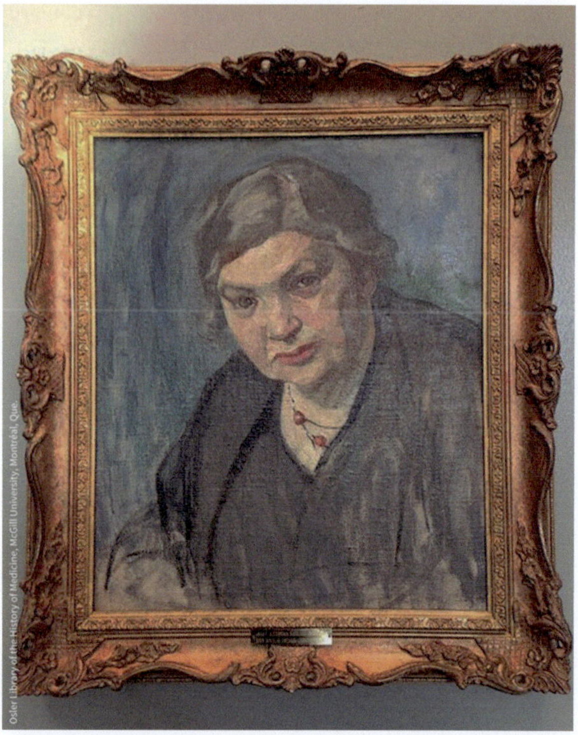


**Fig. 5.3** Portraying Maude Abbott. (Wright JR Jr., Fraser R, Adams A, Hunter M. CMAJ. 2017 Feb 21;189(7):E281-E283. https://doi.org/10.1503/cmaj.160976. No abstract available). The image includes text on the left side: "Osler Library of the History of Medicine, McGill University, Montreal, Que"

[51] Gillett, in Clifford (1989), p. 197.

[52] Wright et al. (2017).

[53] Lomas (2005).

executed one clever experiment after another, and applied powerful analysis, as he took the first ingenious steps to discover how oxygen sustains life. Maude scrutinized her collection of hearts but did no experiments. Her strategy was Big Data's—aggregating lots of data from multiple sources and making sense of it as best as she could. If only in a small way, Abbott anticipated the multicenter studies which constitute the backbone of contemporary clinical medical research. Sociability was her indispensable tool: She procured much of her new data via networking and pushed her nascent field toward the goalpost of new treatments by, in effect, pumping up the team. Abbott's gift was not so much knowledge as ferment.

Abbott primed congenital cardiology's pump but did not twist that tap. As we will learn in Chap. 6, Helen Taussig is referred to as *almost* the mother of pediatric cardiology; the mother of *clinical* pediatric cardiology would have been a better assessment. Helen was only 10 years old, you see, when Canadian Maude Abbott published her landmark review of cardiac malformations in Osler's *Modern Medicine* (1908). Abbott put Morgagni's centuries old clinical-pathological correlation to superb use as she developed a deeper and better organized understanding of congenital heart disease than previously available; she went on to contribute lots more, including what I think of as her Periodic Table of Congenital Cardiology. Abbott's data—although flawed, as we have seen—were enormously useful for others who broke new cardiac ground. Her energy and passion multiplied by many times her seminal observations, making her something like a venture capitalist and bankrolling this embryonic field. For me at least, Maude Abbott was the mother *and* father of congenital cardiology, even if she seldom saw a patient.

But now we turn to Chap. 6 and examine the fruitful if sometimes awkward collaboration of Alfred Blalock, Helen Taussig and Vivien Thomas who take us to the first success at improving the lives of children with complex congenital heart disease.

## References


Abbott ME (1908) Congenital cardiac disease. In: Osler W (ed) Modern medicine: its theory and practice, vol IV, ch. IX. Lea Brothers & Co., Philadelphia, pp 323–425

Abbott ME (1936/2006) Atlas of congenital cardiac disease. McGill-Queen's University Press, Montreal

Abbott ME (1959) Autobiographical sketch. McGill Med J 28:27–152

Bauer DF, Astbury EC (1944) Congenital cardiac disease bibliography of the 1,000 cases analyzed in Maude Abbott's *Atlas*. Am Heart J 27:688–723

Bing RJ (1988) The Johns Hopkins: the Blalock-Taussig era. Pers Bio Med 32:85–90

Bing RJ (ed) (1999) Cardiology: the evolution of the science and the art, 2nd edn. Rutgers University Press, New Brunswick

Blalock A (1946) Physiopathology and surgical treatment of congenital cardiovascular defects. Bull NY Acad Med 22:57–80

Brooks B (2011) An illness in the family: Dr. Maude Abbott and her sister, Alice Abbott. CBMH/BCHM 28:171–190

Brown JW (1939) Congenital heart disease. Staples Press, London

Campbell M (1968) Natural history of persistent patent ductus arteriosus. Brit Heart J 30:4–13

Clifford GJ (ed) (1989) Lone voyagers: academic women in coeducational universities, 1870–1937. The Feminist Press, The City University of New York, New York, NY

Dobell ARC, Van Praagh R (1996) The Holmes heart: historic associations and pathologic anatomy. Am Heart J 132:437–445

Evans WN (2008) The relationship between Maude Abbott and Helen Taussig: connecting the historical dots. Cardiol Young 18:557–564

Fishman AP, Richards DW (1964) Circulation of the blood. Men and ideas. Oxford University Press, New York, NY

Francis WW (1941) Maude Abbott (1869–1940). Bull Hist Med 10:305–308

Freedom RM, Yoo S-J, Mikailian H, Williams WG (eds) (2004) The natural and modified history of congenital heart disease. Blackwell, Elmsford

Hales S (1733) Statistical essays: volume 2. Containing a haemastatick, London, Printed for W. Innys and R. Manby, at the west-end of St. Paul's, and T. Woodward, at the Half-Moon between Temple-Gate, Fleet Street

Keating JM, Edwards WA (1888) Diseases of the heart and circulation in infancy and adolescence. P. Blakiston, Son & Co., Philadelphia

Lomas D (2005) Painting the history of cardiology. BMJ 331:1533–1535

MacDermot HE (1941) Maude Abbott: a Memoir. Macmillan, Toronto

Marquis RM (1987) Congenital heart disease: the ductus as the pathfinder. Br Heart J 58:429–436

Martin CF (1941) Maude Abbott. J Path Bacteriol 52:390–393

Osler W, McRae T (1908) Modern medicine, its theory and practice. Vol. IV, diseases of the circulatory system—diseases of the blood—diseases of the spleen, thymus and lymph-glands. Lea & Febiger, Philadelphia

Peacock TB (1858) On malformations, &c., of the human heart. John Churchill, London. Reprinted in the classics of medicine library. Birmingham: Gryphon Editions, Ltd.; 1981

Perry CB (1937) Discussion on the course and management of congenital heart disease. Proc Royal Soc Med 30:693–700

Rowland I, Charney N (2017) The collector of lives: Giorgio Vasari and the invention of art. W.W. Norton, New York, NY

Taussig HB (1947) Congenital malformations of the heart. The Commonwealth Fund, New York, NY

Taussig HB (1965) On the evolution of our knowledge of congenital malformations of the heart. Circ 31:768–777

Waugh D (1992) *Maudie of McGill: Dr.* Maude Abbott and the foundations of heart surgery. Hannah Institute & Dundurn Press, Toronto/Oxford

White PD (1940) Maude Abbott's contributions to cardiology. McGill Med J 10:32–35

Wright JR Jr, Fraser R, Adams A, Hunter M (2017) Portraying Maude Abbot. CMAJ 189:E281–E283

# Chapter 6
# Collaborators: Taussig, Blalock, Thomas

The Great Hall of the British Medical Association in London is cavernous, and it was packed when two Yankee physicians gave a combined lecture describing their breakthrough treatment for certain types of heart malformations. The year was 1947, and medicine was just turning its attention to matters put on hold during the dark years of WWII. Alfred Blalock (Fig. 6.3), the urbane chief of surgery at Johns Hopkins, and Helen Taussig (Fig. 6.1), almost the mother of pediatric cardiology, as we'll see later, recounted their experience treating hopelessly ill children with a radical new operation. They weren't so much describing a procedure as a revolution in the way that people thought about congenital heart disease. The Blalock-Taussig-Thomas shunt, first performed in late 1944, had cracked open a piñata of new treatment possibilities. International interest in the operation was intense.

Lord Russell Brock, a British surgeon and an early giant in the field, described the scene: "The silence of the audience betokened their rapt attention and appreciation. The hall was quite dark for projection of [Blalock's] slides which had been illustrating patients before and after operation, when suddenly a long searchlight beam traversed the whole length of the hall and unerringly picked out on the platform a Guy's [Hospital] nursing sister, dressed in her attractive blue nursing uniform, sitting on a chair and holding a small cherub-like girl of 2½ years with a halo of blonde curly hair and looking pink and well; she had been operated on at Guy's by Blalock a week earlier. The effect was dramatic and theatrical and the applause from the audience was tumultuous. It was a Madonna-like tableau, a perfect climax to an impressive lecture on an epoch-making contribution and left nothing more to be said by the lecturer. . . . [N]o one there could possibly forget it." Despite his lecture being announced at the last minute, attendees packed and then oozed out of the museum at the College, and amplifiers were set up in adjacent corridors to accommodate the overflow. Blalock generously gave the presentation a second time an hour later for those who missed out. The Baltimore surgeon was also asked to speak


T. J. Kulik, M. Dick, *Reimagining a Child's Heart*,
https://doi.org/10.1007/978-3-031-88608-9_6

at the Royal College of Surgeons, and the same enthusiastic reception awaited him in Paris, later on the same trip.[1]

The interest in and accolades for this pioneering achievement went far beyond the largely professional audiences that jammed into lecture halls. Word of the operation spread literally faster than wildfire, even before its presentation at meetings or publication in medical journals. Patients from far and wide, some of whose operations were financed by their hometown newspapers, poured into Johns Hopkins.[2] Between 1944 and 1951, patients from 46 of the then-48 states (only Nebraska and Delaware were not represented), and 69 souls from the rest of the Western Hemisphere, Europe, and Asia made their way to Baltimore for the operation.[3]

The hype was in some ways too much, and an occasional—perhaps cynical—observer concluded that shameless self-promotion was afoot. At the American Surgical Association's 1946 meeting, the president of the organization, William Darrach, publicly criticized Blalock for the tremendous publicity that followed in the wake of his achievement. Wounded and furious, the newly super-starred surgeon threatened to quit the Association, forcing what amounted to a retraction from Darrach. Mark Ravitch, one of Blalock's many highly accomplished trainees and later his biographer, denied that Blalock deliberately sought to generate this kind of buzz,[4] but it's clear that he and Taussig had a flair for the dramatic. Before the London lecture, at a meeting of the Johns Hopkins Medical and Surgical Society, transcending the customary desiccated disquisition on technical surgical details, they arranged to have some of the "pink and newly active children (which Blalock had operated upon) walk among the audience, carrying stethoscopes for those who wanted to listen to the murmur of the artificial ductus."[5]

What did Blalock and Taussig do, and why the excitement? They identified children with certain types of cyanotic heart disease (more on cyanosis later) who would benefit from a simple surgical rearrangement of their anatomy and effected that rearrangement. Eileen Saxon, who was saddled with a malformation called tetralogy of Fallot, was their first patient. A diminutive (4 kg) and miserable 16-month-old, she had so little oxygen in her blood that her life was reduced to little more than lying in bed under an oxygen tent; Eileen lacked even the wherewithal to eat much. The "shunt" that Blalock crafted increased blood flow to her lungs, and hence the amount of oxygen in her blood. Sufficient oxygen for Eileen to finally leave the hospital and have something, at least for a time, like a normal life. This was not the first successful cardiac operation ever performed, but it was the first *transformative* cardiac intervention. The Blalock-Taussig-Thomas ("B-T-T") shunt was the primogenitor "aortopulmonary" shunt—other surgeons subsequently developed a number

[1] Ravitch (1966), Sellors (1967), Stoney (2004) and Naef (1990, p. 91).

[2] Ravitch (1966), Bahnson (1982), Thomas (1985, p. 97–101) and Stoney (2004).

[3] Taussig et al. (1971).

[4] Ravitch (1966).

[5] Ravitch (1966), Longmire (1991, pp. 110–111), Engle (1997), Stoney (2004) and Neill and Clark (1995, p. 56).

of variants—and its creation was a major landmark in the treatment of congenital heart defects. This artifact was more than innovative therapy for these disabled patients, it was the first intervention for cyanotic heart disease that actually ameliorated the primary physiological derangement—too little oxygen in the blood.

The impact of the shunt on the field was remarkable, as is partly reflected in the inventory of therapy for congenital heart disease, which showed a useful increase in treatments and efficacy over the few years bracketing the B-T-T shunt's introduction. As we have noted, a 1939 textbook by James Brown had fewer than two pages of therapy for congenital heart disease; 8 years later, Taussig's classic *Congenital Malformations of the Heart* (1947) had thirty-two. Most of Taussig's new treatments were not offspring of the shunt (for example, dicumarol and penicillin were introduced after 1939), but sixteen pages address selection of patients for surgery and management around the operation, a sure indication that the B-T-T shunt was quickly entering the standard canon of therapy. And her massively larger sections on anatomy, physiology, and diagnosis (over 500 pages, vs. 235 in Brown's smaller format) affirm that the congenital heart enterprise had impressively lunged forward, certainly due in large part to the stimulus of the new operation. The palette of effective therapy was still limited to a few washed-out colors, as Dr. Taussig unintentionally implied: "The *two most important considerations* in the care of patients with congenital malformations of the heart are: (1) to allow the individual to lead as normal a life as possible, and (2), above all, to surround him with an atmosphere of confident expectation that he will grow up and become a useful citizen."[6] But first morning light edged the horizon.

Another gauge of the B-T-T shunt's disruptive effect is the abrupt and massive increase in the number of scholarly papers on congenital heart disease published the first few years after it made the scene. After decades with academic activity in this domain ticking along at a snail's pace, the number of citations skyrocketed in the 5 years after Blalock and Taussig's seminal report. While some of this activity was likely due to the ending of WWII, the remarkable increase relative to the pre-war years suggests that the galvanizing effect of the shunt was largely responsible.

Eileen Saxon did not have a single ventricle defect, but the B-T-T shunt was swiftly pressed into service for single ventricle malformations as well, and in modified form remains in very active service today. And the fact that its creation narrative must be the most storied in all of congenital heart surgery[7] furnishes another reason to start our journey with this seminal invention.

Following the Blalock-Taussig-Thomas (B-T-T) shunt's 1945 debut, newspapers and magazines ranging from the *Dundee Courier* to the *Daily Mail* on the east side of the Atlantic, and from *The New York Times* to *Life Magazine* on the west, eagerly

[6] Taussig (1947, p. 537).

[7] The 2003 PBS documentary *Partners of the Heart,* the 2004 Emmy Award winning television film *Something the Lord Made*, contemporary newspaper reports of the operation (See *The Blue Baby Operation*, http://www.neonatology.org/pdf/bluebabyoperation.pdf), and prestigious awards given to the shunt's authors, probably qualify the B-T-T shunt as the most talked about of *all* cardiac surgical inventions, excepting the first heart transplant.

circulated the news. New therapies described in medical journals usually only slowly diffuse (if at all) into the public domain, but *The Washington Post* published a brief note on the operation[8] simultaneously with its description in the *Journal of the American Medical Association*. By 1948, *The New York Times* had published four short pieces about patients journeying to Baltimore for the shunt,[9] and the narrative eventually expanded into a lengthy spread in *The American Weekly*. More recently, many professional periodicals have recalled its history, and it figures large in several books for the lay audience.[10] HBO produced a made-for-TV movie of this tale, as did PBS[11]; only a major motion picture and a Broadway show cling to the bucket list of untapped venues.

Why *was* the B-T-T shunt the "sensation of the century," in the words of one surgical historian,[12] commanding even the attention of the general public? Designed to augment blood flow to the lung in tetralogy of Fallot (Appendix 1), the shunt increases the blood's oxygen content in people having too little. It followed in the wake of the operation which had first galvanized cardiac surgery (Chap. 4, yet easily eclipsed it in interest and acclaim. The shunt overshadowed ductal ligation (and repair of coarctation [narrowing] of the aorta, which had just preceded the shunt) partly because of its dramatic visual effect. Increasing oxygen transport rather than merely reducing the ill effects of too little supply, it was a radical departure from the best available therapy. People's color turned from mulberry to pink. More remarkably, before the operation, the patient's muscles received so little oxygen that they could only amble, breathlessly, trifling distances. The shunt mobilized people—now they could walk and play and live a life.[13] In contrast to this striking transformation, the effect of ductal ligation was usually subtle; the patient's color was unchanged, and the effect on exercise capacity was less marked. Gross's operation simply didn't have the same optical impact as the Baltimore innovation.[14]

The B-T-T shunt, for the very first time, engendered hope, hope for something like a normal life. Conventional treatments made patients more comfortable and took the edge off complications. This operation delivered something fundamentally different: *less* need to adapt and *fewer* complications. Instead of dying young—roughly half of those with unoperated tetralogy of Fallot die by 3 years of age, and only one-quarter survive to 10 years[15]—shunted patients now had a pathway to

[8] *The Washington Post*, May 17, 1945.

[9] *The New York Times*, December 4, 1945 (p. 28); November 24, 1946 (p. 50); September 14, 1947 (p. 63); December 13, 1948 (p. 25).

[10] Thomas (1985), Baldwin (1992), Murphy (2015), Morris (2017), Nuland (1989) and Weisse (1991).

[11] Dans (2004).

[12] Meade (1961, p. 361).

[13] Stoney (2004, p. 71) and McNamara (1984).

[14] Surgeon-historian William Stoney considered the B-T-T shunt, along with four subsequent developments, to be one of the five most pivotal operations in cardiac surgery; ductal ligation was not on his list (Stoney 2008, p. xiii).

[15] Bertranou et al. (1978).

adulthood.[16] This innovation transformed patient's boundaries—physical and temporal—from convergent to divergent, causing physicians and their cyanotic patients to *think differently* about the disease. It's easy to see why word of this life-altering procedure, and the expectations it aroused, shot through the community, both professional and lay. The dawn of congenital cardiology had abruptly advanced from ductal ligation's lambent pink fringe into a burning disc levitating on the horizon.

The genesis story of the B-T-T shunt has been oft told, the gist of which has been: (1) *Helen Taussig* (the pediatric cardiologist at Johns Hopkins) has an idea—invent a way to increase blood flow to the lungs, and blue patients with certain malformations will become pinker and more vigorous. (2) Rebuffed by the first surgeon she approaches with this idea, Taussig appeals to *Alfred Blalock*, the newly arrived chief of surgery at Hopkins. (3) Blalock takes Taussig up on her proposal, and sets his crack laboratory technician, *Vivien Thomas*, onto perfecting and testing a shunt. (4) Thomas, toiling many hours in the dog laboratory, sets the stage for its clinical application. (5) Blalock—assisted with advice from Thomas at his right shoulder—performs the first, drama-suffused operation on Eileen Saxon, an indigo slip of an infant. It's a success! (6) Word gets out, and the world rushes to Baltimore for this novel procedure. But this classical version of the tapestry, while mostly correct, is bleached out and missing strands. This narrative is actually more nuanced, complex, and richer.

This chapter is partly about *collaboration*. So too was *Collector of Hearts*, but in a different way. Whereas Maude Abbott's collaborations straddled decades and helped levitate an entire discipline, the B-T-T shunt is a discrete invention, created over a few years. We steal an intimate view of three people cooperating—and colliding—as they create their revolutionary new therapy; teamwork, and team friction, are more clearly limned here than in *Collector*. So is *imagination*, more powerful than calculation but less reliable. It opened the door for the shunt, but failed Taussig and Blalock when the time came to advance to the next level of congenital cardiology—open heart surgery (Chap. 7).

The medical innovator's bane—the paucity of models for testing new therapies—surfaces again; but we also see how the body provides needed assistance in creating new treatments. And I put in a plug for the nameless people who make projects—great and small—actually happen, while people at the top of the chain consume all of the credit.

[16] Of the 779 patients who had B-T-T shunts between 1944 and 1951, 12% died within 2 months; 82% of the survivors had a good or excellent result. Of those surviving more than 2 months, 64% were alive after 15 years (although nearly a third needed additional cardiac operation[s]). 342 patients were alive an average of 24 years after initial surgery (a survival rate of ~44%). (227 of these patients had had a corrective operation after their shunt, so their survival was not entirely due to their initial shunt.) Of patients surviving at least 15 years, ~250 had married, and 161 had children. Of the ~46% of those responding to Taussig's inquiry, 36% were college graduates, nearly half with postgraduate training. The vast majority were gainfully employed (with 16% as a "major executive or professional" or salaried professional or "large concern manager"). Taussig pointed with pride to a patient appointed a professor of law at the University of Kansas before his 30th birthday (Taussig 1971; Taussig et al. 1975; White et al. 1956).

We start with the early histories of the dramatis personae. Alfred Blalock—a gracious son of the South—and Helen Taussig—a tough-minded New Englander—were upper middle-class kids, born only a year apart. Long before their famous collaboration, their lives ran on curiously parallel tracks: Johns Hopkins trained them; their early professional development lagged their most brilliant peers; serious health problems threatened to derail them both; their careers were influenced, albeit in distinct ways, by the same Harvard physiologist. Vivien Thomas, on the other hand, was a black man of working-class stock. Blessed with technical surgical gifts exceeding Blalock's and managerial skills Taussig lacked, he was the project's invaluable foreman. Invisible for too long, Thomas eventually emerged to highlight the critical role of human infrastructure in transforming ethereal ideas into tangible reality.

## Helen Taussig

### *No Diagnosis, No Operation*

Helen Taussig was born in 1898 in Cambridge, Massachusetts of academic gentry[17] Fig. 6.2). Her father Frank was an economist and Harvard professor, an advisor to Woodrow Wilson, and onetime chairman of the U.S. Tariff Commission. Edith, Helen's mother, lacked Frank's prominence, but was hardly unwashed; she had attended Radcliffe and cultivated an interest in education and science. The Taussig home was warm and supportive,[18] but Edith died of tuberculosis when Helen was eleven, leaving her father with the challenge of nurturing Helen and her three siblings. Helen had dyslexia, which had left Frank wondering if she would make it through even grammar school. She later recalled how "extraordinarily patient" her father had been helping her with her studies: "[H]e never *once* complained to me, he never *once* chided me, he never *once* said 'Helen, can't you do better?' or 'What is the matter'?"[19] Afflicted with a mild case of mediastinal tuberculosis as a child, Taussig was frail and attended school only half days for 2 or 3 years.

Despite her reading travails, Taussig made it to and passed her first two college years at Radcliffe. She was an excellent tennis player (once winning the Radcliffe championship), competed in varsity basketball, and participated in student theatrical productions. Finding Radcliffe "a bit" disappointing,[20] Taussig was instantly taken by the University of California at Berkeley when she visited the summer after freshman year. The departure of her father and friends from Cambridge provided

[17] Helen Taussig lacks a comprehensive biography. Joyce Baldwin's slender volume (1992) and an MD thesis (Goodman 1983) come the closest. Taussig's recollections are available: Harvey (1978), Taussig (1965, 1979, 1981, and several others). Former associates also supply insights: Trimble (1953), Engle (1977), McNamara et al. (1987), Neill (1987, 1994) and Bing (1999, pp. 95–99).

[18] Goodman (1983).

[19] Harvey (1978).

[20] Harvey (1978).

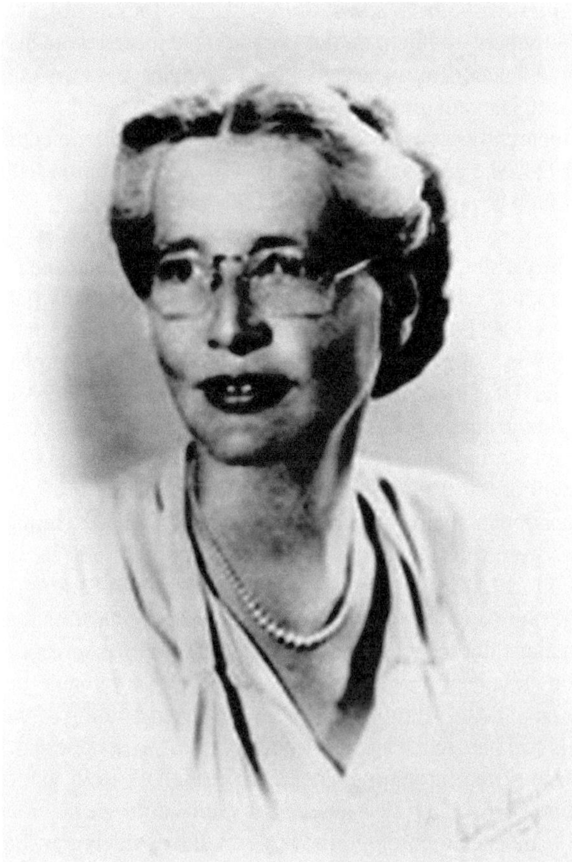

**Fig. 6.1** Helen B. Taussig. MD. (With permission from the Chesney Archives of Johns Hopkins Medicine, Nursing and Public Health)

further motivation to leave home, and she transferred to Berkeley for her last 2 years of college. Still enjoying tennis and theater, Taussig was a heroic walker and hiker, trekking all day outside of San Francisco and even hazarding a winter expedition into Yosemite. Graduating in 1921 with an A.B. degree, she returned to Cambridge to ponder her next move.

Though inclining toward medicine, her future was as yet unmapped as she arrived home. Frank suggested Harvard's new School of Public Health, but when Helen discussed her prospects with its dean, she was unapologetically informed that women were not accepted as degree candidates. On the knife edge between public health and medicine, she swerved toward the latter. A histology course at Harvard in the fall of 1921 marked the beginning of her medical career, followed by anatomy at Boston University's School of Medicine. Alexander Begg, a professor and dean of the school, possibly sensing that Taussig was good for more than the standard curriculum, handed her a beef heart, challenging her to trace the paths of its dimly appreciable bands of muscle fibers. She succeeded only in mutilating the organ. A second project, studying strips of live cardiac muscle *in vitro*, was more gratifying, garnering her a paper in the

*American Journal of Physiology* (1925). Taussig hoped to go to Johns Hopkins' medical school—which, unlike Harvard's, admitted women—and, having heard that "one good" letter from Harvard would secure acceptance, enlisted her father's friend, eminent Harvard physiologist Walter Cannon, to draft a recommendation. The letter apparently proved persuasive, and Hopkins welcomed her as a second-year student in 1924. She invested her free time in the heart station with cardiologist Edward Carter, which began her career in pediatric cardiology.[21]

Graduating in 1927, Taussig was bent on an Osler Medical Internship at Hopkins. Only a single slot was allocated for a woman, and she narrowly lost out to one Vivian Tappan, whose grade point average—which still galled Taussig decades later—exceeded hers by only two-tenths of a point.[22] She completed instead a year's fellowship in Carter's clinic, followed by a pediatric internship lasting a little over a year. The fall of 1930 found Taussig an assistant in the Department of Pediatrics at Hopkins and the director of its cardiac clinic. The clinic was preoccupied with rheumatic heart disease, but Taussig's boss, the legendary Edwards Park, suggested that she expand her portfolio: "'Now, doctor (Park directed, as Taussig recalled), you have got to learn congenital malformations of the heart.' I replied to him in some rather uncomplimentary terms to the effect of 'Dammed, if I will.' He said to me, 'It doesn't matter how you feel, it's going to be forced upon you.'"[23] Park not only insisted that Taussig see all the patients with a congenital cardiac malformation, but that she examine them using a fluoroscope.[24] Intrigued by May Wilson's work at Cornell, Park predicted that this relatively new technology would prove valuable in assessing cardiac malformations. It did. Although the X-rays revealed nothing of the heart's interior, by outlining its contours in a way that a standard chest X-ray does not, Taussig could often infer the type of malformation.[25] It was in the fall of 1935 that that she had this epiphany: "I fluoroscoped a little cyanotic baby and could see no enlargement of the right ventricle . . . the electrocardiogram showed left axis deviation! I made the clinical diagnosis of an absent right ventricle." A month later, another cyanotic baby had an identical malformation and a similar chest X-ray, and "Then and there I realized that malformations of the heart repeated themselves and that similar malformations caused similar changes in the size and shape of the heart. *The key to clinical diagnosis of malformations of the heart had been turned*" (emphasis mine).[26]

---

[21] Taussig (1979).

[22] Goodman (1983, p. 8).

[23] Trimble (1953).

[24] Fluoroscopy is a continuous X-ray image is shown on a monitor; using this modality, Taussig was thus able to get a better three-dimensional picture of the heart than using a plain X-ray.

[25] Taussig (1965, p. 31).

[26] Diagnostic acumen in the mid-1940s was far from perfect. Blalock (1946a) describes a patient dying after a shunt discovered to have a single ventricle, without pulmonary stenosis. In another patient, Blalock could not locate the right pulmonary at operation for shunting; autopsy revealed it was small and abnormally located. Eight of the first 110 patients operated upon had an incorrect diagnosis, not counting those not selected for surgery who could have been (Blalock 1946b). More reliable and granular diagnosis awaited cardiac catheterization, angiography, and echocardiography.

By dint of hard work and penetrating observation (including, all too often, "following the child to autopsy" to confirm or deny a diagnosis), Taussig learned to divine the architecture of what was beating in her young charges' chests. She also acquired a reasonable understanding of the physiology of congenital malformations. Her diagnoses were sometimes incorrect, even fatally so, but were accurate enough, often enough, that she and her surgeon could justify a perilous operation. Since the most effective surgical procedure to spring from the hand of man is worthless if you don't know when to apply it, accurate diagnoses were mandatory for developing the B-T-T shunt. Taussig's diagnostic skill was as important to this invention as the suture fixing the tissues together—no diagnosis, no operation. As near as I can tell, she was the only pediatric cardiologist in the world who had developed this set of tools.

Taussig's maturation into a formidable diagnostician took place despite what could have been a fatal blow delivered to her nascent career. She was going deaf. Certainly, by the time of her faculty appointment and possibly sooner, Taussig started losing her hearing. A clunky hearing aid, slung around her neck, helped. An amplifying stethoscope was pressed into service. She learned to lip-read. But these workarounds being barely satisfactory, Taussig sometimes had to resort to asking people to communicate in writing. Her deafness had set in early in her career, allowing her ample time to pursue a specialty less demanding of one's ears. She chose instead to adapt to her disability, deftly using all available clues to diagnose and monitor the condition of her patients. Silly stuff has been written about Taussig (implausibly) feeling heart murmurs (sounds made by the heart) too faint for others to hear with a stethoscope,[27] but she may well have amplified her sense of touch to derive more information from palpation than most of us. More importantly, she could synthesize multiple types of information into a diagnosis (symptoms, the physical exam, X-ray studies and electrocardiograms), taking into account prior probability (some defects being much more common than others). In any case, this determined and resilient lady turned what could have been, for a mid-twentieth century cardiologist, a washed-out road into a speed bump. If Taussig wasn't the first doctor in her field, she was surely the first *complete* pediatric cardiologist: She could cobble an accurate diagnosis—at least most of the time—and marry it up with the therapeutic power of the cardiac surgeon, thus forming the modern congenital cardiac therapeutic unit.

Taussig did more than deduce the structures of her patient's hearts. Observing children who died when their ductus spontaneously closed at weeks or months of age, she inferred that ductus-supplied pulmonary blood flow could keep a patient with obstruction of flow from the heart to the lungs alive.[28] Why not create an artificial ductus to do the same? Taussig was not the first to figure that a patent ductus can

---

[27] Baldwin (1992, p. 40).

[28] Blalock and Taussig (1945) and Taussig (1965). Richard Van Praagh, however, believes that Taussig was incorrect: It wasn't a patent ductus that kept some of her tetralogy patients pink, but rather a different sort of connection from the aorta to the lungs, aortopulmonary collateral vessels (Van Praagh 2012).

compensate for other defects. In 1777, Sandifort speculated that a patent ductus might prevent cyanosis in tetralogy of Fallot. In the mid-nineteenth century, Thomas Peacock observed the same, as did Maude Abbott at the turn of the twentieth century, and James Brown in his 1939 textbook.[29] No one seems to have tumbled to the idea of *creating* such a communication, which is hardly surprising, given thoracic surgery's primitive status at the time. But in 1940 or 1941, radiologist Paul Swenson suggested to George Humphreys, the chairman of surgery at Columbia-Presbyterian, that an artificial ductus would be helpful in tetralogy of Fallot. Humphreys demurred, fearing *too much* pulmonary blood flow with a surgically created connection. Robert Gross in Boston had created, in dogs, the same connection subsequently used by Blalock and found that the increased pulmonary flow greatly augmented the volume pumped by the left ventricle while reducing flow to the body, a potentially disastrous clinical result. But narrowing the connection would reduce the pulmonary flow to a tolerable amount, which apparently had not occurred to Humphreys.[30]

Both Swenson and Taussig had the same big idea, and both were stuck; her appeal to the preeminent heart surgeon of the day, Robert Gross, had failed to convince him to apply the shunt that he had perfected in the laboratory to a cyanotic human (Chap. 4).[31] Lacking a surgeon of sufficient imagination to turn her conception into a creation, Taussig bided her time.

## Vivien Thomas

### *No Infrastructure, No Operation*

Taussig and Blalock were just edging out of childhood in 1910 when Thomas was born in Lake Providence, Louisiana.[32] Weary of fighting the Mississippi River spring floods, his family relocated to Nashville, Tennessee 2 years later, a move which ultimately proved pivotal for Thomas. His father William was a hardworking master carpenter and contractor, and his mother Mary a seamstress. Thomas shares little of his family life in his autobiography, but implies that his parents were supportive, with high expectations for their children. Vivien apprenticed with his father at age 13, staying in school while learning the craft of carpentry on Saturdays and after school. Summer vacations were no vacation for Thomas; he swung a hammer

[29] Peacock (1858, pp. 110–111), Abbott (1908, p. 379) and Brown (1939, p. 2).

[30] Eppinger et al. (1941) and Shumacker (1982).

[31] In an interview with Vincent Gott (1977) Taussig said that she had asked Gross to build her a ductus in 1939, but in a February 1968 lecture, she recollected that it was the spring of 1940 (Taussig 1968).

[32] Thomas (1985). For biographical details, see also McCabe (1989), Ravitch (1966), Longmire (1991), and Olch (1967). Thomas disagreed with some material in Ravitch's Blalock biography, saying that "I told [Ravitch] that he did not have enough consultation of some of the stuff that he had written" (Olch 1967, pp. 25–26). Thomas did not elaborate on disagreement with Ravitch in that interview, although in his autobiography he writes that Ravitch had wrongly attributed a procedure invented by Thomas to C.R. Hanlon (Thomas 1985, p. 117).

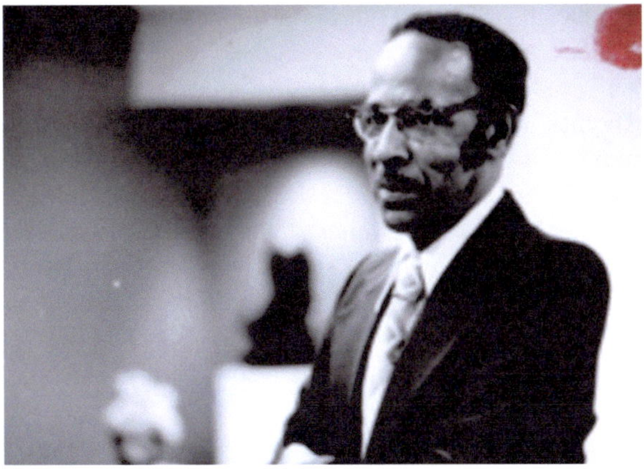

**Fig. 6.2** Vivien Thomas circa 1975. (With permission from the Chesney Archives of Johns Hospital Medicine, Nursing and Public Health)

and ripped pine from seven in the morning until five-thirty at night in the Nashville swelter. His sights were set on Tennessee State College and ultimately medical school. Losing his carpentry job and life's savings when The People's Bank closed its doors in the wake of the 1929 crash, by February 1930 Thomas was scrambling for work instead. A close friend had suggested Alfred Blalock's laboratory at Vanderbilt but warned him that the surgeon was "hell" to work with. Desperate for a wage, Thomas decided to take a chance.

Arriving at the lab at eleven o'clock in the morning on February 10, Thomas found Blalock heading for the operating room, and their interview was delayed for an hour. Later, he found Blalock to be young-appearing and looking for a director of a surgical laboratory. Puffing a cigarette and sipping a Coke, Blalock's greeting was cordial and his manner informal.[33] Thomas shared his background and circumstances, and Blalock described the lab's projects and the job requirements. After touring the facility and quizzing the staff, Thomas found the work sufficiently interesting, and Blalock apparently decent enough, to sign up. The pay was poor ($12 a week against the $20 he had been making as a carpenter), but Thomas saw the job as temporary, something to tide him through the cold winter months until outdoor worked picked up again.[34] As it turned out, Thomas was Blalock's only major domo in his Vanderbilt and Hopkins labs (where the pair moved in 1941). Finding an assistant of Thomas's unusual talents and retaining him for one's professional lifetime is a rare gift, and for Blalock a godsend. Thomas's association with Blalock was surely the single most important factor (outside of Blalock's personal qualities) which made the surgeon's career.

Thomas *was* talented. Those best positioned to evaluate his surgical skills were Blalock's surgical residents who had worked with Thomas in the lab, and they were invariably impressed. William Longmire found Thomas a man of "intellectual resourcefulness and great technical ability".[35] C. Rollins Hanlon's take: a "superb"

[33] Olch (1967).

[34] Thomas (1985), McCabe (1989), Ravitch (1966), Longmire (1991) and Olch (1967).

[35] Longmire (1991, p. 64).

technician, who could develop the details of a procedure only conceptualized by Blalock.[36] Denton Cooley—another resident, with a formidable pair of hands himself—judged Thomas to be a "great" technician.[37] Mark Ravitch proclaimed Thomas' manual skill "legendary."[38] In contrast, consensus has it that Blalock was more of a dogged than brilliant technician.[39] And, as Longmire implied, Thomas brought more than manual dexterity to the operating table. Using "traction" and "anchor" sutures and other strategies to assist himself while operating, he often eliminated the need for a second pair of hands. Finding available surgical clamps unsuitable for the novel procedures he and Blalock were developing, Thomas invented two new types of clamps (one was developed along with Longmire). Working with a machinist, he also built a positive pressure ventilator, capable of providing ether anesthesia.[40]

It is often unappreciated that Thomas's expertise extended well beyond operations and experiments, exceeding the scope ordinarily required of a laboratory technician. Managing the Blalock lab was its own major project: procuring supplies, looking after the welfare of the animals, arranging upkeep of the space and equipment, and supervising other lab personnel were wedged in between long hours of experiments. Thomas trained laboratory technicians, taught medical students and physician's assistants, and helped hone the technical and research skills of surgical residents. In 1950, Hopkins commenced planning a new facility to replace the old Hunterian lab; Thomas was one of only three people dispatched to the Mayo Clinic to study their model research facilities. He also was deeply involved, as we will see, in supporting the clinical enterprise, especially after the B-T-T shunt attracted hundreds of patients to Hopkins. Solving innumerable problems, coping with challenging personalities (surgeons' egos being surgeons' egos), and even drawing blood

[36] Stoney (2008, p. 166).

[37] Stoney (2008, pp. 245, 247).

[38] Ravitch (1966, p. 12).

[39] Longmire (1991, p. 199). Others spoke similarly of Blalock: "not a good technician" (Sanford Leeds; Olch 1973); "insecure as a technical surgeon" "Dr. Blalock realized and acknowledged the fact that technically he was not the greatest surgeon in the world. …he told me that some of the resident staff 'could operate circles' around him" (Thomas 1985, p. 107). Thomas not only observed Blalock's technique, but likely had heard critiques of his boss from surgical residents. William Longmire (a Blalock resident and good friend) confirmed the general impression of Blalock's technical skills by way of only weakly rebutting Blalock's critics: "Dr. Blalock's surgical skill has been questioned but if you could have seen him complete one of these difficult operations you would recognize that the skill was there" (Stoney 2004). Mark Ravitch, another Blalock resident, implies that Blalock was not an outstanding technician, describing him as a "bold, no-nonsense operator, somewhat impatient at times, a little rough…he got into trouble somewhat more often because of his impatience, but then was masterful, and endlessly careful in extricating himself" (Ravitch 1966). Other Blalock trainees have weighed in: "competent, aggressive" (Frank Spencer); "clinical surgeon, and he wasn't really adept and sure of himself all of the time" (Denton Cooley; Stoney 2008, p. 245); "not a brilliant surgical technician, but he was good" (Henry Bahnson; Stoney 2008, p. 187); "a good technician, but not a brilliant technician" (J. Alex Haller; Stoney 2008, p. 260).

[40] Stoney (2008, p. 166) and Thomas (1985, pp. 34, 73–74, 83–84, 97).

from howling kids, Thomas kept a blur of balls in the air for nearly five decades. He was the infrastructure—human infrastructure—upon which Blalock's edifice was planted.[41]

***

## Alfred Blalock

### *No Imagination, No Operation*

Born in 1899 in Culloden, a one-horse Georgia town, Blalock was of a rather different sort of gentry than Taussig.[42] His father George owned and operated a general store, headed a small bank, and owned a large tract of cotton-bearing land with

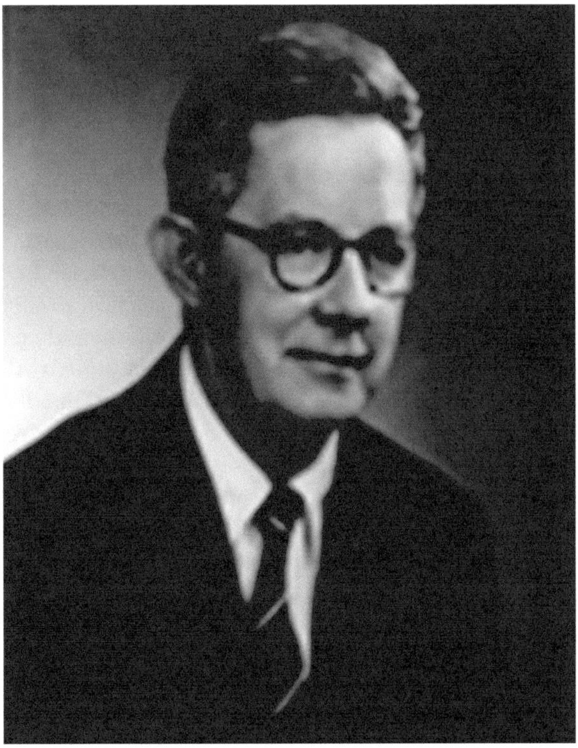

**Fig. 6.3** Alfred Blalock MD. (With permission from the Chesney Archives of Johns Hopkins Medicine, Nursing and Public Health)

[41] Timmerman (2003).

[42] Longmire (1991), Ravitch (1966), Wangensteen (1968), Thomas (1985), Bing (1988), Olch (1967) and Sabiston (1978).

tenant farmers. His mother Martha, at least by one account, was a remote cousin of Jefferson Davis. George was well read but an autocratic and demanding disciplinarian; softer and sweeter, Martha formed something of a buffer between father and children. Despite what sounds like an uncomfortable atmosphere at home—at least one of the children said that the marriage was unhappy—for Blalock, "the environment, in general, was a pleasant one."[43] Moving with his family to Jonesboro, Georgia when he was eleven, Blalock grew up busy and hard-working—cutting grass, running a paper route, milking cows, playing tennis and basketball. Unlike Taussig as a child, he was healthy, though that would change only too soon.

Having taken advanced classes at the Georgia Military college for a year, Blalock entered the University of Georgia at age sixteen as a sophomore. Like Taussig, he played basketball and was an excellent tennis player, winning a letter in the sport. He enjoyed many other extracurricular activities, and was elected to the prestigious Gridiron Club which, despite its name, acknowledged overall excellence. Blalock was "well-rounded" rather than academically precocious. A hardly fulsome letter of recommendation from one of his professors—"I have no hesitation in saying that he is mature enough and his habits of study are sufficiently well formed to be admitted. I hope you will take him."—certainly implies as much.[44] It also mentions that Blalock took up medicine his senior year in college, but a letter from him (1944) suggests longer roots: "My interest in medicine arose at such a young age that I cannot trace its development."[45] Graduating in the spring of 1918, Blalock entered Johns Hopkins medical school in the fall.

Blalock's first year at Hopkins was a "difficult one,"[46] presumably due at least in part to his sheaf of extracurricular interests: tennis and golf, running the school bookstore, and an active social life. (His good friend and onetime roommate, Tinsley Harrison, later a distinguished academic physician in his own right, described him as a "Casanova . . . a Don Juan. Really a ladies' man."[47] The effect of these distractions on his grades soon proved to be a problem. He graduated in 1922.

Like Taussig, Blalock was disappointed in his post-doctoral training prospects. His class standing precluded a general surgery internship, leaving him with a one-year position as a house officer in urology (actually, rotating between urology, surgery, and gynecology). Blalock secured a position as a general surgery resident for the following year, but lost it at year's end, publicly ascribing this to the "too keen" competition on the service.[48] His former trainee and close friend and biographer William Longmire, Jr. tells a sorrier tale. The man slated to become the next year's chief resident was reputed to be aggressive and abusive and was detested by the junior trainees. Joining in a pact, the residents vowed to each other to threaten to

[43] Longmire (1991, p. 29).

[44] Ravitch (1966, p. 638).

[45] Longmire (1991, p. 34).

[46] Longmire (1991, p. 30).

[47] Longmire (1991, pp. 33, 242).

[48] Sabiston (1978).

quit unless a different chief was selected. True to his word, when Blalock met with the acting chief of surgery (J.M.T. Finney) and finding the chief resident assignment unchanged, he declined to sign up for another year and left his office out of a job. Unbeknownst to Blalock, the cabal had collapsed, and his fellow residents had stayed on despite the new chief resident. The Georgian was left hanging. (Ironically, Blalock and the chief resident eventually became close personal friends, perhaps accounting for Blalock's not widely circulating this story.)[49]

Blalock was offered a last-minute externship in otolaryngology by his friend Samuel Crowe, and by virtue of this makeshift arrangement stayed at Hopkins another year. What he really wanted, though, was general surgical training, and when Blalock could not recoup this position the following year, he looked elsewhere. Responding to the entreaties of Tinsley Harrison—then chief resident in medicine at Vanderbilt—he moved to Nashville as chief resident (and instructor) in surgery in July of 1925. Harrison had introduced Blalock to laboratory research during his general surgery training at Hopkins (1924),[50] which proved a seminal turning point for Blalock. Previously having little interest in basic research, the lab occupied much of Blalock's time despite Vanderbilt being primarily a clinical training program. Running experiments until midnight, he finished the day "carousing and raising hell until three or four AM."[51] The intensity and efficiency of his effort paid off: Over a 2 year span, he was an author on nine papers. But his many hours of clinical training, laboratory work, and late-night carousing debilitated Blalock, and soon exacted a shocking toll.

If Taussig's maiden foray into faculty life was unsettled, Blalock's was parlous. In about April of 1927, he was diagnosed with pulmonary tuberculosis. Now a serious but treatable condition, at the time it was often fatal. Lacking effective antibiotics for the causative bug, *mycobacterium tuberculosis*, rest was the primary therapy, and the Trudeau Sanitarium at Saranac Lake, New York was a frequent refuge for east coasters. Blalock checked into Trudeau frightened, yet surely chafing at his enforced absence from his career.[52] He was also disappointed that the staff at Trudeau refused to apply the latest therapy for the disease, intentional pneumothorax,[53] and a year later escaped for a few months in Europe. Blalock mostly visited research laboratories, including the Department of Physiology in Cambridge. He worked

[49] Longmire (1991, pp. 37–38).

[50] Ravitch (1966, p. xxii).

[51] Longmire (1991, p. 45).

[52] At Trudeau, Blalock shared Lea cottage with Canadian surgeon Norman Bethune. Something of an artist, Bethune painted murals in the Lea as he struggled with the psychology of their often lethal disease. Bethune's mural included crude headstones predicting the year of death of his roommates; Blalock's was inscribed 1929, Bethune's, 1932. Bethune survived his TB to have a fascinating career as surgeon and social activist (Nadeau 1940; Zuidema and Sloan 2001; Deslauriers and Goulet 2015).

[53] Pneumothorax therapy involves intentionally introducing a measured amount of air into the side of the chest affected by tuberculosis. The lung on that side collapses, aiding in resolution of the disease.

there under the physiologists' physiologists G.V. Anrep and Joseph Barcroft, co-authoring a paper with the latter.[54] After a bout of pulmonary hemorrhage in Germany, Blalock returned to Trudeau, where pneumothorax therapy was finally performed. Whether because of this treatment, which was repeated at intervals over 30 months, or other factors, Blalock was finally rid of his disease.

Poised on the threshold of a career demanding exceptional physical and emotional reserves, TB was the last thing that this ambitious young surgeon needed. But Blalock's sickness may have been the tinder that lit a fire in his belly, a drive to make important discoveries and make them fast. Colleagues observed that this illness, and the risk of early death implied, impelled Blalock to—as Robert Skidelsky wrote of John Maynard Keynes—"rush through life with a clock ticking in his ear,"[55] anxious that his candle would burn to the butt before he had left any legacy.[56]

Blalock put in hundred-hour weeks at Vanderbilt after returning from New York,[57] acquiring the reputation of an unfailingly considerate and polite slave driver. Vivien Thomas later recalled that "it wasn't anything to work a 16 hour day" if the experiment demanded it.[58] One crude index of Blalock's productivity resides in his curriculum vitae: 228 publications, roughly half of which are reports of laboratory investigations.[59] Blalock pursued a variety of problems at Vandy, but his study of *shock* was, by his own lights, his most important work[60] and presumably what underlay his hope of winning a Nobel Prize.[61] Shock, boiled down, is a state of inadequate oxygen delivery to the body's tissues. Its pathophysiology varies with its cause, of which there are several (for example, trauma, sepsis, heart dysfunction). In Blalock's time, this often-mortal condition was little understood. The traumatic variety—which kills those injured in accidents and on the battlefield—was a cipher, and alternative theories were vehemently debated. Walter Cannon, the author of Taussig's medical school letter (see above), was a proponent of the notion that toxic substances, or deranged neural activity, were pathologic agents in the genesis of traumatic shock. His theory derived from a model which underestimated the fluid loss from the circulation in dogs subject to crush injury. Blalock, using a better-designed and meticulously executed preparation, showed that loss of fluid alone accounts for the primary pathophysiology—there was no need to invoke toxic substances or the nervous system. Blalock's challenge to Cannon initially provoked sharp discussions between the two, but their relationship eventually softened into one of warm regard and mutual respect.[62] Blalock's insight was profound: Fluid replacement—even on the battlefield—is easily done, *if only one knows to do it*. The

[54] Ravitch (1966, p. 16) and Harvey (1982).

[55] Skidelsky (2003, p. 53).

[56] Longmire (1991, pp. 10, 46–47, 175, 188).

[57] Thomas (1985, p. 29).

[58] Ravitch (1966, p. xv), Olch (1967, p. 5).

[59] Ravitch (1966).

[60] Longmire (1991, p. 52), Ravitch (1977a) and Harvey (1982).

[61] Olch (1973), p. 12.

[62] Chambers and Buchman (2000).

number of lives saved owing to the contributions of Blalock (and others, especially surgeon Dallas Phemister) well exceeds the number of people born with cyanotic heart defects, easily making this Blalock's (and Thomas's) most impactful work.[63]

As the volume and quality of his publications swelled, especially those regarding shock, so did his national reputation. Blalock clinched a full professorship by 1938. While his drive and methodical approach were exceptional, they alone cannot explain his rapid success. Consumed by the laboratory during his training and early faculty years, Blalock personally did much of his experimental work. But as his reputation grew, so did his teaching, administrative, clinical, and other professional activities. By mid-1939, Blalock had precious little time for the laboratory.[64] While this progression is typical for successful researchers—such success is often taken to imply managerial expertise, with invitations to move up the food chain—this shift in effort often slashes research productivity. Translating Blalock's investigative creativity into new knowledge ultimately turned on Vivien Thomas' skill and dedication. Thomas (and assistants) performed virtually all of the technical work, and his problem-solving skills meant that little supervision was required. His boss got to live two lives—research, and all the rest—thanks to Thomas: While Blalock was in Washington, DC dispensing expert advice, Thomas's hands were moving inside a dog's chest; as his boss endured endless committee meetings, Thomas was inventing better equipment. Blalock sweated for hours in the operating theater while, simultaneously, critical experiments were completed by Thomas. Without Thomas' intelligence, technical expertise, and resourcefulness, Blalock could never have expanded his oeuvre to more than a fraction of what he ultimately achieved. Thomas didn't merely help Blalock invent the B-T-T shunt, he helped Blalock invent Blalock.

Although his research had secured his fame, Blalock had also established himself as a thoracic surgeon, performing thymectomies, ligating ducti arteriosi, and stripping away constricting pericardium. His métier was not confined to the laboratory; he was a "treating doc" too, displaying all the qualities required for a leader in his field. In 1937, the Henry Ford Hospital in Detroit tried unsuccessfully to attract Blalock as its Surgeon in Chief. A year later, Dean DeWitt Lewis, Chairman of the Department of Surgery at Johns Hopkins, retired, triggering what became a drawn-out search for his successor. A number of prominent surgeons turned the job down, but Blalock leaped at the opportunity when it was finally offered.[65] He moved to Baltimore in 1941 as Professor of Surgery and Director of the Department of Surgery. Vivien Thomas was part of the package, though it's a fair assumption that the recruitment committee hardly knew or cared that he existed.

> The design is mine. The daring, yours.
> –Virgil, the *Aeneid*[66]

---

[63] In 2018, over 60,000 *deaths* due to hemorrhagic shock occurred in the US (Cannon 2018), while only roughly 1100 liveborn infants had tetralogy of Fallot (Apitz et al. 2009).

[64] Thomas (1985, p. 39).

[65] Harvey (1982).

[66] Virgil. *The Aeneid*, Robert Fagles (trans). Book 12, ln. 188, p. 360. New York, NY: Viking Penguin.

Late one morning in 1943, Helen Taussig, armed with 10 years of lessons learned and unflagging determination to rescue her cyanotic patients, trooped to the "doghouse" (the Hunterian surgical research laboratory) to meet with Alfred Blalock and Vivien Thomas. For Taussig, Blalock's arrival at Johns Hopkins was like overdue rain on parched earth. Blalock was young and driven, and having ligated three ducti in Nashville was about as much a cardiac surgeon as anybody. But was he game to dare something new? Deeply concerned about the plight of her azure patients, what Taussig had in mind was a potentially life-changing innovation. In the Hunterian, she laid out, in great detail, the case that surgically augmenting pulmonary blood flow in tetralogy of Fallot would usefully increase arterial oxygen content. She appealed to Blalock to invent an artificial ductus, but as to *how* this might be done, she hadn't a clue. At least that was Thomas' take on the first glimmerings of the B-T-T shunt,[67] even if not Taussig's. She later recalled sketching a blueprint for the surgeon: Park and Blalock had conceived of an operation to treat aortic coarctation by connecting the end of the left subclavian artery to the side of the descending aorta.[68] Taussig—so she said—suggested to Blalock that if that were possible, so too would be a connection between the subclavian and the pulmonary arteries; she also claimed partial credit for the experimental model of cyanosis used as proof of concept for the shunt.[69] But other observers resonated with Thomas. Blalock trainee and biographer Mark Ravitch quotes Park as saying that Taussig had no suggestions as how to increase pulmonary flow.[70] But Ravitch would have had at best second-hand information, and in 1977 he mistakenly stated that the shunt created in Blalock's Vanderbilt lab by Sanford Leeds was an end-to-side connection (it was end-to-end), suggesting his understanding of this topic may have been tenuous.[71] And William Longmire wrote that Blalock remembered that it was Park—thinking of the subclavian-to-aorta operation—who suggested using the subclavian artery for an artificial ductus.[72]

We know that while in Nashville, Blalock, Sanford Levy (who later changed his name to Leeds and moved on to the University of California, San Francisco), and Thomas, using techniques developed by Carrel and Guthrie (Chap. 4, perfected anastomosing the end of the left subclavian artery to the (proximal) end of the left pulmonary artery, hoping to study high pulmonary arterial pressure.[73] While this arrangement *could* be used to increase pulmonary blood flow in tetralogy, an end-of-subclavian to *side* of pulmonary artery connection would be far better. Blalock and Thomas had developed the subclavian-to-*side of aorta* connection noted above in 1942–1943, and it would have been natural for Blalock to use this end-to-side

---

[67] Thomas (1985, p. 80–82) and Olch (1967, pp. 26–28).

[68] Blalock and Park (1944).

[69] Taussig (1965, 1976) and Snellen et al. (1981, p. 162).

[70] Ravitch (1966, vol. I, p. xiv).

[71] Ravitch (1977b).

[72] Longmire (1991, p. 113).

[73] Levy and Blalock (1939) and Thomas (1985, p. 34).

anastomosis (but to the pulmonary artery) to reify Taussig's idea.[74] We do not know, and likely never will, whether Taussig, Blalock, or Park (Thomas made no such claims) first made this modest conceptual leap. But we don't care. What matters is that Taussig conceived a way to reduce cyanosis and sold her idea to a surgeon with enough imagination and confidence to take this idea into the operating room. And, besides, the shunt was neither new when Taussig breeched the doghouse, nor first crafted there (or at Vanderbilt). As we've seen, Robert Gross had previously created exactly the same, using dogs, for long term physiological studies, as had Sanford Leeds in San Francisco in 1943.[75] Indeed, unlike Blalock, who exquisitely detailed how the shunt was constructed,[76] Gross didn't even bother including its technical details in his paper. Blalock and Taussig's seminal advance flowed from the imagination to conceive that *a shunt could be therapy*; their breakthrough was more conceptual than technical.

There is also disagreement regarding who did exactly what in the Blalock lab. Thomas' autobiography implies that he solved many technical problems pretty much on his own, or with trainee surgeons, and his technical virtuosity makes this easily plausible. Sanford Levy stated that the subclavian-to-pulmonary artery end-to-end connections at Vanderbilt was Blalock's idea but were always executed by Thomas and Levy.[77] The technique of subclavian to aorta end-to-side anastomosis was developed, according to Thomas, "completely on my own."[78] And Thomas wrote that he had performed many such shunts in dogs before Blalock first assisted him with the procedure.[79] Longmire's slant was different. "Blalock's custom in his experimental work was to start with an idea or thesis and plan experiments to test it. If the experiment involved an operation, he himself would perform the original procedure with Vivien Thomas's assistance. *After a procedure was established*, Thomas would then carry out as many operations or procedures as were needed to complete the original plan."[80] (Thomas's statement that "I would assist [Blalock] in a particular procedure the first time"[81] is consistent with this, although whether it applies to all new procedures is unclear.) Longmire implies that the technical authorship of the procedures developed in the Blalock lab was Blalock's, although whether this was true for the B-T-T shunt is unstated. But trying to parse credit for the creation of the B-T-T shunt amongst Blalock and Thomas seems to me a fool's errand. They worked together so closely, with so many points of intersection, that the origin of ideas and solutions to technical problems must have sometimes been ambiguous to the principals involved (and even more so to outsiders looking in).

---

[74] Blalock (1946a, p. 66).

[75] Eppinger et al. (1941) and Leeds (1943).

[76] Blalock and Taussig (1945).

[77] Olch (1973).

[78] Thomas (1985, p. 73).

[79] Thomas (1985, pp. 73, 80–104).

[80] Longmire (1991, p. 95), emphasis mine and Ravitch (1966, p. xxiii).

[81] Thomas (1985, p. 34).

Blalock and Thomas had developed a technical solution for increasing pulmonary blood flow roughly 2 years before installing it in an unsealed human chest.[82] A tremendous volume of experimental work, taking over a year, was performed before venturing the first clinical shunt.[83] Why did they sink so many resources into these experiments and delay introducing this life-altering therapy? Blalock felt that he needed *proof of concept* before hazarding this procedure in a child. Today, adding a shunt when pulmonary flow is wanting is like twisting a faucet for a glass of water, but in 1944, the pathophysiology of congenital heart disease was still being pieced together. Doctors imagined that *inadequate oxygenation* of blood in the lungs might at least partly account for cyanosis. If true (which it seldom is), this could minimize the effect of increasing blood flow. Others[84] conceived cyanosis as a problem of the amount of right-to-left shunting, rather than the volume of pulmonary blood flow.[85] Blalock was at first unsure that a shunt would help: "…Dr. Helen Taussig and I became interested in *the question whether increase of the blood supply to the lungs* by the creation of an artificial ductus arteriosus *would benefit* patients with tetralogy of Fallot or pulmonary stenosis."[86] "The most important element of [Blalock and Taussig's] contribution", wrote contemporary heart surgeon Russell Brock, "is the conception of the part played by . . . inadequate pulmonary blood flow. As a result of this, they *postulated* that the cyanosis and disability could be relieved by improving the blood supply to the lungs. . . . The *proof of the correctness of their postulate* lies in the good results of their operation."[87] What is obvious today was only a hypothesis as Blalock contemplated pressing his blade into a child's chest.

Blalock turned to a canine model for proof of concept. Shunting dogs with tetralogy would provide the strongest proof, but Elliott Cutler's problem (Chaps. 4 and 5) was his problem: As dogs do not develop mitral stenosis, at least not very often, neither are they born with tetralogy of Fallot. Alternatively, Blalock and Thomas might have experimentally fashioned tetralogy. This malformation's key features are pulmonary stenosis and a ventricular septal defect, but the latter proved almost impossible to create. Even producing pulmonary stenosis proved difficult: The pulmonary artery was narrowed using thick linen ligature, umbilical (cloth) tape, rubber tubing, bands of ox fascia (tissue), and silver clips. But these materials either ruptured the vessel or cut it through, with the artery reforming around it. And constricting the pulmonary artery alone had no effect on arterial oxygen saturation,

[82] Longmire (1991, pp. 70–71).

[83] Thomas (1985, p. 90).

[84] Nadas and Bing allege that "It is certain, however, that Taussig's idea that an increase in pulmonary blood flow would be beneficial for patients with tetralogy of Fallot was not correct. It was not the diminution in pulmonary blood flow, but the right to left shunt, or the decrease in effective pulmonary blood flow, which was responsible for the cyanosis and clinical symptoms of these patients" (Nadas and Bing, in Bing 1999, p. 96). Taussig was, of course, spot on, and the origin of this woolly thinking by these two brilliant congenital cardiologists eludes me.

[85] Blalock and Taussig (1945), Blalock (1946a, b) and Brock (1951).

[86] Blalock (1946a); emphasis mine.

[87] Brock (1949); emphasis mine.

since—as they later came to realize—without a ventricular septal defect, there was no right-to-left shunt.[88] After many months of failed experiments, they found that sewing the distal end of the right pulmonary artery to the pulmonary vein and removing lobes from one or both lungs resulted in a stable model of cyanosis.[89] Producing only six dogs suitable for trying out a shunt, two had only a "slight" increase in arterial oxygen saturation after shunting, and four had "significant" augmentation.[90] It is hard to imagine a weaker proof of concept: The model bore no anatomic resemblance to tetralogy, its pathophysiology was somewhat different, and the shunt only inconsistently increased the oxygen saturation. Blalock recognized that his data were weak—he claimed only that these results "strengthened the impression" that a shunt would prove useful.[91] And there were other questions. Would a cyanotic patient tolerate anesthesia and incursion into the chest? Could one branch pulmonary artery be temporarily occluded while sewing in the shunt without lethal hypoxemia? Would subclavian artery interruption critically starve the arm it perfused of oxygen? Blalock knew that these questions could find no answer in the laboratory but would only be resolved in the clinical theater.[92] By the fall of 1944, his confidence in the technical feasibility and physiological utility of his shunt was enough for Blalock to approach the parents of a gravely ill child, asking for their permission to try something difficult and brand new, deep inside her chest.

> We walked over to the third or fourth floor where there was the baby that we were going to operate upon tomorrow. I took one look at the patient and thought my God, this man isn't going to operate on this patient.
>
> –William Longmire[93]

Eileen Saxon suffered her first hypercyanotic episode ('tetralogy spell') at 8 months of age. Born 7 weeks early, she weighed just under two and a half pounds, yet like many babies with tetralogy of Fallot, she was pink early on. Eileen's prematurity, not her heart, had obliged her to spend her first 4 months in the hospital. After discharge, she poked along reasonably well, but her father Francis—who bent sheet metal into bombers at the Glenn Martin aircraft plant before enlisting in the navy—had noticed that his daughter got dusky with her bottle, and her growth and activity were lagging. Eileen's first spell occurred on her mother's watch: The oxygen content of her blood plummeted rapidly to a critical level, starving her brain, one of the most oxygen-voracious organs. Her eyes rolling up just as she lost consciousness, Eileen was blacked out until the physiological factors which control oxygen delivery and consumption in tetralogy re-established a precarious balance. Hailing a cab, Dorothy rushed her to the Harriet Lane Home (Johns Hopkins' pediatric hospital),

[88] Thomas (1985, pp. 85–86).

[89] Thomas (1985, pp. 85–89).

[90] Blalock (1946a).

[91] Blalock (1946a).

[92] Blalock (1946a).

[93] Stoney (2004, 2008).

where the diagnosis of "blue baby" was made.[94] Over the next few months, Eileen experienced more spells, her cyanosis increased, and her growth and activity fell. Eventually, she lacked the wherewithal even to take formula. Trapped in an oxygen tent in the Harriet Lane, she was 16 months old and terminally ill at the time of her operation.[95]

Save for her diminutive size (just under nine pounds), Eileen was exactly the sort of patient that Taussig and Blalock had been looking for. Her barely viable physiology put her on a scalpel's edge relative to withstanding the stresses of anesthesia and the operation itself, but it also provided *justification* for taking the risk. "[Eileen Saxon is] the type of child on whom you should try [the shunt,]" Taussig recalled Blalock saying. "You don't do a new operation on a *good* risk; you do a new operation on a patient who has no hope of survival without it."[96] Blalock gathered up William Longmire, then his chief resident, to see Eileen the night before the operation. Longmire was aghast at her size and deep cyanosis; he predicted that when her chest was opened and the left lung collapsed, that would be the end of her. Eileen was, indeed, hanging on by a thread. Blalock had only *assisted* Thomas, and that only once, performing the shunt in the lab. Plans for Blalock to practice as the primary operator had to be cancelled, as Eileen's urgent need for operation preempted the rehearsal. Blalock rolled his first patient into the operating room having never done the shunt as the primary operator.[97] The day was Wednesday, November 29.[98]

Austin Lamont, the first full-time physician anesthesiologist at Hopkins, was scheduled to handle Eileen's anesthesia. Apparently finding the principle of "*primum non nocere*" to trump "desperate times require desperate measures," Lamont cancelled the case the night before. Undeterred, Blalock scrambled and got Merel Harmel, a resident not quite a full year into his training, to step in a day later. (But Lamont, not completely shedding responsibility, was in the operating room, and subsequently provided anesthesia for Blalock's second patient and many to follow).[99]

That this first shunt operation was successful is astonishing, given the primitive conduct of the procedure, not only by twenty-first century standards, but even compared to operations performed shortly thereafter.[100] Anesthesiologists had much less experience with intrathoracic surgery than they do today, inferior anesthetic agents, and fewer medications to adjust blood pressure and other hemodynamic variables. There being no endotracheal tubes small enough for her, Eileen's anesthesia was by open drop ether. Because an anesthesia mask, rather than a tube inserted into the trachea, was used to inflate the lungs, Harmel lacked precise control of lung expan-

---

[94] Thorwald (1971, pp. 14–15).

[95] Blalock and Taussig (1945).

[96] Harvey (1978).

[97] Thomas (1985, p. 91).

[98] Thomas (1985, pp. 97–104), Neill (1987), Longmire (1991, pp. 108–109) and Ravitch (1966, p. xliii).

[99] Longmire (1991, p. 98), Lowenstein and Reeves (2014, pp. 831–832) and Blalock and Taussig (1945).

[100] Blalock and Taussig (1945), Thomas (1985, pp. 91, 94) and Stoney (2004).

sion. Neither Eileen's blood pressure nor her oxygen saturation were measured, the only monitoring being "a finger on the carotid pulse."[101] Blalock performed the anastomosis between the subclavian and pulmonary arteries using straight needles rather than the curved variety that are much easier to work with—a real challenge, even today, in so small a patient. (Thomas custom-made the needles, cutting longer needles down to half an inch and sharpening the tip. Soon thereafter, the Deknatel company was induced to manufacture curved needles with very fine suture, swaged-on rather than threaded through a hole.)[102]

As we've noted, this was Blalock's first go at the anastomosis. Just after arriving in the surgical theater, he sent for Thomas. On seeing his technician climb into the observer's gallery, the surgeon beckoned him closer to the action, to the step stool just behind him. As Blalock crafted the connection between the two arteries, a piece of sewing demanding sub-millimeter precision, he appealed to Thomas for advice: Is the pulmonary artery incision long enough? Are these stitches close enough together? When Blalock began a stitch in the wrong direction, Thomas corrected him.[103] Ninety concentrated and tense minutes,[104] later the sterile drapes were lifted off Eileen: Still having a pulse, breathing, and a little pinker, surgeon and colleagues beheld a minor miracle. Blalock was also gratified to find that her left hand's blood flow was "fairly good." Taussig, who was present as the shunt was created, must have been relieved, but her guard was still up as this tiny pioneer transitioned into the next phase of her tenuous journey.

Intensive care units were as yet to be developed,[105] so Eileen weathered her "stormy" postoperative course on the general floor. She was closely monitored—that is, someone was always at the bedside, not that sophisticated monitoring devices were used—but her minders were often pediatric residents, not seasoned providers. One such resident, Ruth Whittemore, was at Eileen's bedside for two days, catching an occasional nap on an adjacent cot, ever ready to needle evacuate air or blood from Eileen's chest. Routine monitoring of blood gases and other chemistries had yet to be developed, and Eileen was thought too small to have even a single arterial puncture, so her arterial oxygen saturation was never measured. A couple of weeks passed before she picked up steam, and two months later she was discharged from the hospital, a little pinker and gaining good weight.[106]

Fortune smiled on Blalock and Eileen on the day of her shunt. Although Harmel and Longmire recalled that Eileen's color was "dramatically improved" at operation's end,[107] Taussig wrote that, while Eileen was "improved," it was "not until the

[101] Lowenstein and Reeves (2014, p. 831).

[102] Blalock and Taussig (1945) and Thomas (1985, pp. 91, 96).

[103] Thomas (1985, pp. 92–94), Stoney (2004), Ravitch (1966, p. xxxix).

[104] Blalock and Taussig (1945) and Lowenstein and Reeves (2014, p. 831).

[105] Kelly et al. (2014).

[106] Blalock and Taussig (1945) and Neill and Clark (1995, pp. 54–55).

[107] Lowenstein and Reeves (2014) and Stoney (2004).

third child [who had a shunt] did we see a dramatic change."[108] Blalock felt no thrill (a vibration indicating copious blood flow) in the pulmonary artery at the operation's end[109] and, later, heard no continuous murmur (such a murmur would also suggest good shunt flow).[110] Eileen lived only a few months before narrowing of her shunt mandated a second surgery, at which she died.[111] The shunt flow must have been only marginally effective; if Blalock's anastomosis had been but a fraction of a millimeter narrower, the B-T-T shunt's launch would have proven more discouraging than exhilarating.

The report of the first three shunted patients (Eileen and two others) was published in one of medicine's most prestigious journals, the *Journal of the American Medical Association* (*JAMA*).[112] It commenced by summarizing the physiology of cyanotic malformations—information which was required for virtually all of *JAMA*'s readership to understand what had been accomplished. Roughly eight of its nearly fourteen pages are devoted to background material, and a detailed technical discussion of the procedure was was included.

This paper is a masterpiece, immensely appealing for a human quality gone missing from the astringent disquisitions which are today's academic reports. Carefully read, one can sense the authorship shifting from one contributor to the other. The first one and one-half pages were apparently written by the cardiologist, after which she hands off the narrative to her surgical colleague. Taussig marked her territory by eschewing the royal "we" and specifically attaching her initials to the key concept (alleviating cyanosis via increasing pulmonary blood flow) which constituted the shunt's rationale. Blalock's technical contributions were self-evident—no need for him to embed his initials—and the detailed discussion of the surgical considerations reveals the mind of a meticulous surgeon at work. Consistent with the style of the day, the paper was fat in pages but lean of authors. (Today's reports are more concise but often generously larded with authors, sometimes including minimal contributors.) Blalock and Taussig gave co-workers credit where credit was due, and in a manner more apt than adding names to the author list. In the body of the text, Merel Harmel is acknowledged for providing the anesthesia, and encomiums are delivered to six cited pediatric house staff who "provided excellent care . . . (without which) in all probability the child's life would not have been saved." At a particularly trying point in the second case, Blalock's first assistant William Longmire supplied "encouragement [which] played no small part in" Blalock's persisting until the operation was successfully completed. Vivien Thomas was the only participant lacking in recognition—strikingly so, considering his many hours of toil and advice rendered at Blalock's elbow during the operations.

---

[108] Taussig (1981).

[109] Blalock and Taussig (1945).

[110] Ravitch (1966, p. xliii).

[111] Longmire (1991, p. 104).

[112] Blalock and Taussig (1945).

The *JAMA* paper, newspaper articles, talks, and word of mouth splintered the flood gates in Baltimore. Families from across the US and the globe rushed to Hopkins. Between 1944 and 1951, patients from 46 of the then-48 states, as well as 69 others from outside the US, converged on Baltimore; 1037 patients were operated upon in that interval. Fewer than two hundred cardiac operations a year is only a modest caseload for a program today, but for an institution in the 1940s that had previously done virtually no cardiac surgery, the increase in activity was massive. The cardiology clinic was overrun. Many families arrived unannounced, with no place to stay, adding to the strain. Hometown newspapers, angling for a story, raised funds for the operation, and attached reporters to the sponsored patients. "Newspaper reporters, especially local ones" Thomas wrote "were always around. They were in the clinic, in the corridors, and on the patient floors."[113] Physicians from across the globe drove and flew and steamed to Baltimore and packed the observation gallery. Blalock graciously accommodated the visitors, some of whom departed with gifts of hard-to-obtain medical supplies.

Taussig was delighted with the torrent of patients, eager to finally help the previously un-helpable. But the work was exhausting. "After the first few weeks, members of the surgical and pediatric house staff were literally working night and day taking care of these critically ill patients," Longmire confided to his diary (June 18, 1945). "My, what a busy time—time for little else. Much tension in the OR during these cases and doing two a day for many days in a row wears us all out."[114] A section of the children's surgical ward was designated for cardiac patients (the "tet room"), and a recovery and rudimentary intensive care room cobbled together. Even Vivien Thomas was recruited into the fray. Among other duties—including advising Blalock in the operating room, as he had done for the Saxon operation—he was assigned the distinctly disagreeable task of drawing arterial blood from these unhappy kids. Thomas' "very presence on the [hospital] floor would throw the entire floor into an uproar, since it meant that some patient was going to be stuck with a needle. One child would set it off, and in a few minutes every child on the floor would be crying at top voice."[115] Yet others in the shunt's orbit—for example, the people who anesthetized patients who only a few weeks ago seemed too scary to anesthetize—were required to up their game, and they did.[116] The system was stressed and strained in many ways, but this disruptive technology soon put Johns Hopkins cardiac surgery on the map, and Blalock and Taussig on the dais.

The B-T-T shunt inspired a number of variations on the theme, the earliest being developed in Chicago a year later.[117] Today, aortopulmonary shunts are usually constructed using an expanded polytetrafluoroethylene (Teflon) tube inserted between the aorta or branch thereof (usually the subclavian or innominate artery) and the

[113] Thomas (1985, p. 101).

[114] Longmire (1991, p. 109).

[115] Thomas (1985, p. 103).

[116] Harmel and Lamont (1946).

[117] Potts et al. (1946) and Shumacker (1992, pp. 70–74).

pulmonary artery. The "modified B-T-T shunt" serves as a necessary first step toward more definitive rescue for many single ventricles and will likely do so for years to come.

Looking forward to Appendix 1, the shunt was made possible by the body's *spare capacity* and talent for *self-regulation*. Taussig recognized this, acknowledging that her shunt could only be effective in patients whose heart could increase its output enough to accommodate the extra flow to the lungs.[118] Since one cannot coax the cardiovascular system into increasing its output in this setting, its capacity for self-regulation is crucial for the shunt to work. The body has to automatically modify its physiology in yet other ways—for example, adjust its blood volume—that are required for the shunt to be effective. Nature is stingy in providing models of human disease, but she has been generous in evolving a human body clever and flexible enough to accommodate therapeutic interventions.

A film of a 1960 speech of Alfred Blalock's, "Contemplating the Subject of Retirement,"[119] presents a tuxedoed gentleman, handsome and relaxed, looking up now and again from his notes as he delivers Georgia-inflected remarks as suavely as the most polished toastmaster. This surgeon is informal yet confidence-engendering. With a smile faintly tracing his lips, he times his dryly amusing lines perfectly and holds his large and receptive audience utterly captive. Using Sir William Osler's notion that productive professional life ends before middle age as a foil, Blalock's pushback is gentle and measured. This clip is well-worth the ten-minute investment for anyone interested in Blalock, demonstrating better than anecdotes or recollections why he so naturally cultivated the respect and affection of so many in his orbit. This is a thoughtful man, you think, possibly even a wise man, someone you can count on. Evidence of his hard work and tenacity is inscribed in his academic accomplishments, but this speech, given at his 61st birthday celebration before an estimated five to six hundred family members, friends, trainees, and colleagues,[120] implies other personal qualities. Mostly, people found him charming, even charismatic, and as well-mannered and gracious as one might expect of a scion of one of Culloden's best families.[121] Warm and friendly, Blalock was perhaps endowed with an *excess* of probity; many found this man too imposing to get truly close to.[122] Though he wore his fame lightly, his standing among his fellow surgical chiefs was such that a recommendation from him was a virtual guarantee of a plumb training opportunity or a job. His after-dinner performance was perhaps a little misleading: Blalock was high strung,[123] with a quick but *usually* well-managed temper. And

[118] Taussig (1947, pp. 558–559).

[119] Blalock (1960).

[120] Longmire (1991, p. 231).

[121] *Partners of the Heart* (2003).

[122] Blalock trainee G. Rainer Williams' respect for him was so "enormous" that he "could never be completely comfortable with him" (Longmire 1991, p. 217). Harvey Bender, another Blalock resident, recalled "I didn't feel, and I don't think anyone felt, that close to Dr. Blalock. Of all his residents they say that only Bill Longmire called him Al" (Stoney 2008, p. 242).

[123] Longmire (1991, p. 253).

associates have remarked on his plaintive, whiney voice when events went south in the operating room.[124] Recollections of Blalock by those who knew him well suggest that he lacked the sort of capacious and ravenous mind of, say, a Lavoisier. A good friend sized-up Blalock: "[N]ot one of the first class minds I have known, but he was willing to work harder than anybody." Another offered that he was "wise beyond his intellect."[125] I am aware of no documented estimations of Taussig, but available information suggests much the same.

Helen Taussig, on the other hand, in a 1977 interview, could have been your grandmother, save for the doctor-talk.[126] Amicable and voluble, she—unlike Blalock—was perhaps a little past her prime, and seems rather more frail than commanding. Recollections of Taussig are more likely to emphasize her compassion and gentleness with her patients than warmth or graciousness. Yet she formed many strong and durable friendships. The Knights of Taussig, a group of former fellows, stayed in close contact with her long after completing their training. She loved to entertain, both at her Baltimore home on Hollins Lane and at her house at Cotuit on Cape Cod. Frank Taussig had given his daughter a love of place: Helen's childhood summers were enjoyed at the family's home on Massachusetts' scorpion tale, imprinting her forever to the Cape. As an adult, Taussig continued the family tradition of summers there, even structuring her days as her father had: mornings devoted to writing, afternoons reserved for the beach. Friends were often included.[127]

But Blalock's and Taussig's agreeable skins belied cores of sinew. Both were highly jealous of their territory and prerogative. How Blalock disposed of a potential mutiny at Hopkins before he even got the key to his office is illustrative. Shortly before assuming the chair of surgery, he visited Baltimore, announcing that he intended to foreshorten the period of employment of some of the current surgical residents (four of the senior residents had a total of twenty-nine years of house staff training—long-in-the-tooth for then, not now). Upset, the residents hastily huddled and dashed off a letter of protest, which was delivered to Blalock's hotel. Returning to the hotel from a congratulatory dinner, he read the letter and, blood boiling, postponed his return to Nashville. The next morning, Blalock met with each of the residents individually, "curtly repeating the offers he had made the day before on a take it or leave it basis, with no changes."[128]

Taussig, for her part, put elbows out when dealing with the surgeons.[129] Her extraordinary tenacity was never better conveyed than by an incident recollected by Alex Haller. Blalock, assisted by Haller, had performed a taxing operation, taking twice as long as anticipated, on a cyanotic teen. "Dr. Blalock finally was able to

---

[124] Ravitch (1966), Longmire (1991), Thomas (1985), Olch (1973), Weisse (2002) and Stoney (2008).

[125] Longmire (1991, pp. 34, 188).

[126] Gott interview of Taussig (1977).

[127] Baldwin (1992), Neill (1987), Bing (1988), McNamara et al. (1987), Engle (1985) and Weisse (2002).

[128] Ravitch (1966, p. xxxi).

[129] Baldwin (1992, pp. 75–80).

leave the OR to speak with the child's parents. Outside the OR, he and Dr. Taussig locked horns. Through an assistant, she had been keeping tabs on the surgery and was concerned about how one aspect of it had been handled. Dr. Taussig wanted Dr. Blalock to redo part of the surgery. Dr. Blalock was furious. As chief of surgery he believed he knew best. But he decided on a strategy to appease the unrelenting Dr. Taussig. Dr. Blalock stormed into the operating room . . . (just as Haller was completing the skin closure) . . . and pantomimed 'correcting' part of the procedure, while actually making no significant changes."[130]

Many recollections merely allude to this friction, while others are explicit. Cardiologists Richard Bing and Catherine Neil, both at Hopkins at the time, allude to wrangling between "the Professor" (as his residents "respectfully and somewhat affectionately" called Blalock[131] and "the Queen" (the surgeon's nickname for Taussig). Longmire wrote that "a subtle distrust evolved into a thinly suppressed hostility" between the two, and of Blalock's annoyance with Taussig. Charlotte Ferencz, a colleague of Taussig's, wrote that "turmoil, resentments, envy and bitterness" had complicated Taussig's professional life, that for years she was "constantly under siege," but that she had fought back (being "aggressive, defensive, and combative"). (Ferencz did not specify the cause(s) of this turmoil, but one presumes that it was related to her relationship with Blalock's group.)[132] In a late-life interview, Taussig was asked about Blalock, her colleague for over twenty years and dead now for over 20 years. She offered only that he was a very skillful surgeon, a remarkable teacher, was friendly and outgoing, and got a great deal of enjoyment out of life.[133]

Some of this was simply huge egos clashing.[134] Taussig, given the often real or perceived authority gradient between men and women, and surgeons and pediatricians, doubtlessly struggled to maintain equilibrium in her environment. Her deafness, which would disadvantage anyone in her milieu, may have caused her to react more aggressively than she would have otherwise.[135] And Blalock, by some lights, was a bigger part of this problem than he needed to be.[136] Even best friend William Longmire wrote (while providing few details) that Blalock was in what sounds like chronic conflict with many other people and groups at Hopkins,[137] and

[130] Baldwin (1992, p. 77).

[131] Longmire (1991, p. 72).

[132] Bing (1988), Neill (1994), Longmire (1991, p. 114) and McNamara et al. (1987).

[133] Harvey (1978).

[134] Weisse (1991, pp. 65–66).

[135] After Taussig had surgery to improve her hearing, someone asked her if she were a nicer person now that she could hear, and she answered "yes" (Bing 1988; Neill 1994).

[136] Longmire (1991, p. 245).

[137] For example, Longmire (1991) offers these details: Blalock's efforts to block the appointment of his successor went "well beyond the limits of academic propriety" (p. 252) and "aroused considerable resentment" among the faculty (p. 255); his "tenacity and persistence . . . were at times counterproductive in institutional affairs" (p. 279); Longmire implied that there were quite a few people at Hopkins who, for reasons unstated, were critical of him (pp. 96–97).

administrative confrontations with him were "apt to be unpleasant and overly emotional."[138] Taussig's therapeutic conservatism must have been a burr under Blalock's saddle. Harry Muller, one of Blalock's chief residents (1948–1949), had asked Taussig to refer a patient with coarctation of the aorta for repair. She declined. When he asked why, Taussig simply answered—as Muller recalled—that if he didn't like her decision that he could just leave her office. When Muller reported back to his boss, Blalock, with his resident in tow, stomped off to the hospital director and asked permission to develop his own cardiology service within the Department of Surgery. The request went nowhere.[139] But the show still went on, along with the drama. The shunt got created; many lives were enriched and lengthened; cardiac surgeons and pediatric cardiologists trained at Hopkins and then went on to teach the next wave of practitioners.

Enzo Ferrari was never satisfied. When someone asked him what his favorite Ferrari car was, he answered: "The one I haven't built yet." Henry Ford was, and it nearly wrecked his company. Ford was delighted with his Model T, introduced in 1908 and one of history's most successful commercial launches. So satisfied that even in the early nineteen-twenties, with the T no longer competitive with General Motors' more modern offerings, he steadfastly refused to approve an updated version. It was only after the loss of huge market share and the risk of calamity for his company that his son Edsel could finally convince Henry to authorize the design and manufacture of an updated model.[140] More like Henry than Enzo, Taussig was also satisfied, and her contentment with her diagnostic skills and the shunt reveals a surprising lack of imagination. While her satisfaction did not imperil congenital cardiology, had the rest of the field shared her inclination—and failure of imagination—the cost would have been many lost graduations. While her diagnoses were generally accurate, there was obvious room for improvement. Yet it was Blalock, not Taussig, who hired cardiologist Richard Bing to bring cardiac catheterization (a major advance in the diagnosis of heart defects) to Hopkins. Taussig, in fact, at least initially actively opposed his work.[141] Her regard and hopes for open heart (corrective) surgery were no greater. Ake Senning, an early cardiac surgeon, recalled that "When they (Drs. Lillehei and Varco) reported to the New York Academy in 1955 on their correction of Fallot's tetralogy with four of seven patients surviving the operation, our grand lady today, Helen Taussig, was not very happy and said—as far as I remember—'I am unhappy that they had any survivals at all, because now others will try'—and they did."[142] Blalock's imagination was only a little more capacious: He at first opposed open heart surgery. Owen Wangensteen, chairman of surgery at the University of Minnesota, recalled: "It amazed me, at a meeting here in Washington some time in 1955, Walt Lillehei and Dick Varco had talked about

[138] Longmire (1991, p. 279).

[139] Longmire (1991, pp. 114–115).

[140] Collier and Horowitz (1987, pp. 118–122, 124–125).

[141] Weisse (2002, p. 66) and Longmire (1991, pp. 116–117).

[142] Snellen et al. (1981, p. 152).

their experience with the open-heart operation . . . they were assailed in a very emotional manner by Dr. Blalock. Dr. Blalock spotted me in the foyer of the hotel when the meeting adjourned and I, too, got more than a taste of Al Blalock's displeasure."[143] Blalock then turned lukewarm, saying "I am so uncertain at the moment about the relative values of hypothermia, of the mechanical heart lung, and of cross-circulation as adjuvants in cardiac surgery that I will not dwell on the subject. . . . At the moment I am enthusiastic about the use of the cross-circulation,"[144] eventually assigning Henry Bahnson and Frank Spencer the task of introducing this modality to Johns Hopkins. Blalock had chosen well; these surgeons were among the earliest to open the heart, but the center of gravity of congenital cardiology had moved away from Baltimore and toward other centers—such as the University of Minnesota and the Mayo Clinic in the mid-1950s.

Although Taussig's big ideas were spent after the shunt, she made important contributions during the remainder of her career. Though only a decade fresher than Maude Abbott's classic volume, her 1947 landmark textbook *Congenital Malformations of the Heart* (dedicated to her seven-years departed father) was light years ahead of her friend's and served as congenital cardiology's touchstone until well into the 1950s. Taussig contributed enormously as a (*the*, actually) prolific trainer of pediatric cardiologists (123 or 125 by two reports) during the field's initial rapid period of growth and development.[145] She worked at Hopkins until her retirement in 1963, but then continued to publish papers, give talks, and pursue research for years afterward. Taussig never married or had children, but she remained close to her family, and her Knights, for life. She died in May 1986 at age 87, when she drove her car into the path of another leaving a parking lot not far from home.[146] Her honors, awards, and honorary degrees number 68, most notably the Albert Lasker Award (1954), the Eleanor Roosevelt Achievement Award (1957), and the Medal of Freedom of the United States (1964).[147]

Like Taussig, Blalock settled into a productive, if less scintillating, late career. His laboratory work continued, although of low volume and impact. But countless children benefited from his operating room exertions and the talks he gave to future shunt prescribers and crafters outside Baltimore and the US. And his many highly accomplished trainees further multiplied his influence: Twenty-four of Blalock's residents became department chairman or division chiefs.[148] Blalock's home life is largely untouched by his biographers (chiefly Longmire and Mark Ravitch), save that he married Mary Chambers O'Bryan in 1930, and they had three children. The couple remained inseparable until her death in December 1958. Desperately lonely, Blalock married family friend Alice Waters just shy of a year later. Like Taussig, he

[143] Wangensteen (1968) and Olch (1971–1972, pp. 66–67).

[144] Ravitch (1966, vol. II, p. 1760).

[145] Baldwin (1992, p. 70) and Engle (1977).

[146] *The New York Times*, May 22, 1986, p. B16.

[147] McNamara et al. (1987).

[148] Longmire (1991, p. 284).

remained close to his former trainees—the Old Hands—and enjoyed fishing and golf. He retired in the summer of 1964 and was taken by cancer soon thereafter (September). Blalock's career was especially remarkable given his myriad medical infirmities: He had had nine operations (four before the age of forty) and multiple invasive diagnostic tests, not counting the therapeutic pneumothoraces for tuberculosis.[149] The cancer that killed him likely originated in the stump of the ureter remaining after his left kidney was removed when he was 24. Blalock never won his hoped-for Nobel prize, but he did garner the next-best thing, the 1954 Lasker award (with Taussig and Robert Gross). He also received many domestic and international awards and was elected to the National Academy of Sciences (1945).

Vivien Thomas stayed at Hopkins after Blalock's retirement but—to his chagrin—was mostly occupied with supervisory and administrative duties.[150] In February of 1969, at the instigation of (and paid for by) the Old Hands,[151] Hopkins commissioned a portrait of Thomas. The painting's formal presentation was in February 1971—the ceremony being Thomas' "most emotional and gratifying experience of my life"—and it is displayed in the Blalock Building, across from Blalock's portrait.[152] Johns Hopkins provided further recognition of Thomas's exceptional achievements when it appointed him Instructor in Surgery and bestowed an honorary Doctor of Laws in 1976. Thomas shared little of his family life in his autobiography, save that he married Clara Beatrice Flanders in December 1933, and they had two daughters. He retired July 1, 1979. Retirement saw Thomas, at the urging of the Old Hands, commence his autobiography. He completed this invaluable contribution to cardiology's archive shortly before dying in his wife's arms, of pancreatic cancer, in 1985.[153]

As Tinsley Harrison liked to quote: The three stages of research are (1) The planning, "We need to do…"; (2) The work, "You do…"; and (3) The report, "I did…" –Vivien Thomas, *Partners of the Heart: Vivien Thomas and His Work With Alfred Blalock.*[154]

In his biography of Michelangelo, William Wallace called attention to the grossly unfair partitioning of credit given to architects and the essential but "unsung heroes of the building trade," their loyal collaborators. These "skilled and versatile craftsmen who managed men and materials, and capably supervised the day-to-day work" for architects engaged in big projects. Sebastiano Malenotti was indispensable for Michelangelo's renovation of St. Peter's in Rome, which was undertaken when the supreme Italian master was ancient, by sixteenth century standards (in his eighth and ninth decades). "It may seem surprising that such persons, so instrumental to the success of any building project, have remained obscure figures, always

[149] Ravitch (1966).

[150] Thomas (1985, p. 214).

[151] Stoney (2008, p. 265).

[152] Thomas (1985, p. 220).

[153] McCabe (1989).

[154] Thomas (1985, p. 73).

overshadowed by the patron and architect. . . . For the most part, history remembers architects, not building foremen."[155]

As Wallace's observation implies, and the story of William Guthrie countless others confirm, (Chap. 4) "credit where credit is due" is all too often honored in the breech, rather than the execution. Like Sebastiano, Vivien Thomas initially got little recognition for his indispensable contributions, and *even Taussig*, if some observers had prevailed, would have suffered much the same.[156] Longmire thought that Blalock was "overly generous" in apportioning Taussig credit for her role creating the shunt,[157] and unnamed players at Hopkins hankered to cleave her name from the invention.[158] Surgeon-historian Harris Shumaker, Jr. did: He refers only to the "Blalock operation" in *The Evolution of Cardiac Surgery*.[159] But Taussig soon enough secured her share of credit, and Thomas' extraordinary collaboration with his boss was eventually richly acknowledged at Johns Hopkins and in film and other venues.[160] Interestingly, it seems that Thomas was most unhappy about his lack of credit for developing the Blalock-Hanlon procedure, a type of surgery rarely if ever used today, not the shunt.[161] We cannot, of course, afford the workers who split blocks of marble at Carrara the same measure of credit as the sculptor who freed the *David* from that stone. But it's a pity that we so seldom recognize the human infrastructure supporting creative achievements, especially contributors as exceptional as Vivien Thomas. Thank goodness, three decades after Blalock and Taussig overlooked him in their *JAMA* paper, that he has finally been indelibly carved into the shunt's (and Blalock's) story.

In 2016, *The Atlantic* asked its readers and luminaries: What is the greatest collaboration of all time? The answers, some tongue-in-cheek, others not, ranged from conjoined twins to Roosevelt, Churchill, and Stalin saving the Western world. Lennon and McCartney, of course, made their list, but the Hopkins cardiac confederacy did not.[162] Yet theirs is as good an example of collaboration as I can think of in congenital cardiology, maybe in all of medicine. Three people of different backgrounds, perspectives, and skills came together to conjure up what no single one of them possibly could have. Taussig and Blalock lacked the type of dynamic and super-generative partnership as Lennon and McCartney, who threw off song after song people still love. The Baltimore pair evinced more quotidian persistence than inspiration, their imaginative power being unexceptional during most of their careers. But they built something new and groundbreaking, and they applied it to many miserable souls despite friction and head-butting. And this narrative is espe-

[155] Wallace (2009, p. 270).

[156] Timmerman (2003).

[157] Longmire (1991, pp. 113–114).

[158] Olch (1967, p. 24).

[159] Shumacker (1992, pp. 66–68).

[160] Dans (2004), McCabe (1989) and *The Blue Baby Operation* (1996).

[161] Booth and Gordon (1976), Thomas (1985, pp. 117, 123, 127–129) and Goodman (1983).

[162] *The Atlantic* (January/February 2016).

cially delicious because the big cheese(s) don't get all the credit. Scratching just below the surface of the Lasker Prize winners, one discovers the indispensable man who animated Blalock's entire creative program, Mr. Vivien Thomas.

The invention of the shunt also affords us another example of how the paucity of disease models impedes medical innovation. While the shunt was ultimately invented despite the difficulty of developing a model of cyanotic heart disease, had such a model been readily available, time, lives, and resources would have been saved. But on the other side of the cloth, as we note in Appendix 1, the body also aids and abets therapy invention. The viability of the B-T-T shunt hinges on the body's spare capacity and willingness to auto-regulate, to say nothing of its self-healing surgically inflicted wounds. Nature may be demanding, but She's not obdurate.

While congenital cardiology's first inkling of New *Dawn* arrived with Robert Gross's ductal ligation, the B-T-T shunt ascended high enough to cast a shadow. It roiled the field, magnifying its size, its scope, its aspirations. Yet the single ventricle still needed rescue. Malformations causing cardiac overwork, rather than cyanosis—such as holes in the heart or sticky valves—went un-fixed. But advances in cardiac catheterization and angiography in the late 1940s and 1950s delineated these defects in the living patient, implying the possibility of repair. The stage was soon set for congenital cardiology's second disruption.

Open heart surgery opens our next chapter, Breaching the Wall *Open and Dry Hearts*. Congenial cardiology had developed corrective operations—ductal ligations and coarctation repair—but nearly 10 years after the B-T-T shunt, many malformations defied palliation, much less repair. Only by taking a cutting edge to the living heart, opening it and emptying it of blood, could many types of flawed anatomy be seen and repaired. Hijacking the circulation, even if only for a few hours, enables surgical rearrangements of amazing virtuosity, and results vastly more satisfactory than previously imaginable. Thoracic surgeon Leo Eloesser proclaimed that the heart-lung machine—the tool essential for open heart operations—was among "the boldest and most successful feats of man's mind—with invention of the phonetic alphabet, the telephone or a Mozart symphony. Not a Deus ex machina but a machina a Deo; a Promethean fire; leveling from God His secrets to man's understanding; the pulse of the sacred heart; the breath of life."[163] Like Norman Bethune, Eloesser was a surgeon with a strong romantic and artistic bent, which presumably explains his thumping hyperbole,[164] but there is no denying that intracardiac surgery's impact was massively disruptive, accounting for heart surgery's scope and presence today. The pump-oxygenator (heart-lung machine) ultimately substituted for the heart and lungs while the surgeon invaded their space, but its invention wasn't easy. New ideas, and personalities every bit as driven as any we've yet encountered, forced the creation of open-heart surgery. But our next chapter is also about the *range* of personalities—some softer and more tentative than

[163] Eloesser (1970).

[164] Scannell (1983).

others—which underlay this achievement. It also emphasizes the utility, as opposed to limitations, of animal models, on whose back open-heart surgery rode into the operating room.

## References

Abbott ME (1908) Congenital cardiac disease. In: Osler W (ed) Modern medicine: its theory and practice, vol IV, ch. IX. Lea Brothers & Co., Philadelphia, pp 323–425
Apitz C, Webb GD, Redington AN (2009) Tetralogy of Fallot. Lancet 374:1462–1471
Bahnson HT (1982) Surgical treatment of pulmonary stenosis: a retrospection. Ann Thorac Surg 33:96–98
Baldwin J (1992) To heal the heart of a child: Helen Taussig, M.D. Walker and Co., New York
Bertranou EG, Blackstone EH, Hazelrig JB, Turner MD Jr, Kirklin JW (1978) Life expectancy without surgery in tetralogy of Fallot. Am J Cardiol 42:458–466
Bing RJ (1988) The Johns Hopkins: the Blalock-Taussig era. Perspec Bio Med 32:85–90
Bing RJ (ed) (1999) Cardiology: the evolution of the science and the art, 2nd edn. Rutgers University Press, New Brunswick
Blalock A (1946a) Physiopathology and surgical treatment of congenital cardiovascular defects. Bull NY Acad Med 22:57–80
Blalock A (1946b) The surgical treatment of congenital pulmonic stenosis. Ann Surg 124:879–887
Blalock A (1960) Contemplating the subject of retirement [video recording]. Accessed 18 Aug 2024. https://www.ctsnet.org/article/contemplating-subject-retirement-alfred-blalock
Blalock A, Park EA (1944) The surgical treatment of experimental coarctation (atresia) of the aorta. Ann Surg 119:445–456
Blalock A, Taussig HB (1945) The surgical treatment of malformations of the heart. JAMA 128:189–202
Booth M, Gordon G (1976) Interview with Vivien Thomas [audio recording]. Johns Hopkins Medical Archives. Accessed 18 Aug 2024. https://soundcloud.com/hopkins-medical-archives/interview-with-vivien-thomas-1976
Brock RC (1949) The surgery of pulmonary stenosis. Br. Med J 2:399–406
Brock RC (1951) Discussion on the surgery of the heart and great vessels. Proc R Soc Med 44:995–1003
Brown JW (1939) Congenital heart disease. Staples Press, London
Cannon J (2018) Hemorrhagic shock. N Engl J Med 378:370–379
Chambers NK, Buchman TG (2000) Shock at the millennium, I: Walter B. Cannon and Alfred Blalock. Shock 13:497–504
Collier P, Horowitz D (1987) The Fords: an American epic. Summit Books, New York
Dans PE (2004) The physician at the movies. Pharos Autumn:38–41
Deslauriers J, Goulet D (2015) The medical life of Henry Normal Bethune. Can Resp J 22:e32–e43
Duke B, Kalin A (Directors) (2003) Partners of the Heart [documentary film]. Spark Media, Washington, DC
Eloesser L (1970) Milestones in chest surgery. J Thorac Cardiovasc Surg 60:157–165
Engle MA (1977) Dr. Helen B. Taussig, the tetralogy of Fallot, and the growth of pediatric cardiac services in the United States. Johns Hopkins Med J 140:147–150
Engle MA (1985) Dr. Helen Brooke Taussig, living legend in cardiology. Clin Cardiol 8:372–374
Eppinger EC, Burwell CS, Gross RE (1941) The effects of the patent ductus arteriosus on the circulation. J Clin Invest 20:127–143
Goodman GL (1983) A gentle heart: the life of Helen Taussig. Yale Medicine Thesis Digital Library. 2658. Accessed 17 Aug 2024. http://elischolar.library.yale.edu/ymtdl/2658

Gott V (1977) Interview with Dr. Helen Taussig. Accessed 18 Aug 2024. https://www.youtube.com/watch?v=XjManYzgsEQ

Harmel MH, Lamont A (1946) Anesthesia in the surgical treatment of congenital pulmonic stenosis. Anesthesiology 5:477–498

Harvey WP (1978) A conversation with Helen Taussig. Med Times 106:28–44

Harvey AM (1982) Alfred Blalock 1899–1964. National Academy of Sciences Biographical Memoir. Accessed 18 Aug 2024. https://www.nasonline.org/wp-content/uploads/2024/06/blalock-alfred.pdf

Kelly FE, Fong K, Nolan JP (2014) Intensive care medicine is 60 years old: the history and future of the intensive care unit. Clin Med 14:376–379

Leeds SE (1943) The effects of occlusion of experimental chronic patent ductus arteriosus on the cardiac output, pulse and blood pressure of dogs. Am J Phys 139:451–459

Levy SE, Blalock A (1939) Experimental observations on the effects of connecting by suture the left main pulmonary artery to the systemic circulation. J Thorac Surg 8:525–530

Longmire WP Jr (1991) Alfred Blalock: his life and times. Privately printed for WP Longmire

Lowenstein E, Reeves JG (2014) A history of cardiac anesthesiology. In: Enger EI II, Saidman LJ, Westhorpe RN (eds) The wondrous story of Anesthesia. Springer, New York

McCabe K (1989, Aug) Like something the Lord made. Washingtonian, pp 109–111, 226–233. Accessed 18 Aug 2024. http://www.risingpress.org/cnu/mccabe.pdf

McNamara DG (1984) The Blalock-Taussig operation and subsequent progress in surgical treatment of cardiovascular diseases. JAMA 251:2139–2141

McNamara DG, Manning JA, Engle MA, Whittemore R, Neill CA, Ferencz C (1987) Helen Brooke Taussig: 1898 to 1986. JACC 10:662–671

Meade RH (1961) A history of thoracic surgery. Charles C. Thomas, Springfield

Morris T (2017) The matter of the heart: a history of the heart in eleven operations. Thomas Dunne Books, New York

Murphy J (2015) Breakthrough! How three people saved "Blue Babies" and changed medicine forever. Clarion Books, Boston

Nadeau G (1940) A T.B.'s progress: the story of Norman Bethune. Bull Hist Med 8:1135–1171

Naef AP (1990) The story of thoracic surgery: milestones and pioneers. Hogrefe & Huber Publishers, Toronto

Neill CA (1987) Dr. Helen Brooke Taussig May 24, 1989 – May 21, 1986 international cardiologist. Int J Cardiol 14:255–261

Neill CA (1994) Helen Brooke Taussig. J Pediatr 125:499–502

Neill CA, Clark EB (1995) The developing heart: a history of pediatric cardiology. Kluwer Academic Publishers, Dordrecht

Nuland SB (1989) Doctors: the biography of medicine. Knopf, New York

Olch PD (1967, April 20) Interview with Vivien T. Thomas, National Library of Medicine

Olch PD (1971–1972) Interview of Owen H. Wangensteen, Oct. 21 and 22, 1971 and Mar. 5, 1972, and Jan. 28, 1972. National Library of Medicine, Accessed 18 Aug 2024. https://digirepo.nlm.nih.gov/master/oralhist/2935143R/2935143R.pdf

Olch PD (1973, Jan 29) Dr. Sanford E. Leeds discusses the Vanderbilt years of Dr. Alfred Blalock. Interview with Leeds, National Library of Medicine. Accessed 18 Aug 2024. https://digirepo.nlm.nih.gov/master/oralhist/2935108R/2935108R.pdf

Peacock TB (1858) On malformations, &c., of the human heart. John Churchill, London. Reprinted in The Classics of Medicine Library. Birmingham, AL: Gryphon Editions, Ltd.; 1981

Potts W, Smith S, Gibson S (1946) Anastomosis of the aorta to a pulmonary artery. JAMA 132:627–631

Ravitch MM (ed) (1966) The papers of Alfred Blalock, vol I and II. The Johns Hopkins Press, Baltimore

Ravitch MM (1977a) The contributions of Alfred Blalock to the science and practice of surgery. Johns Hopkins Med J 140:57–67

Ravitch MM (1977, Feb 26) Interview with Mark Ravitch, [audio recording]. Johns Hopkins Medical Archive, 1977b. Accessed 18 Aug 2024. https://soundcloud.com/hopkins-medical-archives/interview-with-mark-ravitch

Sabiston DC (1978) Presidential address: Alfred Blalock. Ann Surg 3:255–270

Sargent J (Director) (2004) Something the Lord Made [feature film]. HBO Films, Los Angeles

Scannell JG (1983) Leo Eloesser, M.D.—Eulogy for a free spirit [book review]. Ann Surg 198:235–238

Sellors TH (1967) The genesis of heart surgery. Br Med J 1:385–393

Shumacker HB Jr (1982) Better early than late. Am J Surg 144:170–179

Shumacker HB Jr (1992) The evolution of cardiac surgery. Indiana University Press, Bloomington

Skidelsky R (2003) John Maynard Keynes, 1883-1946: economist, philosopher, statesman. Penguin Books, New York

Snellen HA, Dunning AJ, Arntzenius AC (eds) (1981) History and perspectives of cardiology: catheterization, angiography, surgery and concepts of circular control. Leiden University Press, The Hague

Stoney WS (2004) Bill Longmire and the blue baby operation. J Am Coll Surg 198:653–659

Stoney WS (2008) Pioneers of cardiac surgery. Vanderbilt University Press, Nashville

Taussig HB (1947) Congenital malformations of the heart. The Commonwealth Fund, New York

Taussig HB (1965) On the evolution of our knowledge of congenital malformations of the heart. Circulation 31:768–777

Taussig HB (1968) The first Blalock-Taussig anastomosis [audio recording]. Johns Hopkins Medical Archives. Accessed 18 Aug 2024. https://soundcloud.com/hopkins-medical-archives/the-first-blalock-taussig-anastomosis-by-dr-helen-taussig-1968

Taussig HB (1976) The development of the Blalock-Taussig operation and its results twenty years later. Proc Am Phil Soc 120:13–20

Taussig HB (1979) Difficulties, disappointments, and delights in medicine. Pharos. 42:6–8

Taussig HB (1981) Little choice and a stimulating environment. J Am Med Women's Assn 36:43–44

Taussig HB, Crocetti A, Eshaghpour E, Keinonen, Yap KN, Bachman D, Momberger N, Kirk H (1971) Long-term observations on the Blalock-Taussig operation, I: results of first operation. Johns Hopkins Med J 129:243–257

Taussig H et al (1975) Long-time observations on the Blalock-Taussig operation, VIII: 20 to 28 year follow-up on patients with a tetralogy of Fallot. Johns Hopkins Med J 137:13–19

The Atlantic (2016, Jan/Feb) What is the greatest collaboration of all time? Accessed 18 Aug 2024. https://www.theatlantic.com/magazine/archive/2016/01/what-is-the-greatest-collaboration-of-all-time/419142/

The Blue Baby Operation [digital exhibit archive] (1996) Johns Hopkins Medical Institutions. Accessed 17 Aug 2024. http://www.neonatology.org/pdf/bluebabyoperation.pdf

The New York Times, December 4, 1945, p. 28; November 24, 1946, p. 50; September 14, 1947, p. 63; December 13, 1948, p. 25; May 22, 1986, p. B16

The Washington Post, May 17, 1945

Thomas (1976)

Thomas VT (1985) Pioneering research in surgical shock and cardiovascular surgery: Vivien Thomas and his work with Alfred Blalock. University of Pennsylvania Press, Philadelphia

Thorwald J (1971) The patients. A Helen and Kurt Wolff Book, Harcourt Brace Jovanovich, Inc., New York

Timmerman (2003)

Trimble HO (1953) Award of the 1953 college medal to Dr. Helen Taussig. Dis Chest 24:343–347

Van Praagh R (2012) The Farber-Landing lecture: pediatric pathology—the clinician's "open sesame" and its importance in pediatric cardiology and cardiovascular surgery. Ped Dev Pathol 15:431–449

Virgil The Aeneid, Robert Fagles (trans). Book 12, ln. 188. Viking Penguin, New York, p 360

Wallace WE (2009) Michelangelo: the artist, the man, and his times. Cambridge University Press, Cambridge, UK

Wangensteen OH (1968) Reflections on the Blalock papers. Bull Hist Med 42:357–361

Weisse AB (1991) Medical Odysseys: the different and sometimes unexpected pathways to twentieth-century medical discoveries. Rutgers University Press, New Brunswick

Weisse AB (2002) Heart to heart: the twentieth century battle against cardiac disease—an oral history. Rutgers University Press, New Brunswick

White BD, McNamara DG, Bauersfeld R, Taussig HB (1956) Five-year postoperative results of first 500 patients with Blalock-Taussig anastomosis for pulmonary stenosis or atresia. Circulation 14:512–519

Zuidema GD, Sloan H (2001) Alfred Blalock, Norman Bethune, and the Bethune murals. Surgery 130(5):866–881

# Part III
# Modern Era

# Chapter 7
# Breaching the Wall: Open and Dry Hearts

*Lillehei . . . provided the can-opener for the largest picnic thoracic surgeons will ever know.* —*Denton Cooley (Gott 2005)*

When all four engines of a 747 choked in a cloud of volcanic ash on the way to Jakarta in 1982, the plane glided for 20 minutes until they could be restarted.[1] If our engine chokes, we crash in an instant. Cut blood flow to the brain, and we black out moments later; interrupt its oxygen supply for 3 or 4 minutes, and we are out for good. The heart is the most urgently needed, by far, of our organs. (The lungs are similar, although much less prone to sudden failure than the heart.) The kidneys, liver, and gut are as essential, but can be offline for days, and the rest of the body lives indefinitely after brain death.[2] This pump *must* pump 60/60/24/7/365. And therein lay nascent cardiac surgery's greatest challenge. Open-heart surgery is routine today, but in the 1940s, one could as easily imagine gazing across a confusion of snowy Himalayan peaks from the summit of Everest as peering into the interior of a motionless but living human heart.

By the late 1940s, the New Dawn of congenital cardiology had broken, but only just. The patent ductus and coarctation had yielded to the blade and suture. Severe hypoxia was rendered less so—in some malformations—by the B-T-T shunt. By 1951, an operation to narrow the pulmonary artery in certain defects (to decrease pulmonary blood flow) proved useful palliation but was far from curative.[3] Most defects were uncorrectable, including holes inside the heart (atrial and ventricular septal defects)—sticky and leaky valves such as stenotic mitral and pulmonary valves excepted—remained mostly invulnerable to surgical siege. And some complex malformations, like transposition of the great arteries and most single ventricle defects, could not even be effectively palliated. Roughly 75% of people born

[1] Thornhill (2017).

[2] Shewmon (1998).

[3] Damman et al. (1961).



T. J. Kulik, M. Dick, *Reimagining a Child's Heart*,
https://doi.org/10.1007/978-3-031-88608-9_7

with a cardiac malformation had to wait for modern congenital cardiology—the era of open-heart surgery—for repair or, in the case of the single ventricle, effective palliation.[4]

But people were trying. Russell (later Lord) Brock thrust a thin cutting tool, followed by dilating forceps, through the right ventricle wall to slice and stretch open malformed pulmonary valves. He invented another instrument, also inserted blindly into the heart, for chomping out excess muscle from under the pulmonary valve.[5] But Brock's procedures were risky, and their long-term results left a lot to be desired.[6] The earliest attempts at closing holes in the heart were primitive but incredibly ingenious. One involved blindly passing a heavy suture, dragging a strip of fascia lata (tissue surrounding the muscles of the thigh) with a "good blob" of tensor fascia femoris muscle, into the heart and through a ventricular septal defect, hoping to plug it.[7] Charles Bailey (about more later) employed a similar technique, except using pericardium.[8] For atrial defects, he (and Henry Swan) invaginated both atrial appendages, causing them to meet in the defect, and sewed the tips together, thereby (fingers crossed) occluding the hole. Baily also reported three operations on ventricular septal defects: In one case, the pericardial graft obstructed the right ventricular outflow track and had to be removed. Murray operated upon two ventricular and one atrial septal defect, with unknown effect. Brock's experience with infundibular resection: Eight of eleven patients survived, seven of whom had at least a good short-term result.[9] Robert Gross sewed a sheet of thin rubber, fashioned into an open-topped cone, on the wall of the right atrium. When the atrium was opened into this cone, blood rose up to its pressure level, only a few centimeters, allowing the surgeon to work (blindly) inside the well. This technique was also used at the Mayo Clinic.[10] Bailey tried to spin a silk purse out of "finger" surgery's sow's ear: "Even after the perfection of artificial heart-lung equipment it is probable that (its) inherent risks and dangers . . . will in the aggregate, be much greater than those associated with 'transmyocardial palpatory surgery.'"[11] The opposite proved true. These techniques, and yet others,[12] were not as safe or effective as open-heart procedures and were feckless against complex defects.

Even as a few surgeons poked blindly inside the heart, the early 1950s saw two parallel efforts to breech its walls and drain it of blood, thereby permitting precise surgical manipulations. One theory of the case was to temporarily substitute a

---

[4]This number is derived from the relative incidence of various congenital cardiac malformations (Hoffman and Kaplan 2002), taking into account whether effective surgery (in most cases, correction) could be offered before open-heart surgery; for various reasons, this is only a rough estimate.

[5]Johnson (1970, pp. 100–103).

[6]Swan and Zeavin (1954).

[7]Murray (1948).

[8]Bailey et al. (1952).

[9]Bailey et al. (1952), Swan (1953), Murray (1948), and Brock and Campbell (1950).

[10]Gross et al. (1952), and Romaine-Davis (1991, p. 128).

[11]Bailey et al. (1952).

[12]Johnson (1970, pp. 100–103).

mechanical device for the heart, or heart and lungs, so that the muscle could be opened without compromising blood flow. The alternative approach used hypothermia (cold) to reduce the body's need for oxygen, enough so that the heart could be taken offline for a (very) few minutes while it was opened for repairs. Open-heart surgery using cardiopulmonary bypass (the pump-oxygenator, AKA the "heart-lung machine") permitted lengthier repairs and ultimately prevailed, but for a few years, almost all open procedures were conducted via the metabolism-lowering effect of low temperature. In 1961, Henry Swan—the most prolific practitioner of the ice bath—still considered this modality fine for simple intracardiac operations,[13] even as cardiopulmonary bypass was in full swing in the US and Europe.

*Breaching the Wall* describes how congenital cardiology forced its way into its Modern Era by solving the problem of the open heart. We will see how a meticulous Canadian devoted years to refrigeration research before being scooped in its clinical application by an unknown Minnesotan. Inventing a pump-oxygenator, especially the oxygenator, proved tricky, inspiring one impatient surgeon to turn to moms and dads for oxygenators for their child's heart surgery. But this controversial expedient was only a stop-gap, and ultimately a machine was developed to temporarily substitute for both the heart and lungs. The garage-inventor will take some inspiration here: A young physician, anything but an engineer and working on a shoestring, quickly perfected a better pump-oxygenator than a long-laboring team of IBM engineers. And we meet a new personality type. We've encountered many people, certain to their core of the rightness of their calling, whose activities were deeply informed by this conviction. But people lacking such sublime certitude—whom I think of as not *all-in*—have also advanced congenital cardiology's ball. Although open-heart surgery was most famously the product of the wholly committed, it also evolved on the backs of two personalities just a little outside the fray. Finally, we amble down an avenue seldom seriously explored, asking whether gutsy pioneers sometimes went *too* far in their generative zeal. Advancing cardiac surgery demanded daring and risk-taking—for both patient and doctor. When looking back to open-heart surgery's earliest days, considerable allowance must be made for activities—especially subjecting patients to novel and risky surgery—that would later no longer stand the light of day. And we do. G. Wayne Miller, for example, in *King of Hearts* wrote that Charles Bailey—probably the most aggressive of the early heart surgeons—was "just this side of reckless."[14] But Miller was too generous, if typical, in his forbearance: The Philadelphia surgeon *was* reckless, at least at times. While understandable—after all, Bailey had almost supernatural talent and conviction and acted out of a sense of mission—looking past beyond-the-pale behavior is incomplete history, if not bad history. We briefly explore this corner of the nascent open-heart world and ask a corollary question: Early on, did the field *need* a certain wildness in order to advance?

---

[13] Swan and Paton (1961).

[14] GW Miller (2000 p. 57).

We begin at the beginning, with the technique which enabled the first successful open-heart repair—hypothermia with circulatory arrest (stopping all blood flow in the body), decreasing the need for oxygen for a short period.

A young Einstein famously pondered, deeply, what would happen if he chased a beam of light. Like countless scientists before and after him, he was driven by a burning curiosity. Medieval artists were inspired to magnify and render undeniable the glory of God; modern artists hope to create new ways of self-expression (and remuneration). Economists confect theoretical constructs, often more elegant than reflective of the current facts on the ground. Medical doctors are motivated differently. They don't glorify God, chase beauty, aim to express themselves in novel ways, or weave clever theories. Not all are curious, and those who are, largely pursue knowledge not for its own sake but rather toward practical ends. Medical doctors, like engineers, seek to solve practical problems. They are focused on restoring the wild type (see Appendix 1). Fame and fortune are, variably, part of the equation, but mostly doctors are driven to make their patients better.[15] The germinal histories of our pioneers assert this: Their first step down a road of discovery and creation was impelled by patients they were powerless to help. We will learn that surgeon John Gibbon—the inventor of the first heart-lung machine—pursued his 23-year obsession thanks to a woman whom he could have saved if only he had had such a device. The story of Francis Fontan and his eponymous procedure is similar. Ditto for Helen Taussig. Though not inspired by any particular patient, her motivation clearly lay in the many lavender souls she treated and deeply empathized with. Blalock, it seems to me, was primarily urged to craft his shunt not for the shear satisfaction of solving a technical problem, or the notoriety it would bring (although this may have played a role), but mostly to improve people's lives. Wilfred G. Bigelow's story is no different.

Bigelow was a surgeon—and Canadian-to-the-core—not to be confused with his father Wilfred A., a general practitioner and surgeon in rural Manitoba.[16] In 1941, Bigelow *fils*, then a resident in Toronto General Hospital, crossed paths with a young man from the Canadian Northwoods with frostbite-inflicted gangrene of his fingers. The unpleasant task of the amputations fell to Bigelow. Contemplating this unfortunate fellow's plight, Bigelow scoured the literature on frostbite, finding few Canadian reports and the European papers hard to access.[17] How precious little was then known about effective treatment is embedded in the story of Maurice Herzog and Louis Lachenal on the Annapurna massif in 1950. These two French high-altitude climbers had experienced the exhilaration of having attained its highest peak, the first summiting of an 8000-meter mountain, but their hands and feet suffered severe frostbite on their descent. Fellow climbers applied the initial treatment: rubbing, slapping, and beating their frozen extremities with a rope. Suffering yet

[15] There have been and are physicians whose creative portfolios are situated far outside the zone of therapy creation and application, but relatively few.

[16] Bigelow (1984), and Cooper (2010, pp. 107–108).

[17] Bigelow (1942, 1984, p. 11).

more exposure as they descended further, they finally reached the expedition's physician, Jacques Oudot (a French vascular surgeon). He injected—with considerable difficulty—novocain into their brachial and femoral arteries. Herzog's distraught description of this excruciating exercise pierces deeper than any of his many other mountainside tribulations. He howled and sobbed miserably as Oudot searched for his arteries with the needle, having never before experienced such excruciating pain.[18] Though Oudot's treatment was well-intentioned—in some sense heroic, considering that he was working inside a tiny tent at 20,000 feet—by current lights it was pointless and even harmful. Gentle handling and rapid warming of the effected parts are currently emphasized; for severe frostbite, the medications used and their application are very different than Oudot's.[19] Herzog ultimately lost his toes and most of his fingers. Bigelow's impression was correct: The field *was* wide open for improvement. He immersed himself in the available literature and wrote a nice review,[20] but soon got entangled in WWII, serving with the Royal Canadian Army Medical Corps. Frostbite was put on ice.

Actually, in the army, Bigelow still thought about cold, but in a different way. Observing soldiers who lost limbs because reconstruction of severed arteries could not be performed in the field, he wondered if cooling a limb, thus slowing its metabolism, would preserve its viability until the repair. He got as far as having a cooling cabinet built, but too near the end of the war to press it into service.[21] After discharge, he trained for a year as a vascular surgeon with Blalock and turned his sights onto congenital cardiology, especially the problem of accessing the interior of the heart. Bigelow knew of concurrent efforts to invent a "heart-lung" machine, but he was put off by these clunky contraptions of uncertain utility. It was in 1946 that Bigelow "awoke one night with a simple solution to the problem, and one that did not require pumps and tubes—*cool the whole body, reduce oxygen requirements, interrupt the circulation, and open the heart*. The idea undoubtedly sprang from my five-year interest in frostbite and local cooling of the body."[22]

Though Bigelow did not construe it in quite this way, he contemplated using hypothermia to solve a problem of *interface* (see Appendices 1, 2, and 4). Pumping fluids and adjusting the gases they contain was ancient technology at the time. But a heart-lung machine has to pump and exchange gasses from a finicky and dangerous fluid—blood. Bubble oxygen through blood, and it foams. Red blood cells rupture if roughed-up. Blood clots form on artificial surfaces, then break off, clogging arteries and mechanical devices. *If* Bigelow could exploit a natural characteristic of the body—a hypothermia-induced reduction in oxygen requirement—to interrupt the circulation for a useful length of time, these interface problems would disappear. But cold was cloaked with many unknowns: How low to go on the thermometer?

---

[18] Herzog (1997, pp. 245–247).

[19] Poole and Gauthier (2016) and Hickey et al. (2020).

[20] Bigelow (1942).

[21] Bigelow and Lanyon (1944).

[22] Bigelow (1984, p. 40).

Would the body, or individual organs (especially the brain), be injured? And even if the interface were agreeable, would hypothermia yield enough open-heart time for the surgeon to complete his work? Only animal models could answer these and many other questions. Bigelow started cooling dogs upon his return to Toronto in 1947.

Interest in the biologic effects of cold has a centuries-long provenance. Liverpool physician James Currie published his observations, more disquieting than enlightening. James Hunter in the 1780s had observed cold's effect on a variety of organisms.[23] In 1804, immersing people in cold water for up to 45 minutes, Currie slipped a thermometer under their tongue and assessed their pulse using his finger. Experiment VII was typical: when one Richard Sutton was exposed to 40 °F (4.4 °C) salt water, his temperature "sunk, as usual, on his immersion, but to an unusual degree. It did not stop until it got to 83° (28.3 °C), which might be accounted for by the extraordinary chattering of his teeth, admitting some contact of the air." He suffered for 35 minutes before being hauled out and warmed, none the worse for wear.[24] A year later, Scottish surgeon George Kellie told the story of a young man—apparently dead but actually not—suffering from hypothermia on the end of Leith pier. This case report was the lead-in for a lengthy dissertation on hibernation and cold-induced torpor. Drawing parallels between the two, he suggested that in both cases torpor followed from depressed respiration and its effect on the blood.[25] Neither thought about either hypothermia or hibernation in terms of oxygen consumption or metabolism.

Hypothermia in homeotherms—that's us—and hibernation in hibernating animals are often conflated, although they are in many ways distinct. One big difference is that when homeotherms are cooled, they defend their temperature by constricting skin blood vessels, shivering, and releasing metabolism-increasing hormones. But these states are similar, in that body temperature and oxygen consumption are reduced in both.[26] In 1832, physiologist Marshall Hall showed hibernation to reduce the body's need to breathe: "A hedgehog which had been so lethargic in an atmosphere of 40 °F as not to awake for food during several days, was immersed in water of 42 °F. It moved about and expelled air from its lungs. It remained under the water during 22½ minutes. It was then removed. It appeared uninjured." But when a *non-hibernating* hedgehog was immersed, "It expired in three minutes."[27] Like Kellie, he drew a direct line between depressed respirations and hibernation, but he didn't connect cold with depressed metabolism.

Cold hibernators also differ from cold homeotherms in that the former can remain comfortably numb for months, while the clock quickly runs out the safe time for hypothermic homeotherms. And hibernators tolerate much colder body

[23] Hunter (1786, pp. 87–112).

[24] Currie (1804, p. 209).

[25] Kellie (1805).

[26] Henderson (1966).

[27] Hall (1832, p. 345).

temperatures, as low as nearly freezing, while the risk of death rises as the mercury falls below 25 °C in homeotherms.[28] But the confidence intervals around the lowest survivable body temperature are wide. Humans passed out in the cold after excessive libations have survived rectal temperatures as low as 24 °C.[29] And even lower. In 1999, a 29-year-old Norwegian skier fell in a waterfall gully and was trapped under ice for 40 minutes; she was clinically dead when rescued. Her core temperature fell to 13.7 °C during her complex resuscitation, but she survived with few if any residua.[30] In 2001, international attention was riveted on Erika Nordby, a 13-month-old who wandered into a frigid Edmonton night clad with only a diaper. Found hours later, her temperature had dropped to about 16 °C, and she was pulseless for roughly 2 hours before being resuscitated. Despite her profound hypothermia and loss of circulation, Erika recovered fully.[31] And in 2006, a strange story emerged from Japan: Mitsutaka Uchikoshi, a 35-year-old civil servant, was injured while hiking on Mount Rokko. After 24 days on the mountain, unconscious for all but one, his temperature had fallen to 22 °C before a passing climber stumbled across his inert form. It is not known how long Uchikoshi was that cold. He apparently recovered well.[32]

While it was tantalizing to think that hypothermia offered a relatively simple, even elegant solution to the problem of the open heart, Bigelow had only an idea, not a tool. Indeed, it wasn't even certain how cooling alters oxygen demand, delivery, and utilization. Experience with hypothermia in cancer and schizophrenia treatment had left its effect still undefined. Increases, decreases, and no change in metabolism had been reported.[33] How cold is too cold? How long can the circulation be safely interrupted at a given temperature? How should the surgeon adjust, in hypothermic patients, various physiological variables such as venous and arterial pressures and blood chemistries? And what are its harmful effects, and how might they be minimized?

Bigelow launched his research program in 1947 in the basement of the Banting Institute at Toronto General Hospital.[34] Like Blalock, he directed a team of researchers, but a rather larger one: lab technicians, eight fellows (between 1947 and 1953), and collaborators and advisors from other disciplines. At first, they refrigerated dogs in a cold room but, tiring of coats and gloves, quickly turned to cooling blankets, ice bags, and cold-water immersion. Eliminating shivering, they soon discovered, was not enough to reduce oxygen consumption—pharmacologic release of

---

[28] Henderson (1966).

[29] Pembrey (1904).

[30] Gilbert et al. (2000).

[31] Wikipedia, "Erika Nordby."

[32] McCurry and Jha (2006).

[33] Coincident with Bigelow's foray into hypothermia, Smith and Fay (1940) treated cancer with local, or total body cooling to as low as 74 °F (23.3 °C), for days at a time. Dill and Forbes (1941) targeted schizophrenia, using cooling blankets to refrigerate patients to as low as 25.5 °C for up to 48 hours.

[34] Bigelow (1984, pp. 44, 192).

muscle tone was required. Mature dogs could be safely taken to 20–23 °C, and newborns even lower. Only after hundreds of experiments did they finally cool dogs, arrest their circulation, and incise their hearts (1949). Thirty-nine animals were operated upon, and half survived. Bigelow stuffed 3 years of experiments into a talk—its climax being a movie showing off an empty canine heart—presented to an interested but largely skeptical audience at the 1950 American Surgical Association meeting at the Broadmoor Hotel in Colorado Springs.[35] Though no one knew it at the time, this meeting proved pivotal for inchoate open-heart surgery: Two of hypothermia's earliest and most important practitioners (F. John Lewis and Henry Swan II) eagerly absorbed Bigelow's thesis and soon commenced research programs of their own. Bigelow (a cautious Canadian, so not yet ready for Homo sapiens) worked two more years amassing data and honing their craft before reaching a tipping point: Eking their way up the evolutionary ladder to just shy of humans, they studied monkeys instead of dogs. All but one of twelve cooled to 16–19 °C, with the heart opened for 15–24 minutes, survived. Just as important, they fared well neurologically, suggesting that the cold-brain interface was reasonably benign.[36]

In 1952, 5 years after setting up his basement lab, Bigelow was finally ready for Toronto General's operating room. Thinking younger patients more suitable than older and having only enough time to repair simple defects (8–10 minutes), Bigelow looked for a child with an atrial septal defect or pulmonary valve stenosis. But his was an adult hospital. The adjacent Hospital for Sick Children was where the kids were, but its head cardiologist, John D. Keith, and surgeon, William Mustard, were contemplating an open-heart program of their own and in no mood to share.[37] Mustard later stated that Keith, recognizing the risk of heart-lung bypass, referred only cyanotic patients, for which nothing could be done. This might suggest that Keith was reluctant to refer the simpler—and usually less in need of early correction—defects that Bigelow was looking for.[38] Unbeknownst to Bigelow as he cast about for his first patient, F. John Lewis was completing his own canine research with hypothermia. On September 2, he was first off the mark, executing the world's first successful open-heart operation. Dismayed at losing priority, Bigelow was nevertheless gratified to see his idea transformed into therapy and later operated upon adults using cold.[39]

But Bigelow knew all too well that the meager time purchased by refrigeration seriously limited its utility, leaving the problem of the open-heart largely unsolved.[40] Intrigued by groundhogs, which are good for 3 °C and up to 2 hours of circulatory arrest, Bigelow became absorbed in probing the biology of hibernation.[41] He secured

[35] Bigelow (1984, pp. 42–65).

[36] Bigelow and McBirnie (1953).

[37] Goor (2007, pp. 201–202).

[38] Goor (2007, p. 187).

[39] Bigelow (1984, p. 56) and Waddell et al. (1957).

[40] Goor (2007, p. 202).

[41] Bigelow and McBirnie (1953).

a ready supply of the furry critters by excavating the world's only groundhog farm and mustered a formidable research retinue, including a raft of fellows, technicians, collaborating chemists, physical chemists, physiologists, and pharmacologists. The National Research Council of Canada funded his work (as did the Defense Research Board) and provided direct consultation. Bigelow's team was anything but mom-and-pop, but 10 years of multidisciplinary exertions failed to pry loose the groundhog's secret, ultimately dooming hypothermia's long-term open-heart prospects.[42]

## F. John Lewis: All-in?

One of the best things about Harris Shumacker, Jr.'s *The Evolution of Cardiac Surgery* is its images of physicians, almost all cardiac surgeons, including many of its legends. Of 112 pictures, in 103 the subject is nattily attired in coat and tie (or the equivalent); one sports a tie but no coat; three are in surgical scrubs. Only three are coat and tie-less, but in one a sleek leather vest imparts a soupcon of formality. Arrayed against those of his peers, John Lewis' photograph[43] is a little jarring: Wearing hair longer than the vast majority of his peers and a mustache (also a rarity in surgeons of the era), Lewis had donned only a light-hued mock turtleneck. The picture doesn't lie. As Ake Senning, a contemporary cardiac surgeon, put it, John Lewis was different.[44]

Floyd John Lewis (Fig. 7.1) was born in tiny Waseca, Minnesota in 1916. Pure Gopher, his undergraduate and medical schooling were at the University of Minnesota, as was his surgical training. Owen Wangensteen, famous for his conviction that laboratory research is integral to training academic surgeons, was Minnesota's chief of surgery at the time.[45] Wangensteen also ruthlessly promoted surgical innovation—meaning new procedures of certain risk but uncertain efficacy—executing end-runs around impediments as required. "As a department chairman," he explained to one interviewer, "I have often considered it my responsibility to get around inflexible rules, without meaning. I hesitate to think of how many infractions of rules I have committed during my tenure—but all to the good of my

[42] Bigelow (1984), pp. 66–87. Hypothermia is currently used as an adjunct to cardiopulmonary bypass in neonatal heart surgery, and in select cases of adult cardiac surgery (see Chap. 11). Scientists still puzzle over the biology of hibernation but have probed surprisingly deep into its machinery. For example: Heat and cold are sensed by the skin using "transient receptor potential" channels. The channels primarily involved with the feeling of warmth (TRPV1) are also stimulated by capsaicin, the chemical giving peppers their heat; the TRPM8 channel, which is most relevant to feeling cold, is also activated by menthol (Cerri 2017). If a truly prolonged state of "suspended animation"—several hours—could ever be achieved, might this eventually supplant the pump-oxygenator?

[43] Shumacker (1992, p. 223).

[44] Cooper (2010, p. 116).

[45] Wangensteen (1969).

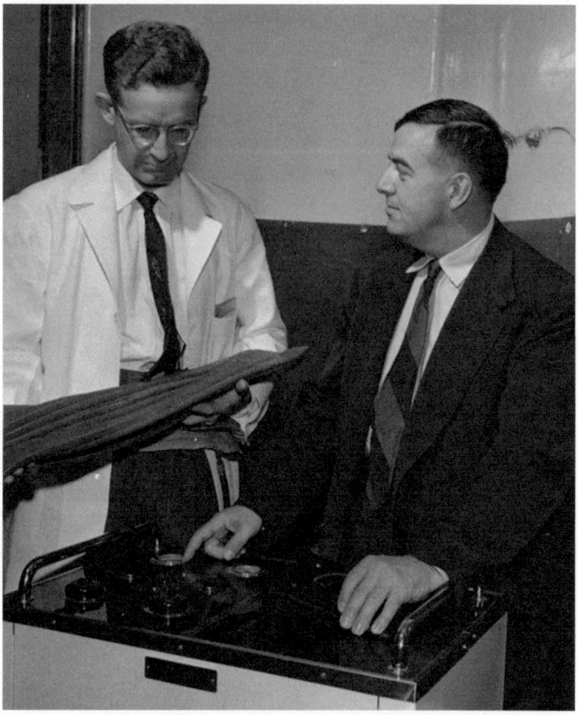

**Fig. 7.1** F. John Lewis (looking a little like Alfred Blalock) and mentor and colleague Richard Varco. (With permission form the University of Minnesota Archives)

men, my department, and the school, I believe."[46] At his residency's end, Lewis signed on as faculty into this environment where imaginative and bold envelope-pushing was encouraged and resolutely supported by the chief.

But Lewis was more of a philosopher—or perhaps better put, an unusually broad and reflective thinker—than a surgeon-cowboy. He generated a list of great books and worked his way through most of them,[47] a flair for quality writing rubbing off along the way. His 1986 speech (discussed below), his *Science in Surgery* (which includes quotes from James B. Conant and Alfred North Whitehead),[48] and a letter to Daniel Goor, a cardiac surgeon who trained with Walt Lillehei at Minnesota, are studded with thought-provoking observations expressed with a taut elegance.[49] At least by retirement (his early and middle years are mostly a blank), Lewis drew, painted, wrote books and essays, and plunked away at the piano. He activated larger muscle groups as well, spending countless hours exercising, hiking, mountain climbing, sailing, and cycling.

What matters most is that he was *historically* different: Lewis, for the very first time, closed a hole in a "dry heart" (Wangensteen's concise gloss) and discharged

46 Olch (1971–1972), p. 63.

47 GW Miller (2000, p. 74).

48 Lewis (1965).

49 Goor (2007, pp. 19–20).

the patient with a pulse. Having heard Bigelow's 1950 talk in Colorado Springs,[50] Lewis soon set about doing the needed laboratory research to apply this concept to humans. In 39 hypothermic dogs, he opened the heart, created an atrial septal defect, then used circulatory arrest to mend the hole days or weeks later. For the last ten who had defect creation, nine survived, with identical numbers for defect closure. Ninety percent survival, Lewis felt, authorized the use of "refrigeration"[51] in a child. Five-year-old Jacqueline Johnson was his first patient, "underdeveloped, sickly" and weighing only 29 and a half pounds, apparently due to an atrial septal defect.[52]

September 2, 1952, was Lewis' day of living nervously. Johnson's temperature plummeted to as low as 26 °C, and her circulation was interrupted for 5½ minutes as Lewis' hands flew, the entire operation taking less than an hour.[53] Jacqueline was discharged after 11 days of uneventful convalescence. The good doctor described his signal feat using only eighteen lines appended to the tail-end of a lab research paper.[54] This breakthrough would have been the first glint of a dazzling career for many another surgeon, but not for Lewis.

He was partly a victim of history's river, of which he took a wrong branch. Concurrent with his early success, C. Walton Lillehei, a colleague and best friend, was fixing to *bypass* the circulation rather than briefly interrupting it. Lillehei's cross-circulation research (discussed later) had begun by late 1952,[55] and in March 1954—by which time Lewis had done only about eleven operations—Lillehei executed his first such operation in a person. Cross-circulation, allowing a much longer interval of open-heart than hypothermia, enabled repair of more complex and consequential malformations. While this stream would soon run dry, at the time it seemed more promising than refrigeration, as least to Wangensteen. William Buckley, an anesthesiologist involved in cross-circulation, recalled that "Lillehei had struck upon a method you could see right away was going to revolutionize the whole field of cardiac surgery. . . . It was clearly recognized that we were doing revolutionary things. I think Lewis saw the handwriting on the wall and realized

[50] GW Miller (2000), Goor (2007), and Stoney (2008, p. 87). However, in an interview with David K.C. Cooper, Lewis recalled that he had heard about hypothermia from a colleague (Cooper 2010, p. 23).

[51] Lewis letter to Wangensteen, September 12, 1952. University of Minnesota Archive. http://gallery.lib.umn.edu/exhibits/show/openheart/item/3214

[52] Cooper (2010, p. 117). "Apparently," as it is unusual for an atrial septal defect to cause this much disability in a child.

[53] Also at the operating table was Richard Varco, an important contributor in open-heart surgery's earliest days (Cooper 2010, pp. 206–212) and Mansur Taufic.

[54] Lewis and Taufic (1953). Lewis interrupted the circulation by ligating the azygos vein, using loops of heavy silk suture to temporarily occlude the superior and inferior vena cava, and clamping the aorta and pulmonary artery. For subsequent operations, the pulmonary veins were also temporarily occluded (Lewis et al. 1954).

[55] A letter dated February 24, 1953, from Lillehei to Sigmamotor, the manufacturer of the pump he used for cross-circulation experiments, indicates that he was engaged in such research by at least late 1952 (University of Minnesota Archives. http://gallery.lib.umn.edu/exhibits/show/openheart/item/3228)

ultimately that the track that he was on was not going to lead to anything lasting." Wangensteen saw the same and diverted most of Lewis' research funding to Lillehei.[56] In theory, Lewis could have redirected his efforts to the just emerging cardiopulmonary bypass surgery, but one hardly imagines that there was room for these two—even if best friends—occupying the same space in the same outfit.

Chemistry and the politics it influences also percolated underfoot. Wangensteen was extraordinarily close to Lillehei—his protégé was like a son to him—which must have influenced how Wangensteen partitioned resources and other support between the two.[57] And Lewis put people off. Daniel Goor, one of Lillehei's trainees beginning in 1965 (so rendering his observation second hand), wrote that Lewis had become bitter, often making sarcastic comments about members of the surgery department, including Wangensteen.[58] He didn't suffer fools gladly and was hard for most anyone to get close to. Surgeon Norman Shumway, a highly accomplished heart transplant surgeon and Lewis protégée, wrote that Lewis was his "mentor and inspiration," but that no one knew him even well enough to call him "F"; he also wrote that Lewis "could not tolerate second rate individuals or dilettantes in medicine . . . [which] did not help his career to say the least."[59] A man apart, Lewis had little talent for team building.[60] Thomas Starzl, the famous liver transplant surgeon who trained at Northwestern during Lewis' tenure, wrote that Lewis' "stiletto thrusts [delivered at conferences] were remembered with a smile long after by his friends, and brooded over permanently by the victims."[61] At one point he cut anesthesiologists out of his procedures: "Lewis would put in the arterial and venous lines, administer some thiopental and curare . . . intubate the patient, connect the patient to his homemade respirator, then go out to scrub."[62]

It was perhaps inevitable that his wings would get clipped. Lewis was "booted out by Wangensteen"[63] in 1955 to St. Paul's Ancker Hospital, where he served as

---

[56] Goor (2007, p. 212).

[57] Goor (2007, p. 61), GW Miller (2000, pp. 217–218). A letter from Wangensteen to Richard Varco (Sept. 10, 1952) indicated Wangensteen's support for Lewis doing more open-heart cases, but a letter from Lewis to Wangensteen on July 30, 1953, indicates that Wangensteen had recently denied Lewis permission to do open-hearts (University of Minnesota Archives. http://gallery.lib.umn.edu/exhibits/show/openheart/cold/operative-first)

[58] Goor (2007, p. 212–213).

[59] Shumway (1996, 1999).

[60] Cooper (2010, pp. 125–126).

[61] Starzl (1992, p. 60).

[62] Shumway (1996).

[63] Goor (2007, p. 213).

director of postgraduate surgical education.[64] Escaping this backwater in 1957,[65] he moved to Northwestern University Medical School, expecting to 1 day ascend to the chair of surgery. This promotion was never in the cards, nor even many more dry hearts. His second patient in Chicago died, the victim of an incomplete diagnosis. Compounding this disaster, the child's father was a prominent Chicago banker. He soon drifted out of surgery and into biomedical engineering. Lewis achieved some success in that domain, playing a major role in establishing the country's first biomedical engineering department,[66] but was "fairly chronically dissatisfied"[67] and resigned from Northwestern in 1976 at age 60.[68] Lewis moved to Santa Barbara, California,[69] where he died on September 20, 1993.

Why is John Lewis more than a footnote but less than a chapter in congenital cardiology? History's stream didn't drown Lewis; he was easily intelligent and skilled enough to tackle cardiopulmonary bypass surgery, should he have tried. Nor Wangensteen's preference for Lillehei stopped other open-heart frontiersmen build fine programs elsewhere. Minnesota was an incubator non-pareil for open-heart surgery in the 1950s, but not unique; Denver, Houston, and other cities were hard on Midwestern heals. John Kirklin, for example, left the Mayo Clinic in 1966 to build a leading open-heart program at the University of Alabama at Birmingham, no one's idea of a medical mecca at the time.[70] And if Lewis' acerbic style didn't lubricate gears, neither did it freeze them. From before Galen to Lavoisier to now, history is replete with trenchant and aloof but indelible personalities. Lewis *was* hobbled by his lack of aptitude for team building, since attracting patient referrals and entraining a supporting cast were needed to scale up his initial success. But I decipher this career interrupted as being the product of a deeper imperfection. As for many of us, Lewis' oeuvre was largely the issue of the strength of his belief in his work and in himself. It seems to me that he didn't *believe in* surgery, at least not enough, to be *all-in*. Not enough to force his way forward, whatever the obstacles, not enough to

[64] Many letters (in the University of Minnesota surgical archives) between Lewis and Wangensteen after John's having left Minneapolis reveal a cordial and even warm relationship on both sides; in fact, Wangensteen on multiple occasions invited Lewis to stay with his family when in town. Lewis, for his part, often solicited advice from his former mentor and boss—usually regarding job prospects—and appears to have genuinely appreciated the advice proffered. These letters do not suggest personal animosity as a reason that Wangensteen pushed Lewis out of the University.

[65] Miller states that it was the deaths of two patients with ventricular septal defects in Minnesota that led to Lewis' defecting from cardiac surgery (GW Miller 2000, pp. 112–113), but if Cooper is correct, Lewis was still doing at least some cardiac surgery after he left Minnesota.

[66] Preston (1994)

[67] Goor (2007, p. 213). Lewis' letter to Wangensteen on June 29, 1960, indicated that he was doing no general and very little cardiac surgery, partly because his hospital (Passavant) had no pediatric service. Other letters suggest that his days were mostly occupied by laboratory research.

[68] Goor (2007, p. 214).

[69] Cooper says that it was in the spring of 1977, at age 59, that he moved to California (Cooper 2010 p. 127); Preston states that Lewis moved to Santa Barbara at age 61 (Preston 1994).

[70] Roberts (1998).

insist that he have his way—and that this lack of perfect commitment was rooted in John Lewis being uncomfortable in his own skin.

In October 1988, Lewis spoke at the C. Walton Lillehei Surgical Symposium in Minneapolis, one of those present at the creation who shared recollections of open-heart surgery aborning. The speeches were the usual fare—history via anecdote with occasional references to the symposium's honoree. Lewis' was different. Subtle and allusive, it rewards the careful eye; every word demands attention. He offered anecdotes, in the guise of an "imagined" rather than a named surgeon. The imaginary surgeon[71] was "Not Walt, but perhaps someone like him and the way we were back then."[72] Lewis was thoughtful and introspective, self-critical, and skeptical. "Beyond its sound and enduring technical center, surgery (acquired) a scientific *patina*" (my emphasis); the imaginary surgeon "helped train enough surgeons to perform about twice as many [operations of various kinds] as were actually needed"; "A type of ambiguous ethics was built into his work, but the medical ethicist who was to build an edifice to these soft, plastic, philosophic bricks came much later. Do not get nervous, friend; only a creative spirit drives technique and action."[73] Unnecessary surgery and innovation unfettered by ethical constraints? You seldom hear this kind of talk out of the mouths of surgeons, especially at a festschrift honoring one of its most aggressive practitioners. This could be a man who eventually soured on his profession; Shumway speculated that Lewis was predestined to become somewhat disillusioned with surgery.[74] But maybe, in his deepest unconscious recess, he was *never* truly comfortable with his métier.[75]

David K.C. Cooper interviewed Lewis in 1990 and concluded that he had lost interest in medicine long before retirement, noting that Lewis' autobiography[76] confessed that he was never suited to a surgical career.[77] Lewis stated that he chose medicine because "this was the only science that I could think of at that time. It didn't occur to me that I could become a physicist or chemist. . . . I sometimes wish

---

[71] Goor surmises that the "surgeon" is Wangensteen, but this is surely incorrect; the illusory "surgeon" must be Lewis and Lillehei.

[72] Goor (2007, p. 214).

[73] Lewis (1989).

[74] Shumway (1996), Goor (2007, p. 220), and Cooper (2010, pp. 117–118, 130).

[75] Unhappy at Northwestern, Lewis appealed to Wangensteen to help him find another job. Despite heroic efforts, Wangensteen was unsuccessful, for the reason he offered to Lewis in his letter of October 18, 1960: "I have enquired, of men in institutions where you visited and where you were looked upon as a potential candidate, why they did not select you. Almost invariably, an answer like this was forthcoming. Members of the faculty who saw you believed that you joked about everything and were serious about nothing." In letter of reply (October 21, 1960), Lewis admitted that his wife and a couple of friends concurred with this observation. In another letter, Wangensteen offered Lewis this advice for a job-hunting visit to Salt Lake City: "[M]ay I suggest that you exhibit real and an unfeigned enthusiasm for the position" (November 2, 1965). (Letters from the University of Minnesota surgical archives).

[76] Lewis' autobiography was apparently never published, but he gave Cooper a copy of the manuscript.

[77] Cooper (2010, p. 130).

that I had followed in that [physics] direction." He said that if he had it to do over again, he would live a different kind of life.[78] The contrast with other founders of cardiac surgery could not be starker. Charles Bailey "would repeatedly state that it was his 'Christian duty' to offer surgical solutions to endless, hopeless conditions. He was actually a missionary cardiac surgeon."[79] We soon see that Walt Lillehei was nearly as zealous. Even less fervid surgeons displayed formidable resolve and persistence. Gross's first ductal ligation despite his boss's explicit (and professionally dangerous) opposition, and Blalock's hazarding case after high-risk case (nearly one fourth of his first hundred patients died)[80] were *all-in*, exemplified. Perhaps the philosopher in Lewis found surgery a little too messy to be so committed, but I suggest that there is a better explanation.

Lewis was a battalion third surgeon in the 3rd Infantry Division. He claimed that "I never did too well in the army," and that the army was "mostly a terrible bore and altogether it was a bad experience. . . . [I]t was, in a way, a shameful time of life."[81] What he *didn't* mention was that having been inducted as a first lieutenant he was discharged as a captain, awarded three Bronze Stars, the Combat Medical Badge, and the Victory Ribbon.[82] Why? Sheer modesty? Was Lewis, like many another vet, disinclined to share his war experiences? Or, as I believe more likely, too uncomfortable in his own skin to be proud? Lewis was perpetually engaged in efforts at self-improvement, perhaps belying, Cooper muses, deep-seated feelings of inadequacy.[83] His exertions at writing books (mostly unpublished), at painting, at piano playing confirmed, to Lewis, that he was only a "duffer."[84] Like some people aching to run away from their stationary life, Lewis engaged in a great deal of physical activity. "If I keep [working out], maybe I'll be in great shape about the time I have reached the end of my mortal rope—a *bizarre, wrinkled, well-muscled specimen*."[85] This sorry imagined image of Lewis, by Lewis, suggests that he was only marginally endowed with a key requirement for a successful surgeon, especially one living on the frontier—a powerful ego. Whether my unlicensed mechanistic analysis is correct or not, it seems clear that Lewis represents a different psychological breed than the innovators we've admired up until now.

Lewis refrigerated first, but Henry Swan II refrigerated most famously. Son of a prominent Colorado family, Swan went East for school,[86] returned home to practice, and was recruited to the University of Colorado School of Medicine in 1946 as its

[78] Cooper (2010, pp. 121, 128).

[79] Goor (2007, p. 159).

[80] Harmel and Lamont (1946).

[81] Cooper (2010, pp. 121–122).

[82] Preston (1994).

[83] Cooper (2010, p. 129).

[84] Cooper (2010, p. 218).

[85] Cooper (2010, p. 130); emphasis mine.

[86] Prep school at Philips Exeter Academy, undergraduate at Williams College, medical school at Harvard, and residency at Boston's Peter Bent Brigham and Boston Children's Hospitals (National Library of Medicine, Henry Swan).

first full-time surgical faculty member. He flew to the chief of surgery (1950) but was a hapless aviator. His *New York Times* biographer (Robert McG. Thomas) noted that "[Swan] became easy to spot at medical conferences. He would be the one wearing a cast on one body part or the another, colleagues said, the result of one of the three air crashes he survived."[87] His aerial mishaps were the stuff of endemic gossip in the surgical community.[88] In a letter of remembrance in *Annals of Thoracic Surgery*, a surgeon friend deadpanned that Swan "had a reputation *non pareil* in small plane aviation."[89] (The Civil Aeronautics Board eventually revoked Swan's license).[90]

Like Lewis, Swan's immersion in hypothermia began with Bigelow's Colorado Springs talk. Also like Lewis, he swiftly commenced laboratory research, eventually studying over 300 dogs.[91] Swan's first human open-heart operation—the eight-year-old boy was cooled in a tub of ice—was performed in February 1953.[92] By 1956, he had done 111 operations,[93] and 265 by 1958,[94] as compared to Lewis' 65.[95] The sheer volume of surgery only partly explains Swan's celebrity; like other pioneers we've encountered, he was a showman. In 1955, the Colorado State Medical Society received a complaint about "recent personal publicity of Henry Swan II. M.D." The medical society found no breech of medical ethics, though it allowed that "opinions as to the good taste and propriety of the articles under discussion would vary tremendously among different segments of our population."[96] As had happened in Blalock's Baltimore, doctors world-wide came to Denver lay their own eyes on an eerie scene: patients etherized, *and frigid*, upon a table.

But hypothermia's trajectory was different than that of cardiopulmonary bypass. The latter still orbits, while hypothermia described a parabola which plummeted back to earth hardly a decade after launch. Swan rode that curve higher than anyone else, but with his dismissal as chairman in 1961, his surgery quickly came to ground.[97] But this was of little consequence: Cardiopulmonary bypass had largely eclipsed hypothermia, with or without Henry Swan. The field had moved on.

---

[87] *The New York Times*, Aug. 4, 1996, p. 41.

[88] Goor (2007, p. 229).

[89] Rainer (1996).

[90] Letter from Lyman A. Brewer, III, MD to Bruce C. Paton, MD, dated April 29, 1982, in Henry Swan Papers, U.S. National Library of Medicine, accessed February 3, 2020.

[91] Cooper (2010, p. 135).

[92] Swan (1953).

[93] Swan and Blount (1956).

[94] Swan (1958).

[95] Lewis (1958).

[96] Letter to Henry Swan from Harold E. Haymond, M.D., Chairman of the Board of Supervisors, Colorado State Medical Society, February 22, 1955 (National Library of Medicine, Henry Swan).

[97] Why Swan was fired as chief is murky. His fight with the dean over money was presumably relevant (Goor 2007, pp. 232–233; Cooper 2010, pp. 139–140). Tom Starzl (a surgeon who had arrived in Denver over a year after the firing) speculated—presumably on the basis of $n^{th}$ hand information—that the rupture was due to marital troubles affecting Swan's reputation, com-

The first successful open-heart procedure used hypothermia to briefly escape the need for an interrupted flow of blood, but the idea that a machine might temporarily *substitute* for the heart and lungs predates refrigeration. The concept of pumping blood or other fluids into a part of the body to sustain its function dates back at least to LeGallois in the early eighteenth century. In the mid-nineteenth century, Charles Edouard Brown-Sequard weirdly demonstrated artificial perfusion's potential by pumping his own blood into the arm of a dead prisoner, activating the stiffened muscle.[98] Russian Sergei Brukhonenko performed an even more macabre experiment, preserved in a stark 1940 Soviet Film Agency movie narrated by J.B.S. Haldane, a highly respected British physiologist who witnessed some of the experiments. A dog's severed head is kept alive by bubble-oxygenating venous blood taken from the head, then pumping it back. It responds to light and sound and licks a citric acid solution daubed to its mouth. In mock response, George Bernard Shaw's (an ardent antivivisectionist) take on the isolated dog head: "I am greatly tempted to have my head cut off so that I can continue to dictate plays and books independently of any illness, without having to dress and undress or eat or do anything at all but to produce masterpieces of dramatic art and literature."[99] Also, another dog by Brukhonenko was bled dry and dead for 10 minutes, revived using a heart-lung machine; a few days later, it is as animated and happy as any other dog on the planet.[100] Brukhonenko applied for a patent for his heart-lung machine in 1936, though it was never used clinically. Brukhonenko suffered an unfortunate fate: His papers were mostly published in obscure journals; he was ignored, and his impact on the problem of open-heart surgery was minor.[101]

Charles Lindbergh—famous for his trans-Atlantic flight and infamous for his controversial politics—had envisioned mechanical circulatory support for open-heart surgery in 1929. (His sister-in-law needed repair of a faulty heart valve.) He approached Alexis Carrel (see Chap. 4), hoping to pursue this in his Rockefeller laboratory, but Carrel deflected Lindbergh onto the simpler problem of tissue perfusion.[102] These—and many other—similar ideas and exercises[103] were like fifty chicks pecking once at their shell. What it took to hatch cardiopulmonary bypass was one chick pecking fifty times. John H. Gibbon, Jr. (Fig. 7.2) was that chick.

In February of 1931, a middle-aged woman recovering from gall bladder surgery threw a blood clot into her lungs. Large clots can kill, but clot-removal operations were perilous, and her surgeon (Edward Churchill) hoped that she might squeak by.

---

pounded by erratic behavior, culminating in Swan's (once) diverting an insurance payment from the hospital to himself (Cooper 2010, pp. 139–140). Regardless of the why, it was a sad finish for the man who took Colorado's department of surgery from nowhere to one of the best-regarded in the country.

[98] Shumacker (1992, pp. 243–248).

[99] Krementsov (2009).

[100] Konstantinov and Alexi-Meskishvili (2000) and Krementsov (2009).

[101] Konstantinov and Alexi-Meskishvili (2000).

[102] Dennis (1989).

[103] Shumacker (1992, pp. 243–248).

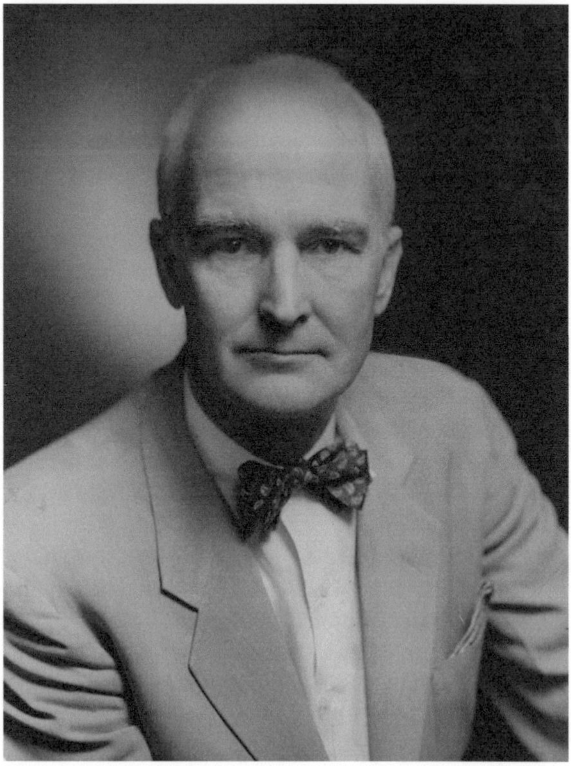

**Fig. 7.2** John H. Gibbons MD. (Courtesy of the Siegman Archives at Thomas Jefferson University, Philadelphia)

Gibbon, then a surgical research fellow at the Massachusetts General Hospital, was dispatched by Churchill to the operating room and fixed at her side for fifteen excruciating hours, taking and recording her pulse, respirations, and blood pressure every 15 minutes. Just as her pulse finally gave up, Churchill slash-opened her chest, removed the clot, and clamp-closed the pulmonary artery incision, all in "6 minutes and 30 seconds." But his lightening clot extraction was too late. That long night ended with the woman's death, but also with the birth of an idea for Gibbon: He imagined that with a cardiorespiratory support device he could have saved her life.[104] If hardly new, this time the idea found a tenacious host. For Gibbon, the problem of cardiopulmonary bypass was "constantly in the back of my mind" for the next 3 years.[105] And he was not alone—heart-lung bypass was in the air in the late 1940s. Clarence Dennis and colleagues at the University of Minnesota had commenced similar work, as had groups in Europe.[106] Only a few years later, yet more surgeons were bent on inventing devices of their own.

---

[104] Gibbon (1978) and Romaine-Davis (1991, pp. 21–22).

[105] Gibbon (1978).

[106] Johnson (1970, pp. 145–146) and Dennis (1989).

Gibbon's quest began in 1934 at the Massachusetts General Hospital, later continuing at the University of Pennsylvania, and finally at Philadelphia's Jefferson Medical College.[107] As we note in Appendix 4, inventing a safe and effective pump-oxygenator was largely a problem of *interface*, especially with one of the body's most important tissues—blood. The knottiest problem was oxygenating venous blood and simultaneously removing carbon dioxide, while leaving the red blood cells intact. Nature has evolved a magnificent solution: a network of miniscule blood vessels (capillaries) forming a dense network around tiny air sacs (alveoli) in the lungs. Oxygen diffuses from the air into the blood, and carbon dioxide vice versa, over an enormous surface area—140 m$^2$, or 70% of a singles tennis court.[108] Today, "membrane" oxygenators work on the same principle, but this technology was unavailable in Gibbon's day. Blowing tiny air bubbles through blood is an obvious solution, but foaming and residual bubbles (which block small blood vessels) proved a daunting problem until anti-foaming agents were developed. Gibbon sprayed venous blood onto a vertical rotating drum, the thin blood film exchanging gas with oxygen blown past. This worked well-enough for cat-sized flows, but it provided too little for a human.

Twelve years after he had started pecking, Gibbon hit a wall. He had built a promising device but one still not ready to run, primarily because of the oxygenator. But he got lucky. Thanks to a freshman medical student at Jefferson, he was given entrée into IBM, met with its Director of Research, and shared with him the exciting work completed thus far.[109] The director and Thomas Watson, Sr., the redoubtable chairman of IBM's board, were suitably impressed and made a major commitment to the Philadelphia team. IBM engineers were heavily engaged with the project from 1946 through 1954, and the company eventually built three progressively more refined iterations of a pump-oxygenator. The Model III was built at a cost of approximately \$79,650 in 1954 (\$766,000 in 2020 dollars).[110] General Motors also joined the open-heart crowd, building pumps for Forest Dodrill, a surgeon at Detroit's Harper Hospital.[111]

Gibbon and his engineer partners eventually sent blood down batteries of screens, which increased the surface area and added turbulence, enhancing gas exchange, and overcoming flow limitations. The oxygenator and circuit were designed to avoid

---

[107] As was the case for Blalock and Bigelow, multiple people not so well known as Gibbon played important roles in the heart-lung machine's development, including his wife Maly; in fact, Gibbon's actual hands-on contribution is easily exaggerated (Cooper 2010, pp. 155–161; Goor 2007, p. 173). For the technical history of Gibbon's pump-oxygenator, see Romaine-Davis (1991) and Gibbon (1978).

[108] Knudsen and Ochs (2018).

[109] Gibbon (1978).

[110] Romaine-Davis (1991, pp. 69–137).

[111] GM built four pumps for partial bypass for open-heart operations for Detroit's Harper Hospital between 1951 and 1956; the first operation was done in 1952. An oxygenator was added in 1954. The pumps bear a striking resemblance to auto engines, although not to the V-12 variety, which they have nevertheless been likened to (Steinquist 2018; Dodrill and Gerisch 1952).

injuring fragile red blood cells. They concocted a way to carefully control the rate of blood withdrawal, lest the wall of the vena cava (from which the blood was drawn) be sucked into the cannula. Dogs died of multiple emboli until a metal filter was added. Feedback devices were invented to monitor and adjust pressures and flows, and pH measurements were used to adjust the flow of carbon dioxide into the oxygenator. To keep the blood warm, the works were enclosed in a temperature-controlled box. Later iterations included a nitrogen-pressurized cabinet to exclude explosive anesthetic gasses.

Gibbon's first patient was a 15-month-old girl thought to have an atrial septal defect (February 1952). One can imagine this operator's sinking feeling when, having opened atrium, he found that the septum was…*intact*. The stress of cardiac surgery, especially with a weakened heart, is mitigated by the beneficial effect of repair, but if nothing is fixed, the patient is even more precarious after operation than before. Gibbon's patient died, and a patent ductus was discovered at post-mortem. His next patient, an 18-year-old woman *with* an atrial defect, was the world's first to survive an open-heart operation on cardiopulmonary bypass (May 6, 1953). After two deaths in July, Gibbon put open-hearts on hold for a year, but after the moratorium ended and yet another death, he abandoned cardiac surgery for good.[112] Why the abrupt exit after finally reaching his goal? Some say that was Gibbon's plan from the start—create the device but leave the operations to others.[113] But many felt that Gibbon just wasn't tough enough to deal with the deaths which were inevitable at this primitive stage of the game, and that he quit discouraged. Gibbon[114] was an all-in surgeon, but not an all-in *cardiac* surgeon.[115]

Gibbon's post-cardiac career was devoted to thoracic surgery, teaching, and administration. He spent so much time on the road giving lectures and serving in professional organizations that in Philadelphia he acquired the sobriquet "the visiting professor."[116] Despite his turning his back on heart surgery, and the fact that others more forcefully enhanced the field, Gibbon received enviable recognition for this work, including the 1968 Lasker Prize. Gibbon retired in 1967 as head of the Department of Surgery at Jefferson Medical College and Hospital. His handling of

---

[112] Gibbon had become a founding member of the club of early cardiac surgeons bedeviled by inaccurate or incomplete diagnoses. As we've seen, Blalock and Lewis were so afflicted, as was Clarence Dennis, whose attempt at bypass surgery predated Gibbon's but failed due to an inaccurate diagnosis (Dennis et al. 1951; Jepson et al. 2017). One of the two patients had an incomplete diagnosis: There was a ventricular septal defect in addition to an atrial septal defect (Romaine-David 1991, p. 130). Gibbon did a total of six open-heart cases with only one survivor (Lillehei in Arensman and Comish 1993 pp. 11–12).

[113] Shumacker (1999, pp. 180–181, 216) and Romaine-Davis (1991, p. 144).

[114] Lillehei and Kirklin both visited Jesse Edwards, then the world's most expert congenital cardiac pathologist, to learn the structure of their patient's heart defects as they embarked upon open-heart operations (Frye 2015, pp. 208, 213), but apparently Gibbon made no such effort to refine his appreciation of cardiac malformations (Cooper 2010, p. 154).

[115] Shumacker (1999, p. 9), Johnson (1970, p. 149), Goor (2007, pp. 174–175), Cooper (2010, pp. 154, 157, 209), Stoney (2008, p. 90), Romaine-Davis (1991, pp. 143–144) and Kirklin (1989).

[116] Romaine-Davis (1991, p. 146).

his own heart disease may offer a précis of his reservations about cardiac surgery. Suffering a myocardial infarction in July 1972 and anginal episodes afterwards, despite repeated entreaties from friends he declined to seek a coronary artery bypass. He died February 5, 1973, at age 69, of an acute infarction while playing tennis with his wife Maly (Fig. 7.3).[117]

Gibbon wasn't the first to connect a pump-oxygenator to a human. Clarence Dennis was the first to hazard an intracardiac repair using a similar machine (April 1951). Incising the heart of a 6 year old girl thought to have an atrial septal defect, he was chagrined to find a more complex malformation, and his patient succumbed to an inadequate repair.[118] The "pump" was first *successfully* used by Turin's Mario

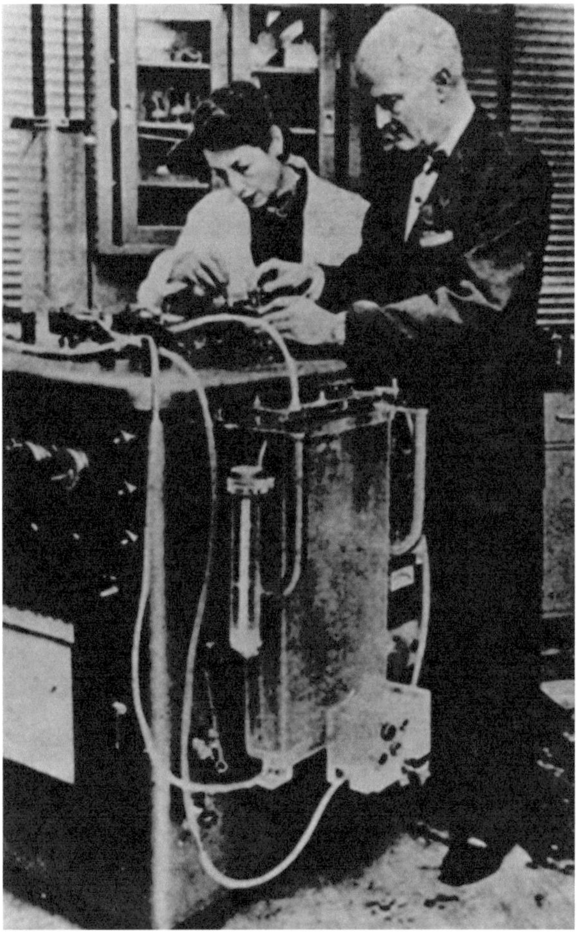

**Fig. 7.3** John and Mary Gibbon with an early cardiopulmonary pump. With permission from the Seignam Archives at Thomas Jefferson University, Philadelphia, PA, USA

[117] Shumacker (1999, pp. 277–279).

[118] Dennis et al. (1951), Lillehei (1982), Jepson et al. (2017), Goor (2007, p. 186), and Shumacker (1992, p. 255).

Dogliotti in August 1951 when he used cardiopulmonary bypass, not to repair a defective heart, but while resecting a large mediastinal tumor.[119] By 1952, Gibbon and Dennis had promising devices but discouraging results, and neither promoted their work.[120] In fact, there wasn't much for them or anyone else *to* promote. Between 1951 and early 1954, 18 cardiopulmonary bypass cases were reported, with only one survivor.[121] John Lewis had had success using refrigeration but wasn't much into horn-blowing either. As we have learned, Henry Swan eventually achieved international renown for his hypothermic repairs, but he was only beginning to gather steam in early 1953. Besides, hypothermia was mostly good for defects that usually produce symptoms only relatively late in life. More interesting malformations, desperate for early repair—such as large ventricular septal defects and tetralogy of Fallot—require more time to fix than hypothermia affords. Despite widespread interest and ingenious effort on both sides of the Atlantic, cardiac surgery was only slowing creeping up to operating temperature by the winter of 1954. But that was soon to change. Between March 1954 and May 1955, Walt Lillehei (Fig. 7.4) turned up the burner and open-heart surgery rose to a full boil.

Born in 1918, the eventual "father of open-heart surgery"[122] had a pretty conventional upper-middle class upbringing. His dad, a prosperous dentist, and his mother, a nurse, raised their son in Edina, an upscale Minneapolis suburb. Lillehei was precocious.[123] He could read better than his grade school peers and liked to; he entered

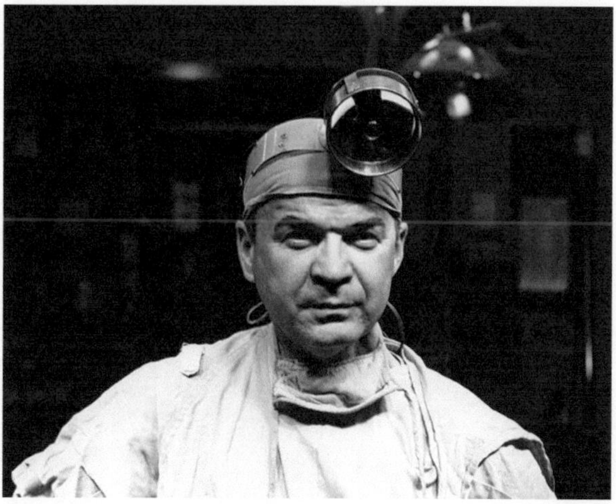

**Fig. 7.4** C. Walton Lillehei. (With permission from the University of Minnesota Archives)

[119] Shumaker (1992, p. 255).

[120] Dennis (1989) and Goor (2007, pp. 172, 180–181).

[121] Arensman and Comish (1993, pp. 11–12).

[122] Cooley (1999).

[123] GW Miller (2000), Goor (2007, pp. 47–63), Stoney (2008, pp. 83–87) and Cooper (2010, pp.182–184).

college before his 16th year. And blessed with superior mechanical intuition, if converting a BB gun to 22-caliber in junior high school and cobbling a functioning motorcycle out of a jumble of parts serve as reliable evidence. And, most notably, he was endowed with a self-formulated and tenacious sense of right and wrong. His biographer, G. Wayne Miller, writes of the time in high school when Lillehei crashed his Ford Model T while trying to use inertia to fling a recalcitrant friend off its running board. Ten years later, while an army captain in Oran, Lillehei expropriated an American Military Police truck, surrendering it only after an MP in a speeding jeep pulled alongside and pointed his .45 at him. "I didn't necessarily believe in signs that said, 'don't do this or don't do that,'" Lillehei told Miller, "If I had a reason to do it, I usually did."[124] We've seen pioneers with a surfeit of drive and persistence in the previous chapters, but none with Lillehei's disregard for the rules of the road, or the opprobrium of peers. Lest one form the impression that he was some sort of sociopathic bogey—nothing could be further from the truth. Lillehei was warm and friendly, and extraordinarily good with his patients. He happily performed operations pro bono for the impecunious and was generous in other ways. But there was a corner of his psyche refractory to important (i.e., promoting self-survival) external signals. Lillehei's immunity from self-doubt greatly leveraged his uncanny inventive bent, but his self-insulation from certain social norms eventually proved troublesome. Innumerable anecdotes indicate Lillehei's disregard for rules and convention, not just for medical dogma, for example: He drove for 12 months without a driver's license after his was revoked, and he freed other investigators' dogs from their cages so that he could use the cages for his own animals. Lillehei surreptitiously cleaned out the contents of his laboratory—including equipment owned by the University—before leaving for his new position at Cornell and had the gall to leave a red rose on the naked floor. Anesthesiologist and colleague Joseph Buckley quoted Lillehei: "What others think is not important. I just do it." And Walt's brother Richard recollected that "Walt was always in trouble. . . . [H]e never did the thing that was expected of him."[125]

The University of Minnesota was Lillehei's choice for college and medical school, after which he served nearly four army years in North Africa and Italy. Enlisting (along with his friend John Lewis) in the reserves in 1942, more for adventure than patriotic expression, Lillehei found plenty of the former, as he later (unlike Lewis) dilated upon at length.[126] After being discharged as a lieutenant colonel with multiple commendations—a Bronze Star, a Bronze Arrowhead, and a European Theater Ribbon with five battle stars[127]—he commenced training under Wangensteen (October 1945). Like Alfred Blalock, at the tail end of his training (1950), Lillehei developed a potentially lethal illness. A parotid lymphosarcoma was discovered,

[124] GW Miller (2000, p. 22) and Goor (2007, pp. 54–55, 126).

[125] Goor (2007, pp. 126–127) and GW Miller (2000, p. 202).

[126] Goor (2007, pp. 52–57), Stoney (2008, pp. 83–86).

[127] GW Miller (2000, p. 28).

and with it dismal prospects for survival.[128] The tumor and suspicious tissue extending from his head into his chest was resected, no holds barred, by a seven-surgeon team, including Wangensteen and Lewis. Lillehei's recuperation consumed a miserable 4 months, but against considerable odds he never suffered any recurrence.[129] Vincent Gott, later one of Lillehei's residents, sensed that he—like Blalock—was driven by his possibly limited time to chisel his mark.[130]

Closed-heart and general surgery occupied Lillehei's clinical time as a fledgling faculty member. His laboratory work was mainly cardiovascular—studying physiological and other effects of experimental arteriovenous fistulas (a side-to-side connection of an artery to the adjacent vein). In March 1951, Lillehei and his family motored off on a busman's holiday, visiting most of the brain trust of early US heart surgeons.[131] While his career was already strongly inclined in cardiac surgery's direction, it was Dorothy Eustice, a patient with an atrial septal defect, mitral stenosis, and severe heart failure who finally froze its arc. Lillehei met Dorothy during one of her many hospitalizations and was immediately taken with this unfortunate young woman, bedridden and fragile, yet undefeated and quietly full of life. Lillehei got to know Dorothy over the course of subsequent admissions and inspected her flawed pump shortly after she died.[132] If only he could have opened Dorothy's heart, Lillehei mused, he could have saved her, fixing the arc of his career from that point on.[133]

Lillehei thought the same as other would-be open-heart surgeons at the time,[134] but also differently. Like everybody else, he aimed to open the heart long enough for lengthy repairs, but he was skeptical of cardiopulmonary bypass, at least that currently available. Present at Clarence Dennis' first operation, Lillehei was dismayed by the behemoth of a bypass machine and the village (16 people) needed to run it. He developed "a 'gut feeling' that many of the problems of extracorporeal circulation had to be related to the enormous complexity of the equipment and methods that had evolved."[135] While casting about for a simpler strategy, a surprising new discovery—the azygous flow concept (or principle)—radically changed the way

[128] Goor, on the basis of a communication with Dr. James Plath at the Mayo Clinic, states that reexamination of the tissue at the Clinic in the early 1980s indicated that it was actually benign, revealing only atypical inflammation (Goor 2007, p. 62). But the diagnosis of malignancy had been confirmed at four different pathology labs in 1950 (GW Miller 2000, pp. 35–36).

[129] GW Miller (2000, pp. 41–47).

[130] Fye (2015, p. 212).

[131] GW Miller (2000, pp. 49–57) and Goor (2007, p. 62).

[132] Cooper (2010, p. 185).

[133] This is Miller's impression of Lillehei's confirming heart surgery as a career (GW Miller 2000, pp. 62–64), but his research, road trip, study of dead hearts (including off-hours at autopsy), and the existing atmosphere at Minnesota suggest that his cardiac career was pretty much set by the time he met Eustice.

[134] Shumacker (1992, pp. 266–267), Fye (2015, p. 204), Lillehei (1982) and Arensman and Comish (1993, pp. 9–30).

[135] Lillehei (1982).

Lillehei thought about bypass. The concept is simple: Organ function (especially the brain's) can be preserved for at least 30 minutes with blood flow only a fraction (roughly ten percent) of normal.[136] Conventional wisdom had had it that something close to normal cardiac output was needed, which—as we saw with Gibbons' oxygenator struggles—complicated inventing a suitable bypass circuit. Delivering lower flow would technically be advantageous by reducing the amount of blood leaking into the heart from its own veins on bypass. Lillehei saw this as "the sword that would eventually sever the Gordian Knot of complexity that had garroted perfusion technology"; others were less convinced.[137]

How might one exploit low flow? Lillehei imagined: Connect a tube to the azygous vein and pump its blood through a lobe of the lung (for oxygenation and carbon dioxide removal), then retrieve the oxygenated blood from a pulmonary vein and pump it into the aorta. When his collaborators—surgical residents Morley Cohen and Herbert Warden, and Richard DeWall (of which more later)[138]—tried this in dogs, it worked when everything was perfectly aligned. But the circuit was prone to kinking, and when lung outflow was impeded, it filled with fluid. There was too little space in the open chest for a reliable circuit. While grappling with this fickle setup, Lillehei's team tumbled to the idea that they needed something akin to an artificial placenta for gas exchange: rather than working with a lung in the narrow confines of the chest, direct the venous blood to a gas-exchanger outside the body. Where the idea of an ersatz placenta originated depends upon whom you read. Morley Cohen thought it was probably his; Miller attributes it to Herb Warden; Richard DeWall thought it was more-or-less a corporate notion; Lillehei makes no specific attribution.[139] This was exactly what Gibbon and others hoped to do, except that Lillehei was thinking low flow and a biological rather than mechanical oxygenator. This idea, already tried elsewhere,[140] quickly morphed into "cross-circulation," where one dog serves as the oxygenator for venous blood taken from a second dog on bypass. Lillehei had intended to use this only as an interim measure to gain experience with open-heart surgery pending the arrival of suitable mechanical equipment, but found that dogs so supported survived more often, and recovered more quickly, than those on Dennis' machine. The donor dog somehow corrected abnormalities—metabolic or other—induced by an artificial circuit. "The differences were truly astonishing, and for the first time the thought entered my mind that this might be the simple clinical method for which we were searching."[141]

Cross-circulation was studied and perfected over 2 years, using hundreds of dogs. Lillehei even cross-circulated skilled hunting dogs, assessing their moves

---

[136] Lillehei (1982) and Cooper (2010, p. 186).

[137] Arensman and Comish (1993, p. 13) and Weisse (2002, pp. 98–99).

[138] DeWall (2011), Cooper (2010, pp. 185–187), Stoney (2008, pp. 100–111).

[139] Cooper (2010, p. 186), GW Miller (2000, p. 91), DeWall in Stoney (2008, p. 103), Goor (2007, p. 23) and Lillehei (1982).

[140] Lillehei et al. (1955a, b, *Surgery, Gynecology & Obstetrics*) and Shumacker (1992, pp. 256–265).

[141] Lillehei (1982, p. 9).

after recovery to be certain that they had lost none of their edge.[142] And he knew that opening the heart was only the prelude—what he did inside was where the rubber would hit the road. It's hard to describe how complex the heart actually is, especially from the perspective of a surgeon who is allowed only a small incision without mortally damaging the pump. Its nooks and crannies hide some varieties of ventricular septal defects. It is prone to damage by errant stitches or rough handling. The geometry of the hearts' valves can be distorted by nearby manipulations. While Lillehei had examined plenty of normal hearts, it was those malformed that he would encounter in the operating theater. Pointing his Buick 90 miles south to the Mayo Clinic, Lillehei and his team (Varco, Cohen, and Warden) consulted with Jesse Edwards (see Chap. 8), at the time the world's foremost cardiac pathologist, and scrutinized many specimens in his extensive collection. By January 1954, Lillehei's scrupulous preparations were complete, and he was ready for his first patient.[143]

Today, subjecting a living volunteer donor to a major operation to remove tissue for transplantation is well-accepted; kidneys, lobes of liver and lung are so transferred. But not in Lillehei's day. The idea of putting a healthy person at risk, especially for a novel and risky procedure, was beyond the pale for many. "The first operation with a potential for two-hundred percent mortality" was cross-circulation's tag line, at least for its skeptics.[144] When word of Lillehei's plans for Gregory Glidden, a one-year-old boy with a ventricular septal defect, rippled through the University Hospitals, opposition quickly materialized. Cecil Watson, the Chief of Medicine, and Irving McQuarrie, his pediatric counterpart, appealed to the hospital director to forbid the operation. But Wangensteen was more persuasive (or powerful), and the surgery proceeded as planned on March 26[145] (Fig. 7.5). The repair went smoothly, and the donor father was unharmed. For several days, things looked good, but Gregory died 10 days postoperatively of pulmonary complications. Lillehei contrived to operate his next two patients in close succession—25 days apart—and when Watson and McQuarrie were out of town.[146] Both patients lived, and the donors suffered no serious complications. Taking a page from the Baltimore collaborators a decade previous, at the press conference trumpeting Lillehei's success, four-year-old Pamela Schmidt was proudly rolled-out to charm the assembled crowd. The news exploded worldwide.[147]

Over the next 15 months, 45 patients were operated upon using cross-circulation, with surprisingly good results considering the era and the defects: 17 patients died in the hospital and six later, with six re-operations and 49% 30-year survival. The

[142] Goor (2007, p. 4), Lillehei (1982) and GW Miller (2000, p. 95).

[143] GW Miller (2000, pp. 109, 116–118).

[144] Goor (2007, p. 4) attributes this to Willis Potts, but Vincent Gott heard from Lillehei that it was Conrad Lam (Gott in Stoney 2008, p. 333).

[145] Goor (2007, pp. 3–5). Miller reports only Watson's opposition (GW Miller 2000, pp. 119–122).

[146] Goor (2007, pp. 9–10).

[147] GW Miller (2000, pp. 146–147).

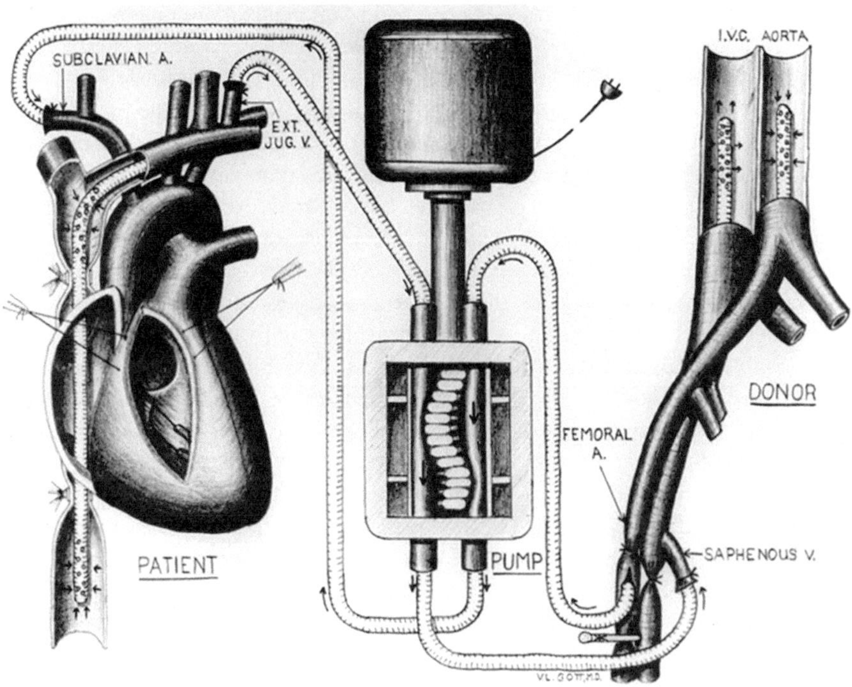


**Fig. 7.5** Lillehei's cross-circulation. (With the permission of the University of Minnesota Archives)

malformations were ventricular septal defect (27), tetralogy of Fallot (or variant) (10), complete atrioventricular canal defect (5), patent ductus (with exploratory ventriculotomy) (1), infundibular pulmonary stenosis (1), and pulmonary stenosis, atrial septal defect, and anomalous pulmonary venous return (1).[148] Parents were usually the donors, but also sundry other relatives and several "volunteers," including at least one penitentiary inmate.[149] But the surgical community was of two minds about cross-circulation. The reaction was at best mixed when Lillehei's experience was presented to the American Association of Thoracic Surgeons in Montreal (May 1954),[150] and to the American College of Surgeons in Atlantic City the same year.[151] Blalock's critique of Lillehei's talk at the American Surgical Association meeting in Philadelphia (1955), while faintly complementary, averred that the "ultimate answer" would be a pump-oxygenator, not cross-circulation.[152] The reaction at

[148] Lillehei et al. (1986).

[149] Lillehei et al. (1986) and GW Miller (2000, p. 163).

[150] Goor (2007, p. 10) and GW Miller (2000, pp. 149–151).

[151] GW Miller (2000, pp. 153, 155–156).

[152] Lillehei et al. (1955a, b), Fye (2015, p. 218), Shumacker (1992, pp. 264–265), Cooper (2010, p. 190), GW Miller (2000, p. 176).

home was often sour,[153] and Wangensteen had to intercede more than once to keep Lillehei's open-heart activities from being stymied.[154]

Critics assailed cross-circulation because it entailed risk to the donor, even if small. While no donor died, two did suffer serious adverse events. The donor mother for the twelfth case required open-chest cardiac massage, although she apparently recovered fully. The donor for the fourteenth suffered a massive air embolus before even being cannulated. She was resuscitated but suffered severe and permanent neurological injury.[155] Still, it's hard to see why donor risk should have caused so much offense. Then, and now, adults willingly subject themselves to medical hazard for different reasons, including for the (rather abstract) sake of advancing medical knowledge. It is hard to imagine a more compelling motivation than trying to save one's disabled or dying child. And donors (at least the parent donors) were not truly non-combatants. The ill health of the child made them, in a very real if different sense, unhealthy as well. They took a small risk hoping to improve both their child's health *and* their own wellbeing. However, opposition was also rooted in the operation's unreliability. At one point, Lillehei had a bad stretch, where only one of seven patients survived, which was bound to leave a bad taste in the mouth of nurses and doctors on the scene. News of the tragic air embolus, in the words of a surgeon visiting the University Hospitals at the time, caused a "sense of grief and horror [to pervade the hospital]."[156] And his flagrant self-promotion—"Lillehei seemed to be everywhere, speaking and showing films about the breakthroughs in his operating room."[157]—surely offended many.

But a few surgeons, such as John Kirklin at the Mayo Clinic,[158] saw what others did not.[159] The young Minnesotan had shown that repair of more challenging defects was possible, and in hearts seemingly too sick to withstand surgery.[160] Even for those firmly fixed on eventually obtaining a mechanical device, Lillehei's example

---

[153] Goor (2007, pp. 10–11).

[154] Per an interview with Peter Olch, Wangensteen fought multiple administrative battles to keep the cardiac program moving ahead: "I was called upon by Drs. Cecil Watson, Professor of Medicine and John Anderson, Professor of Pediatrics, to justify our aggressive intracardiac program. . . . I interceded for Dr. Lillehei and his associates on more than one occasion. . . . My support stopped administrative efforts at placing a restraining hand upon the activities of our cardiac surgeons" (Olch 1971–1972, p. 68).

[155] One recollection mentions only the neurologically injured donor (Shumway in Stoney 2008, p. 430) but Goor (2007, pp. 11–12) and Stoney (2008, p. 33) write of a second case. In 1955, Lillehei built an exhibit describing forty-one cross-circulation operations. The donor cardiac arrest with successful resuscitation is briefly described ("profound hypotension requiring thoracotomy—complete recovery"). The neurologically injured patient went unmentioned (Lillehei et al. 1956).

[156] GW Miller (2000, p. 152) and Starzl (1992, p. 42).

[157] Fye (2015, p. 217).

[158] Kirklin (1989) and Goor (2007, p. 33).

[159] But in an interview with Allen Weisse in 1999 (Weisse 2002, pp. 95–103) Kirklin seems to deny that Lillehei much influenced his open-heart program at the Mayo Clinic, which used the pump-oxygenator before Lillehei.

[160] Lillehei (1982).

was a heartening proof of concept. One can argue that the Minnesota cross-circulation operations were *the* major breakthrough for open-heart surgery, and many have.[161]

But Blalock would be proved correct—cross-circulation was not the answer, as Lillehei soon realized. Donor risk aside, human oxygenators were bound to be more cumbersome and expensive than using a machine. And cross-circulation could not be used for large patients (Lillehei's oldest and heaviest was 14 years old and weighed 37.7 kg) or, with low flow, for long procedures.[162] In early 1954, Richard DeWall, a young family practitioner interested in cardiology, approached Richard Varco with an idea for an artificial mitral valve. He was invited to join Lillehei's lab and later charged with creating an oxygenator simpler and more practical than Gibbon's. This tyro inventor, not much good at math or engineering in college,[163] ignored Lillehei's advice and bubbled oxygen through blood, experimenting to find bubbles of precisely the right size. His breakthrough device was simple and clever—miniscule spheres of oxygen stream up a column of blood in a cylindrical tower; the oxygen-rich blood empties into a slanted tube, then slides down a coiled ramp, shedding bubbles along the way (Fig. 7.6).[164] Crucially, the inside of the tubing was coated with a silicone antifoaming agent which completed the bubble extraction, and DeWall was not the first to use this antifoaming agent in a blood oxygenator.[165]

DeWall's use of Dow Corning Antifoam A—an agent created for use in jet aircraft fuel systems—affords us a glimpse of how very different medical innovation was in his day.[166] DeWall and Lillehei expropriated it for their oxygenator, without the preliminary spade work mandatory today, judging from a letter Lillehei sent to the Medical Director of Dow Corning (September 14, 1955): Dear Sir: "We have been using . . . your antifoam substance A [for cardiopulmonary bypass]. In animal experiments we have been unable to detect any toxicity using much larger than needed quantities of the antifoam substance. The same appears to be true in the *17 human operations* that we have done. However, since we have been recommending this substance to other surgeons for this use, *I would appreciate any information that you might have as to the possible toxicity of the antifoam substance used in this way*."[167] Only after infusing (albeit small amounts) of this agent into 17 people does Lillehei inquire whether the manufacturer has any toxicity data! Open-heart

[161] Cooley (1999), Cooley in Stoney (2008, p. 249), Kirklin (1979), Goor (2007), the title of Chapter I; Shumacker (1992, p. 244–245), Cooper (2010, p. 190) and Lillehei (1982).

[162] Lillehei et al. (1986).

[163] Stoney (2008, pp. 100–103).

[164] Lillehei and DeWall (1958).

[165] Clark et al. (1950).

[166] Stoney (2008, p. 107).

[167] University of Minnesota Department of Surgery Archives; emphasis mine. http://gallery.lib.umn.edu/exhibits/show/openheart/item/3313

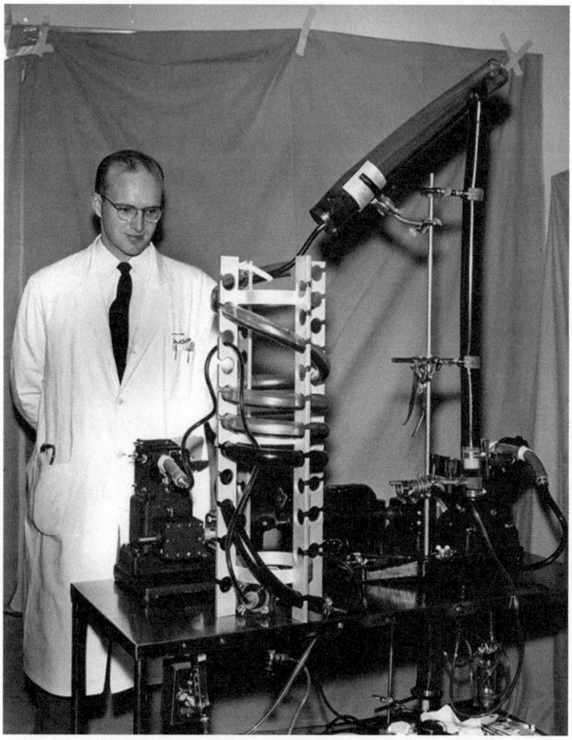

**Fig. 7.6** Richard DeWall and his bubble oxygenator. (With the permission from the University of Minnesota Archives)

pioneers were pretty much free to invent and deploy devices as they saw fit—the US Food and Drug Administration only started regulating medical devices in 1976.[168]

Far simpler and cheaper than Gibbon's IBM circuit, DeWall's took only about 6 months to develop, and was pressed into service in May 1955.[169] By early December, Lillehei had operated upon 37 patients using the DeWall-Lillehei oxygenator.[170] An even simpler iteration, inexpensively produced commercially, was invented by DeWall in 1956 and saw wide use.[171] Gibbon's much more complicated and expensive device was much less successful, although John Kirklin's group at the Mayo Clinic did build and use a modified version.

Lillehei rocketed to the top of cardiac surgery, propelled by drive and imagination, and daring, to say nothing of collaborators who greatly multiplied his efforts. He won the Lasker Prize in 1955 and achieved international celebrity. Lillehei was

---

[168] US Food and Drug Administration. A History of Medical Device Regulation & Oversight in the United States.

[169] DeWall (2011) and Cooper (2010) states it took a little more than a year to perfect his bypass device (p. 193).

[170] GW Miller (2000, p. 184).

[171] Vincent Gott was also involved, but he (perhaps too generously) gives the credit to DeWall (Gott in Stoney 2008, p. 336).

an indefatigable healer; he had opened a thousand hearts by August 1960.[172] He was also an inventor, and facilitator of other inventors, of surgical procedures and, later, devices such as implantable pacemakers and heart valves. This dynamic son of the Midwest was a showman, devoting huge road time peddling his craft and name. What Lillehei wasn't, was an administrator.[173] He didn't like that sort of thing, especially the meetings and detail work, or that organizations gummed up the gears of guys like him or tried to. More fatally, he was a lousy politician. Lillehei made many enemies along the way and didn't much care. He was oblivious to the politics permeating his environment: For Lillehei, politics were like the nineteenth century physicist's ether, fundamental to the structure of the universe but mostly undetectable. But when Wangensteen's retirement loomed in 1966, Walt petitioned hard for the position. Transplant surgeon John Najarian was chosen instead, and the insulted Lillehei quickly decamped to Chief of Surgery and Chairman of the New York Hospital-Cornell Medical Center's Department of Surgery. Leaving his family in the Twin Cities, he was in New York by December.

The move proved unwise.

By March of 1968—only 4 months into his tenure—Lillehei was on thin ice, and his fate was sealed by 1970 (though Lillehei hadn't a clue of his perilous situation).[174] In March, he was informed that his chairship would be terminated on June 30. G. Wayne Miller, and Lillehei's trainee and friend, Daniel Goor, attribute Lillehei's rapid flame-out partly to a culture clash between the innovative and scientifically oriented surgeon and a conservative and antiquated Cornell. But they and others also identified personal deficiencies, including poor quality surgery, inattention to administrative matters, and needless provocations that surely made Lillehei's flame-out inevitable.[175] Further ammunition for his detractors was provided by his exuberant lifestyle, including an expensively redone office, flashy clothes, an E-type Jaguar, wild penthouse parties, and rumors of special lady friends. Lillehei was allowed to stay at Cornell as surgical faculty, but even as he operated in New York, events were unwinding in Minnesota that would hound him for a decade.

Lillehei had assumed little if any obligation to track his income—at least not in any conventional way—for tax purposes, and he had little compunction about filing tax returns. Even entreaties from the IRS were insufficient motivation for him to file overdue documents, which—predictably—eventually provoked an investigation. In April 1972, he was indicted in St. Paul for tax evasion, then convicted, fined, and sentenced to 5 years parole and 6 months of community service. To what extent he had behaved fraudulently, as opposed to negligently, is debatable, although he had clearly claimed inappropriate deductions.[176] But his utter disregard for the

[172] GW Miller (2000, p. 197).

[173] Goor (2007, pp. 64, 71–73, 75), Cooper (2010, p. 201), GW Miller (2000, p. 223).

[174] Goor (2007, pp. 77–79, 84), GW Miller (2000, p. 224).

[175] Goor (2007, pp. 78–87), GW Miller (2000, pp. 220–224) and Cooper (2010, pp. 201–202).

[176] GW Miller (2000, pp. 228–236) and Goor (2007, pp. 88–98).

unpleasant but unavoidable need to render unto Caesar was unequivocal.[177] Lillehei rejected the jury's verdict, telling the presiding judge that he was guilty only of poor judgment, carelessness, and "good honest mistakes," none of which are criminal acts.[178] Fired from Cornell, he returned to St. Paul on December 31, 1973.

Lillehei's censure was broad. Previous friends and colleagues became former; invites for speaking at domestic meetings evaporated (but not for those abroad); he was no longer welcome at his old institution.[179] The wages for Lillehei's otherness were rare achievement and fame; they were also a decade of isolation and cold shoulders.[180]

It took a personage as self-confident, influential, and generous as John Kirklin to bring him in from the cold: "Walt Lillehei, with Dick Varco, really began this modern era of cardiac surgery with cardiopulmonary bypass. . . . [Walt] always was and still is a great hero of mine, because of his enormous ability and warm friendship . . . he was one of cardiac surgery's greatest innovators . . . Dear colleagues: *May I depart from my text to ask this great pioneering cardiac surgeon to stand to your applause. Walt Lillehei, may we see you?*"[181]

Thus commenced the rehabilitation of C. Walton Lillehei, bestowed by John Kirklin—as highly respected and influential a heart surgeon as there ever will be—as he delivered the Presidential Address at the American Association for Thoracic Surgery's 1979 meeting.

His rehabilitation was ultimately crowned by the foundation of the Lillehei Surgical Society in 1985; the C. Walton Lillehei Symposium in 1988; and a Lillehei professorship and the Lillehei Heart Institute, both at the University of Minnesota.[182] Walt Lillehei died in July 1999.

> Charles Bailey did "all sorts of cockeyed experiments with horrendous mortality. . . . In one way, he experimented unreasonably, but I think you needed people who were willing to do that sort of thing to get heart surgery going."
>
> –Robert Frater[183]

I remember walking out of Boston Children's Hospital with Aldo Castañeda years ago. Aldo is a retired congenital heart surgeon, one of the greats, whose surgical training and first faculty position were at the University of Minnesota during the Lillehei era.[184] Referring to the early days of cardiac surgery at Minnesota, he cocked his head a few degrees and indicated—his exact words escape me—that some of the activity was pretty sketchy from the ethical standpoint. He didn't

---

[177] Goor (2007, pp. 88, 94).

[178] GW Miller (2000, p. 236).

[179] Kirklin (1989).

[180] GW Miller (2000, p. 238) states that Lillehei's Minnesota medical license and his membership in the American College of Surgeons were both suspended; Goor indicates not (2007, p. 106).

[181] Kirklin (1989); emphasis mine.

[182] Goor (2007 pp. 135–139).

[183] Cooper (2010, p. 82).

[184] Vida et al. (2006).

elaborate, and I didn't press, but this left a 30-year impression. Aldo told David Cooper, in the context of Lillehei, that that era's surgeons needed "a certain touch of immorality,"[185] and John Lewis' talk at the Lillehei Symposium suggests that they had it. Other locals found Lillehei's ethical standards wanting, including physiologist Maurice Visscher.[186]

But what do immorality or "ambiguous ethics" (Lewis) mean in this context? Published accounts of Lillehei's earliest open-hearts indicate that the patients needed intervention (though one obviously has to reply upon the surgeon's report). For example, cardiac catheterization data for his first eight ventricular defect patients indicate that they did, indeed, meet contemporary criteria for closure; one patient had only a small defect but poor exercise tolerance and a history of frequent pneumonias.[187] (It is possible that some unreported patients did not.) And Lillehei had ample reason to believe that he could improve the patient's condition, that the operation wasn't merely an "experiment." The quality of informed consent is impossible to judge at this distance, but since informed consent only began to take modern form in the 1960s, it would be unfair to apply contemporary standards in any case.[188] What set Lillehei apart wasn't "a touch of immorality," but rather his willingness to countenance the loss of lives, at his very hands, that otherwise would have struggled on indefinitely. (Unlike Eileen Saxon (Chap. 6), these patients were not in death's maw on their way to the operating room.) Lillehei's appreciation of maiden-voyage risk was smothered by optimism, and he was absolutely convinced that *open-heart surgery*—as a general concept—was on the near horizon. He knew, and accepted, that crosses would be planted along the way. John Kirklin, using a pump-oxygenator even before Lillehei, was the same: He prospectively planned on doing eight cases (four died), *regardless of the outcomes*, before taking a deep breath.[189]

But Lillehei's cross circulation project had a dark side, even if one accepts parent donors as ethically acceptable. As we've seen, at least one prisoner was used as a donor. Even considering the ethical gulf between the 1950s and today, Lillehei's explorations with government officials for using prisoners is disturbing. The surgeon wrote to Jarle Leirfallom, commissioner of the Department of Public Health, inquiring whether prisoners might be used as donors for cross circulation procedures: "It was my thought, which has probably occurred to you, that this project might fit into your rehabilitation program since it would seem to me that any man who would volunteer to do this so that another individual might have a chance to live a normal life could not help but acquire some increased sense of responsibility for the rules and laws of an organized society" (October 22, 1954). In his reply (October 29, 1954), Leirfallom was noncommittal but quoted the medical director's (Dr. Cameron) opinion: "I am sure that if the proposition of volunteering to be the

---

[185] Cooper (2010, p. 201).

[186] Goor (2007, pp. 68–69).

[187] Lillehei et al. (1955b).

[188] Jones (2013, pp. 152–156).

[189] Kirklin (1989).

donor . . . were properly presented to the prisoners there might well be some volunteers. Further, I am inclined to agree with Dr. Lillehei that participation in such a procedure [sic] might do a great deal for the prisoner as well as the patient. I would favor it." (Cameron cited prisoners' personal satisfaction derived from *donating blood* during the war as a basis for his statement.) Leirfallom promised further consideration of the project. To compare giving blood to serving as an open-heart donor, to contort the self-interest of the surgeon into the self-interest of the incarcerated "volunteer," by people showing no genuine concern for the welfare of the prisoners, is chilling stuff.[190] And that fact that arrangements were made to use "girls" from the Shakopee Reformatory as donors lowers the temperature even further.[191]

Setting ethics aside, it seems to me that Lillehei was afflicted by something like the ultra-persuasive Steve Jobs' "reality distortion field," except in this surgeon's case it was *his* reality that was distorted, not that of those around him.[192] Lillehei was so eager to use his new hammer that he saw nails where other reasonable (and better informed) people saw screws. Consider his take on ventricular septal defects. In June of 1962, a thoracic surgeon in Johannesburg wrote Lillehei asking whether he thought it "necessary to operate on ventricular sepal defects," and "what is (their) likelihood of spontaneous closure?" Lillehei replied quickly, advising surgery for all patients with such defects (allowing that those less than 2 years old doing well could be deferred until older). His answer to the question of spontaneous closure: "This can be answered in one word, negligible."[193] Today, we seldom close small ventricular septal defects, and this is hardly new. In his 1957 textbook, Alexander Nadas observed that "at least in childhood, these patients do extremely well" and expressed no enthusiasm for surgical remedy.[194] Taussig (1960) and Howard Burchell, a highly-respected adult cardiologist (1957), advised the same.[195] Even in 1978, when cardiac surgery was considerably safer, yet other cardiologists advised that many small defects be deferred for operation until such time that operative mortality is lower.[196] While it is conceivable that Lillehei had only moderate or large defects in mind, this seems unlikely. Indeed, he seemed of two minds on whether even miniscule holes should be closed: "One might argue whether (the very smallest

[190] University of Minnesota Archives. https://gallery.lib.umn.edu/exhibits/show/openheart/cross/alternative-methods

[191] Regarding donors from the Shakopee Reformatory: Letters from Lillehei to A.C. Gillett, Correctional Programs Supervisor, on Dec. 20, 1954, and Feb. 7, 1955, indicate that such arrangements had been made (University of Minnesota Archives. http://gallery.lib.umn.edu/exhibits/show/openheart/cross/alternative-methods)

[192] Isaacson (2011, pp. 117–119).

[193] Letter from Denis Fuller to Lillehei, dated June 23, 1962. Lillehei's reply letter is dated July 13, 1962. Both letters are from the University of Minnesota surgical archives, accessed online, March 16, 2020. In his letter, Lillehei said that he would not close a defect with a "marked left to right shunt," but surely he meant "marked *right to left* shunt."

[194] Nadas (1957, pp. 310–313) and Engle (1954).

[195] Taussig (1960, pp. 681–682) and Burchell (1957, p. 979).

[196] Keith et al. (1978, p. 364).

pinhole defects) need surgery at all, but there is a known increase in susceptibility to bacterial endocarditis although this is not an important risk." Lillehei's spontaneous closure statement—implying that there is no escape from the need for closure by waiting—was inconsistent with the concurrent, published experience of multiple cardiologists who actually saw these patients.[197] Interestingly, Helen Tausig, however, (erroneously) believed that small defects never spontaneously closed.[198]

Lillehei's letter reflected on one level, an honest difference of opinion. Nadas and colleagues—some of the world's most respected pediatric cardiologists—wrote in 1961 that "Surgeons, in their considerable enthusiasm, have recommended early repair of these defects for a variety of reasons. To stem the tide of indiscriminant operation, cardiologists have pointed to the benign nature of small defects (and other factors arguing against surgical correction)."[199] But it also reveals *attitude* rather than data, reflex rather than cogitation. There was no real justification then, and still none 50 years later, for closing most small defects.[200] It was as though Lillehei's newfound technical sufficiency spawned a distortion field which spurned nuance and corporate experience. Lillehei's Medical Progress paper in the *New England Journal of Medicine* (1958) advocates closing "all ventricular septal defects associated with any significant degree of shunt." But what is significant? He makes no effort to quantify this, possibly due to lacking firm data, but more likely—I believe—to leave widely-open indications for surgery. He also states "the inescapable conclusion that few patients born with an isolated ventricular septal defect survive beyond the pediatric age group without corrective management." People who actually followed these patients knew better. Indeed, Lillehei was little interested in collaborating with cardiologists, as recollected by Jim Moller, a pediatric cardiologist at Minnesota during Lillehei's tenure (personal interview, May 22, 2020), and confirmed by the paucity of cardiologist co-authors on his early papers. (Contrast this sorry lack of acknowledgement and collaboration with, to give only one example, John Kirklin's publications and recollections.)[201]

Charles Bailey's "distortion field" was even more overpowering. His first crack at ventricular septal defect repair using his closed technique was in a 26-year-old man with a heart murmur. This fellow had "no special cardiac symptoms," a normal cardiac examination save for the murmur, an essentially normal electrocardiogram, and a chest X-ray showing only "mild fullness of the pulmonary artery and conus." Angiography showed only possible enlargement of the right ventricle. Bailey didn't even have a fixed diagnosis (ventricular septal defect versus pulmonary stenosis)

---

[197] See Nadas (1957 p. 310), Evans et al. (1960) and Nadas (1961).

[198] Taussig (1960, p. 673).

[199] Nadas (1961).

[200] Exactly what constitutes a "small" ventricular septal defect (VSD) is inside baseball stuff not important here. Suffice it to say that Lillehei's letter seems to advocate operating upon essentially all such defects, which would include many currently not thought to need repair. An exception may be the development of bacterial endocarditis at the site of the VSD; after antibiotic treatment, many cardiologists currently recommend surgical closure.

[201] Weisse (2002).

when he opened the chest and inserted his finger into the right ventricle. Feeling a small hole, he thought he had closed a defect, though offering no proof. No indication of *need for operation* was offered: There were no symptoms and an essentially normal cardiac evaluation, save for the noise in his chest.[202] And this was his *first* (reported, at any rate) human operation of that kind, which any reasonable person would have thought to be of significant risk. His third case was a 27-year-old man, asymptomatic until 3 weeks before operation, when he apparently developed "quite severe" difficulty breathing with exertion and palpitations (perception of an irregular heart rhythm). But the story is fishy: Cardiac catheterization showed only a small ventricular septal defect, unlikely to produce severe (or any) symptoms. Bailey nevertheless attempted closure, the patient convalesced smoothly and was said to be asymptomatic 3 months later. A post-operative catheter study revealed that the hole was only partly closed, but Bailey pointed to its reduced size and increased arterial oxygen saturation (92% before, 92.6% after surgery[203]; the apparent increase being within error of the measurement and negligible in any case) as evidence of "physiological improvement." These examples of questionable, at best, operations are only two, and one might argue that it is unfair to apply modern indications for operation to 1950s surgery. But Bailey's *peers* had serious reservations about his practice. Gibbon considered him "beyond the pale" and a "wild man."[204] Cardiac surgeon Tony Dobell "saw some appalling things too; huge risks were taken. . . . He probably pushed (closed heart surgery) beyond where it should have been pushed." Still, Dobell allowed that such behavior was the norm of the era.[205] Dwight Harken thought Bailey was "unethical and irresponsible" with a "lack of respect for human life."[206] But lest you form too disparaging an impression of Bailey, like Lillehei he was headstrong and knew only his own compass, but willingly paid a high personal price to go Sinatra's *My Way*. In the final analysis, Dan Goor considered Bailey "an outrageously great human being."[207]

Some, like Robert Frater, a cardiac surgeon who trained during the era of Bailey and Lillehei, have suggested that "experimenting unreasonably" was actually indispensable for cardiac surgery to vault from Dawn to Modern. That a dash of recklessness was needed, given the human stakes involved. One can point to the example of Gibbon, who built a heart-lung machine but wasn't tough or wild enough to make it work with humans, as proof. But I think that history suggests otherwise. The chief protagonists were courageous and daring but—at least as nearly as I can tell—steady and careful. Bigelow was, from all angles, cautious and conservative, and

[202] Bailey et al. (1952).

[203] The preoperative study showed pulmonary artery pressure = 20–22/6; left ventricular pressure = 90–94/2; right atrial pressure = 6; systemic and pulmonary flows, respectively, = 4.8 and 6.2 liters/minute. Three months post-operatively, the flows were systemic = 4.7 and pulmonary = 5.7 liters/minute.

[204] Cooper (2010, pp. 153, 81).

[205] Stoney (2008, p. 217).

[206] Cooper (2010, p. 98).

[207] Weisse (2002, pp. 72–92) and Goor (2007, pp. 144–164).

had missed out on claiming first use of hypothermia by insisting on patients for whom the operation made the best sense. But he subsequently did employ refrigeration clinically, and one senses would have used it earlier had he had pediatric patients. While Bailey was the very first to crack open a mitral valve (see Chap. 4), Dwight Harken and Lord Brock were hard on his heels. While the latter two were difficult personalities,[208] neither had a reputation for outlandish surgery. John Kirklin, the very model of probity, used cardiopulmonary bypass before Lillehei. While acknowledging Lillehei's contribution, he said that he would have proceeded without Lillehei's example.[209] Even the earliest broadly-successful cardiac surgeons—Gross and Blalock—were daring but sober in their practice. If not as appealing as the idea of the rogue gunslinger bringing rough justice to the wild west, this is good news. The cowboy's era is vanishing. A more rigorous ethical environment, with public reporting and other oversight procedures, has largely supplanted it, and innovation will need to proceed in this context. The history of cardiac surgery suggests that such constraints will not body-block its continuing evolution.

Cardiac surgery's leap into its Modern era entangled many more people and events than available space in this chapter. Indeed, thinking back to the Blalock-Taussig-Thomas shunt, which sprung up virtually out of nowhere, I am struck with how perfectly *sui generis* was the Baltimore group's breakthrough, as contrasted with the diversely prosecuted open-heart project. But the events and people in *Breaching the Wall* are central and essential to the story: new ideas, seemingly endless laboratory research, and new technology.[210] The human factor—imagination, courage, persistence, and even craziness—was woven into the fabric. But not always relentless drive and determination. We've admired people who were *all-in*, ferocious in their determination and saturated in conviction; and we've encountered innovators who weren't. John Lewis' is a story of invention—daring invention—dissociated from single-mindedness and religious zeal, unhitched to any sense of destiny or duty. Gibbon relentlessly pursued his lifesaving machine but peeled off at what most surgeons saw as the next step, perfecting it in clinical use. Both—like many others not scratched into history—added bricks to the wall, even if no capstones. Prone to drama and sudden life-altering moments, by its very nature cardiac surgery has acquired something of an exotic image, especially regarding its formative years. This is the wild west ma'am, and only swashbucklers dare to poke their noses into them thar dangerous hills. But congenital cardiology's advance from Early Days to New Dawn, and finally into the hills of the Modern Era, was almost entirely thanks to tough and determined and courageous, but prudent and measured, pioneers.

---

[208] Cooper (2010, pp. 52–64, 101–103).

[209] Weisse (2002).

[210] A number of major developments directly related to further advances in open-heart surgery are not discussed, such as echocardiography, miniaturization of surgical instruments, and magnification of the surgical field with loupes, along with improvements in surgeons' understanding of cardiac pathology and surgical technique.

We are closing in on our final chapters about single ventricle palliation. But before we get to those decisive chapters, we must take a look at three singular figures who always have a word, if not the last one—the pathologists—who were instrumental in defining the congenital heart anatomy for our surgical inventors. Let us continue on with *Collectors of Hearts – Reprise*.

## References

Arensman RM, Comish JD (1993) Extracorporeal life support. Blackwell Scientific Publications, Boston

Bailey CP, Glover RP, O'Neill TJE (1952) Transmyocardial palpatory surgery of the heart. Can Med Assn J 66:529–535

Bigelow WG (1942) The modern conception and treatment of frost-bite: a survey and discussion of the literature. Can Med Assoc J 47:529–534

Bigelow WG (1984) Cold hearts: the story of hypothermia and the pacemaker in heart surgery. McClelland and Stewart, Toronto

Bigelow WG, Lanyon ECG (1944) Some uses for dry cold therapy, and a proposed cooling unit. Br Med J 12:215–217

Bigelow WG, McBirnie JE (1953) Further experiences with hypothermia for intracardiac surgery in monkeys and groundhogs. Ann Surg 137:361–365

Brock RC, Campbell M (1950) Infundibular resection or dilation for infundibular stenosis. Br Heart J 12:403–424

Burchell HB (1957) Clinical problems related to surgical repair of intra-cardiac defects with the aid of an extracorporeal pump-oxygenator. Circulation 16:976–987

Cerri M (2017) The central control of energy expenditure: exploiting torpor for medical applications. Annu Rev Physiol 79:167–186

Clark LC, Gollan F, Gupta VB (1950) The oxygenation of blood by gas dispersion. Science 111:85–87

Cooley DA (1999) In Memoriam. C. Walton Lillehei, the "father of open heart surgery". Circulation 100:1364–1365

Cooper DKC (2010) Open heart: the radical surgeons who revolutionized medicine. Kaplan Publishing, New York

Currie J (1804) Medical reports, on the effects of water, cold and warm, as a remedy in fever and other diseases, whether applied to the surface of the body, or used internally. McCreery, Liverpool

Damman JF Jr, McEachen JA, Thompson WM Jr, Smith R, Muller WH Jr (1961) The regression of pulmonary vascular disease after the creation of pulmonary stenosis. J Thorac Cardiovasc Surg 42:722–734

Dennis C (1989) A heart-lung machine for open-heart operations: how it came about. Trans Am Soc Artif Organs 35:767–777

Dennis C, Spreng DS Jr, Nelson GE, Karlson KE, Nelson RM, Thomas JV et al (1951) Development of a pump-oxygenator to replace the heart and lungs; an apparatus applicable to human patients, and application to one case. Ann Surg 134:709–721

DeWall RA (2011) The origins of open heart surgery at Minnesota 1951. J Thorac Cardiovasc Surg 142:267–269

Dill DB, Forbes WH (1941) Respiratory and metabolic effects of hypothermia. Am J Physiol 132:685–697

Dodrill FD, Gerisch RA (1952) Temporary mechanical substitute for the left ventricle in man. JAMA 150:642–644

Engle MA (1954) Ventricular septal defects in infancy. Pediatrics 14:16–27

Evans JR, Rowe RD, Keith JD (1960) Spontaneous closure of ventricular septal defects. Circulation 22:1044–1054
Fye WB (2015) Caring for the heart: Mayo Clinic and the rise of specialization. Oxford University Press, Oxford, UK
Gibbon JH Jr (1978) The development of the heart-lung apparatus. Am J Surg 135:608–619
Gilbert M, Busund R, Skagseth A, Nilsen P, Solbø JP (2000) Resuscitation from accidental hypothermia of 13.7° C with circulatory arrest. Lancet 355:375–376
Goor DA (2007) The Genius of C. Walton Lilllehei and the true history of open heart surgery. Vantage Press, New York
Gott VL (2005) Lillehei, Lewis, Wangensteen: the right mix for giant achievements in cardiac surgery. Ann Thorac Surg 79:S2210–S2213
Gross RE, Watkins E Jr, Pomerantz AA, Watkins E, Goldsmith EI (1952) Surgical closure of defects of the interauricular septum by use of an atrial well. N Engl J Med 247:455–460
Hall M (1832) XVI. On hibernation. Phil Trans 122:335–360
Harmel MH, Lamont A (1946) Anesthesia in the surgical treatment of congenital pulmonic stenosis. Anesthesiology 5:477–498
Henderson AR (1966) Induced hypothermia is not "artificial hibernation". JAMA 198:1074–1078
Herzog M (1997) Annapurna: first conquest of an 8,000 meter peak. Morin N, Smith JA (trans). The Lyons Press, New York
Hickey S, Whitson A, Jones L, Wibbenmeyer RC, Fey R et al (2020) Guidelines for thrombolytic therapy for Frostbite. J Burn Care Res 41(1):176–183
Hoffman JIE, Kaplan S (2002) The incidence of congenital heart disease. J Am Coll Cardiol 39:1890–1900
Hunter J (1786) Observations on certain parts of the animal œconomy. London. Reprint: Miami: HardPress; 2019
Isaacson W (2011) Steve Jobs. Simon & Schuster, New York
Jepson BM, Mackay-Bojack S, Moller JH (2017) The first cardiac operation using cardiopulmonary bypass. Ann Thorac Surg 103:e339–e340
Johnson SL (1970) The history of cardiac surgery, 1896–1955. The Johns Hopkins Press, Baltimore
Jones DS (2013) Broken hearts: the tangled history of cardiac care. The Johns Hopkins University Press, Baltimore
Keith JD, Rowe RD, Vlad P (1978) Heart disease in infancy and childhood, 3rd edn. Macmillan Publishing Co., Inc., New York
Kellie G (1805) Case of torpor from cold, and some general observations on the effects of diminished temperature upon the living system. Edinb Med Surg J 1:302–313
Kirklin JW (1979) A letter to Helen. J Thorac Cardiovasc Surg 78:643–654
Kirklin JW (1989) The middle 50s and C. Walton Lillehei. J Thorac Cardiovasc Surg 98:822–824
Knudsen L, Ochs M (2018) The micromechanics of lung alveoli: structure and function of surfactant and tissue components. Histochem Cell Bio 150:661–676
Konstantinov IE, Alexi-Meskishvili VV (2000) Sergei S Brukhonenko: the development of the first heart-lung machine for total body perfusion. Ann Thorac Surg 69:962–966
Krementsov N (2009) Off with your heads: isolated organs in early Soviet science and fiction. Stud Hist Phil Biol Biomed Sci 40:87–100
Lewis FJ (1958) Hypothermia for open heart surgery. Am J Cardiol 2:287–291
Lewis FJ (1965) Science in surgery. J Med Ed 40:983–989
Lewis FJ (1989) Mid-century invention recalled. J Thorac Cardiovasc Surg 98:814–816
Lewis FJ, Taufic M (1953) Closure of atrial septal defects with the aid of hypothermia: experimental accomplishments and the report of one successful case. Surgery 33:52–59
Lewis FJ, Varco RL, Taufic M (1954) Repair of atrial septal defects in man under direct vision with the aid of hypothermia. Surgery 36:538–556
Lillehei CW (1982) A personalized history of extracorporeal circulation. Trans Am Soc Artif Int Organs 28:5–16

Lillehei CW, DeWall R (1958) Design and clinical application of the helix reservoir pump-oxygenator system for extracorporeal circulation. Postgrad Med 23:561–573

Lillehei CW, Cohen M, Warden HE, Read RC, Aust JB, DeWall RA, Varco RL (1955a) Direct vision intracardiac correction of the tetralogy of Fallot, pentalogy of Fallot, and pulmonary atresia defects. Report of first ten cases.

Lillehei CW, Cohen M, Warden HE, Ziegler NR, Varco RL (1955b) The results of direct vision closure of ventricular septal defects in eight patients by means of controlled cross circulation.

Lillehei CW, Cohen M, Warden HE, Read RC, Aust JB, DeWall RA et al (1956) Direct vision intracardiac surgical correction of congenital heart defects. AMA Arch Surg 72:728–735

Lillehei CW, Varco RL, Cohen M, Warden HE, Patton C, Moller JH (1986) The first open-heart repairs of ventricular septal defect, atrioventricular communis, and tetralogy of Fallot using cross-circulation: a thirty year follow-up. Ann Thorac Surg 41:4–21

McCurry J, Jha A (2006, Dec 20) Injured hiker survived 24 days on mountain by 'hibernating.' The Guardian. Accessed 19 Aug 2024. https://www.theguardian.com/world/2006/dec/21/japan.topstories3

Miller GW (2000) King of hearts. Times Books, Random House, New York

Murray G (1948) Closure of defects in cardiac septa. Ann Surg 128:843–852

Nadas AS (1957) Pediatric cardiology. W.B. Saunders Co., Philadelphia

Nadas AS, Scott LP, Hauck AJ, Rudolph AM (1961) Spontaneous functional closure of ventricular septal defects. N Engl J Med 264:309–316

National Library of Medicine Henry Swan. Profiles in Science. Accessed 19 Aug 2024. https://profiles.nlm.nih.gov/spotlight/hp

Olch PD (1971–1972) Interview of Owen H. Wangensteen, Oct. 21 and 22, 1971 and Mar. 5, 1972, and Jan. 28, 1972. National Library of Medicine. Accessed 18 Aug 2024. https://digirepo.nlm.nih.gov/master/oralhist/2935143R/2935143R.pdf

Pembrey MS (1904) Remarks upon temperature. Br Med J 27:475-477

Poole A, Gauthier J (2016) Treatment of severe frostbite with iloprost in northern Canada. CMJA 188:1255–1258

Preston FW (1994) Floyd John Lewis, 1916-1993. Trans Am Surg Assn 112:398–399

Rainer WG (1996) Henry Swan II, MD [letter to the editor]. Ann Thorac Surg 62:1565

Roberts WC (1998) John Webster Kirklin, MD: a conversation with the editor. Am J Cardiol 81:1027–1044

Romaine-Davis A (1991) John Gibbon and his heart-lung machine. University of Pennsylvania Press, Philadelphia

Shewmon DA (1998) Chronic "brain death": meta-analysis and conceptual consequences. Neurology 51:1538–1545

Shumacker HB Jr (1992) The evolution of cardiac surgery. Indiana University Press, Bloomington

Shumacker HB Jr (1999) A dream of the heart: the life of John H. Gibbon, Jr., father of the heart-lung machine. Fithian Press, Santa Barbara

Shumway NE (1996) F. John Lewis, MD: 1916-1993. Ann Thorac Surg 61:250–251

Shumway NE (1999) C Walton and F. John Lewis. Ann Thor Surg 68:S34–S36

Smith LW, Fay T (1940) Observations on human beings with cancer, maintained at reduced temperatures of 75°–90° Fahrenheit. Am J Clin Path 10:1–11

Starzl TE (1992) The puzzle people. University of Pittsburgh Press, Pittsburgh

Steinquist P (2018, Jan 18) When Detroit muscle powered a breakthrough in heart surgery. The New York Times. Accessed 19 Aug 2024. https://www.nytimes.com/2018/01/18/business/detroit-michigan-heart-general-motors.html

Stoney WS (2008) Pioneers of cardiac surgery. Vanderbilt University Press, Nashville

Swan H (1953) Surgical closure of interauricular septal defects. JAMA 151:792

Swan H (1958) The current status of open heart surgery. Postgrad Med 23:127–131

Swan H, Blount SG Jr (1956) Visual intracardiac surgery in a series of one hundred eleven patients. JAMA 162:941–946

Swan H, Paton BC (1961) The current status of hypothermia in cardiovascular surgery. Prog Cardiovasc Dis 4:228–258

Swan H, Zeavin I (1954) Cessation of circulation in general hypothermia, III: technics of intracardiac surgery under direct vision. Ann Surg 139:385–396

Taussig HB (1960) Congenital malformations *of the heart*. Commonwealth Fund, Harvard University Press, Cambridge, MA

The New York Times (1996, Aug 4) p 41

Thornhill T (2017, June 16) Why a plane can still make the runway from 38,000ft even if all the engines fail: Pilots reveal the surprising distances airliners can GLIDE (and that they do it on almost every journey). Daily Mail. Accessed 19 Aug 2024. https://www.dailymail.co.uk/travel/travel_news/article-4603876/Pilots-reveal-distances-airliners-GLIDE.html

US Food and Drug Administration A history of medical device regulation & oversight in the United States. Accessed 20 Aug 2024. https://www.fda.gov/medical-devices/overview-device-regulation/history-medical-device-regulation-oversight-united-states

Vida L, Sade RM, Stellin G (2006) Aldo R. Castanẽda. Cardiol Young 16:221–228

Waddell WG, Fairley HB, Bigelow WG (1957) Improved management of clinical hypothermia, based upon related biochemical studies. Ann Surg 146:542–559

Wangensteen OH (1969) Presidential address: we cannot escape history. Ann Surg 99:193–197

Weisse AB (2002) Heart to heart. The twentieth century against cardiac disease. An oral history. Rutgers University Press, New Brunswick, NJ

Wikipedia. Erika Nordby. Accessed 19 Aug 2024. https://en.wikipedia.org/wiki/Erika_Nordby

# Chapter 8
# Collectors of Hearts—Reprise—Edwards, Van Praggh, Anderson

> There are few subjects which have attracted more attention in the profession than the irregularities in the development of the heart and large vessels. ... It might thus appear that there was scarcely any hope for a new work in this department of pathology
>
> –Thomas B. Peacock, *On Malformations &C, of the Human Heart: With Original Cases*, 1858[1]

The heart's anatomy is subtly complex, far more than can be readily appreciated or explained, even without considering the Byzantine malformations that afflict it. A common one is the ventricular septal defect—a hole in that wall of muscle. The surface area of the interventricular septum is roughly two square inches in a eight pound baby—the weight of many infants undergoing repair of this defect—yet there are *seven* fairly distinct locations where such a hole may occur, depending upon how you classify them, with different implications regarding the likelihood of spontaneous closure, surgical accessibility, potential for causing aortic valve leakage, and risk to the electrical conduction system of the heart posed by surgical closure. Holes in the *atrial* septum and adjacent tissue are a little less diverse in location, but still pose traps. Years ago, I saw a young man referred for cyanosis for whom Robert Gross (Chap. 4) had closed an atrial septal defect when he was a child. Gross had made the mistake of sewing a flap of tissue called the Eustachian valve to the top of the defect, thus directing inferior vena cava blood into the left atrium. Gross' view of the atrial septum was unobstructed when he placed the errant stitches; he was confused by the anatomy, as have been other surgeons, before and since.[2] Perhaps the heart's subtle complexity is best reflected in the experience of one of the world's most accomplished cardiac morphologists: "I certainly understand cardiac morphology far better, even within the last 3 years, than I did 10 years ago. That has been exclusively through the availability to do virtual dissections."[3] Robert Anderson

[1] Peacock (1858), pp. v-vi.

[2] Desnick et al. (1976).

[3] Goreczny et al. (2018).





T. J. Kulik, M. Dick, *Reimagining a Child's Heart*,
https://doi.org/10.1007/978-3-031-88608-9_8

had examined thousands of hearts, written hundreds of papers, and given countless lectures and teaching sessions before a new way of displaying malformed hearts afforded him a *yet better* understanding of this many-splendored—and tricky—pump.

Actually, treacherous. We've seen that diagnostic errors have bedeviled practitioners since congenital cardiology's New Dawn. In fact, in cardiac surgery's early years, mortality as often stemmed from mistaken morphology as other technical problems. A major cause of inaccurate surgery was related to the limited ways of *imaging* the heart and blood vessels, such techniques being relatively crude even into the 1970s. And a full appreciation of the relevant physiology lagged behind open-heart surgery, which also accounted for failed operations. But a tenuous appreciation of normal and—especially—abnormal cardiac structure was also operative. As surgeons waded into ever more complex defects, morphologists (and others) uncovered their subtle features, and technical misadventures have fallen apace. Morphologists are like cartographers, mapping out features of the seacoast where mariners could put in, and the location of reefs and shoals needing to be avoided.

Their lineage penetrates to medicine's bedrock. Classical Greeks, and people more ancient, examined the heart's interior. Vesalius' revolutionary *De humani corporis fabrica* (1543) included images of hearts cleaved open but compared with his exquisite drawings of the hand's many bones, they are leaden and lacking fine detail.[4] But Vesalius had no clear concept of the heart as a pump, and little reason to precisely map its interior. (Hands, on the other hand, got broken, slashed, and crushed; what their bones looked like mattered.) After Harvey, details were of greater interest, and the quality of rendered hearts improved dramatically.[5] In the eighteenth century, for example, Morgagni and Senac (Chap. 1) transformed careful inspection of cardiac malformations into theories of cyanosis. Peacock (1858), surveying the considerable body of morphological description already available, admitted that yet more might—almost—be superfluous, even while offering a well-illustrated volume of his own (Chap. 3). Yet others did the same, with even crisper images. Though the illustrations were superb, morphologists were not yet prodded by the need to provide surveys for surgical excursions, and a coherent body of work had yet to emerge. This changed with Maude Abbott (Chap. 5), one of congenital cardiology's chief instigators as it sidled from Early Days into New Dawn. She collected malformed hearts and systematically classified them, connecting anatomy to physiology, and clinical characteristics to outcomes. Her work was a lodestone for those trying to situate themselves in this remote corner of the medicine.[6]

In fact, anatomists have always been zealous teachers. Their insights have been disseminated via books and papers, but even more effectively by hands-on teaching; numberless practitioners have literally learned at their feet. In the sixteenth century, the University of Padua's magnificent anatomical theater was a teaching machine,

[4] Saunders and O'Malley (1982).

[5] Evans et al. (2009).

[6] Abbott (1936), pp. x–xi.

with ascending circles of students craning for a view, powered by the anatomist. The frontispieces of Realdo Columbo's *De Re Anatomica* (1559 and Andreas Vesalius' *De humani* proudly display a jumble of observers with the peacock anatomist—as much as the cadaver—the center of attention. Rembrandt's painting—the *Anatomy Lesson of Dr. Nicolaes Tulp*—(1632) was less crowded, and some of the onlookers apparently more concerned with being observed than observing, but the anatomist-teacher still cuts an impressive figure. Admittedly, instruction was mostly what these people were paid for; there was no Venice Institute of Health supplying grants for anatomical research at Padua. And anatomical demonstration was also used to demonstrate proof of new theories, especially if influential people were in the audience.[7] But there must be more to it than that; these folks seem often to have an almost maniacal compulsion to preach their gospel. That was Maude Abbott, to a tee (Chap. 5). We soon discuss four modern morphologists who were cut from the same cloth. Maurice Lev's teaching activities were the stuff of legend; while at the Hektoen Institute in Chicago, he rode the local six medical school circuit "carrying a bucket full of hearts and arriving at least 1 h before the scheduled lecture, even on the coldest winter days," and for years eagerly hauled hearts to countless professional meetings for yet more hands-on.[8] Jesse Edwards was a superb teacher, training over five hundred people ranging from students to professors.[9] Robert Anderson has logged countless miles of opportunities for hands-on sessions, lectures, and videos; with the COVID-19 pandemic, he parlayed Zoom lectures into an even wider audience.[10] Richard Van Praagh was just as ardent, if less widely traveled, as we will see.

Abbott, straddling congenital cardiology's first two eras, produced neither the quality nor the quantity of analysis needed for the Modern Era's open-heart excursions. For that, we look to the late 1940s and beyond, when the literature was speckled with anatomical description, some by morphologists, and others by cardiologists and surgeons. I find four full-time morphologists especially interesting, beginning with Maurice Lev. Born in 1908 in Missouri, he got his medical degree at Creighton University in Omaha, and his pathology training at Chicago's Michael Reese Hospital. Working at multiple institutions over his nearly 50-year career, Lev is best known for elucidating the pathways of the heart's nearly invisible electrical conduction system. In the days before cardiac pacemakers, closing a ventricular septal defect was dancing with the devil: A surgeon's needle or suture can stun or kill the conducting tissue, abolishing a viable cardiac rhythm, all too often killing the patient. His work, showing where stitches can be placed without injuring these pathways, was literally life-saving. Lev was also interested in structural defects and paid special attention to the *intrinsic shapes* of the right and left atria, and the right and left ventricles. Up until then, people had focused on the *relative positions* in the

[7] French (1994), pp. 20.

[8] Bharati (1994).

[9] Roberts (1998).

[10] Goreczny et al. (2018); American Association of Clinical Anatomists (2024).

chest of these chambers; Lev realized that taking into account their distinctive shapes yielded new insights, thus setting the table for a more sophisticated way to contemplate cardiac malformations.[11]

But as important as Lev was, many think of Jesse E. Edwards as *the* preeminent early modern morphologist. Trained as a pathologist, Edwards was first a cancer researcher, but after joining the Mayo Clinic in 1946, he was enmeshed in what would soon be the world's most dynamic cardiac unit.[12] Like Abbott, Edwards became a collector of hearts, but even more prodigious, eventually acquiring over 22,000 (though many had acquired, rather than congenital, defects). He was at the Mayo Clinic from 1946 until moving in 1960 to St. Paul's Charles T. Miller Hospital (now United Hospital), where he worked well into his eighties.[13]

Edwards' contributions often exceeded his predecessors in both quantity and quality. For example, he and a collaborator examined 28 cases of "persistent common atrioventricular canal" (a common heart defect) and culled additional cases from the literature, amassing 109 hearts (the largest previous case series was only five).[14] This paper was limited to morphology, but Edwards also produced a large volume of detailed clinicopathological correlation, including a book on congenital heart disease in 1954 and two in 1965, the last of which included angiograms (the cutting-edge imaging at the time). Most of Edwards' congenital work was not truly original, but it was still highly useful elaboration on previous observations.[15] His was supremely practical stuff, created for cardiologists to understand the anatomy and clinical manifestations of cardiac disease, and for surgeons to get their bearings as they set about re-sculpting these malformations.

In the 1960s, one might have thought, given Edwards' and other's myriad studies, that the final word on the subject, or something close, was in. That cardiac morphology, over 300 years after it mattered, was finally a closed book. If so, one would have been wrong.

In 1982, Anton Becker and Robert Anderson published a paper disputing Edwards' (and others') terminology for the "persistent common atrioventricular canal," based upon what they believed was a more refined understanding of the embryology and anatomy of the defect.[16] The journal's editor apparently felt the

[11] Bharati (1994); Lev (1966).

[12] The Mayo Clinic had arguably the deepest bench of any cardiac unit in the 1950s. A partial list of exceptional contributors (besides Edwards) includes John Kirklin, one of a trio of foundational open-heart men (along with Lillehei in Minneapolis and Denton Cooley in Houston); Earl Wood (physiologist); and Howard Burchell, Jeremy Swan, and Jim DuShane (cardiologists). See Roberts (1998) and Fye (2015).

[13] Freedom et al. (2004) Roberts (1998).

[14] Wakai and Edwards (1958).

[15] There are exceptions: Edwards' brilliant embryologically based scheme for understanding abnormalities of aortic arch branching, and his novel and immensely influential observations regarding pulmonary vascular disease are important original contributions related to congenital heart disease.

[16] Becker and Anderson (1982).

need to justify publishing yet another installment of cardiac morphology's perpetual wrestling match: "Many of us undoubtedly react with consternation to the persisting fluidity of the nomenclature for congenital heart disease.… It seems remarkable, after nearly 40 years of increasingly intense interest in the management of patients with congenital heart disease, that much printed space should still be given to discussions of what to *call* the major categories of anomalies." Yet he allowed that the controversy was justified on two grounds: first, that the morphology of such defects is "exceedingly" complex and still being worked out, and second, that one needs an "accurate and adequate" name to understand a given malformation. Despite eons of effort, cardiac morphologists were still grappling with the most apposite names for, and the best ways to think about, malformations. These arcane debates most conspicuously took the form of "transatlantic taxonomic warfare" conducted between two of modern cardiac morphology's most extraordinary contributors.[17]

The organizers of the second International Symposium on Surgical Heart Disease, held at New Zealand's Green Lane Hospital in February 1972, asked Richard Van Praagh to opine on the genetic implications of surgery for congenital heart disease. They hadn't a clue of what they were in for. Musing on the possible consequences of "genetic pollution" resulting from repairing otherwise fatal defects, the 42-year-old cardiac morphologist launched his musings in full by exploring the roots of human motivation, settled into a conventional discussion of the genetics of cardiac defects, then soared off into a highly controversial, contentious and discredited field: "In order to understand why a concern about eugenics seems fully justified, it is necessary to know something about where we are in space-time." He then briefly reviewed thirteen billion years of celestial events and one-hundred thousand years of human development. He concluded that, since we have three to five billion years before the sun "swells up, becomes a red giant and incinerates the earth," there is time enough for humans to pollute their genes. Why bother worrying about this? By escaping from earth to a planet orbiting a cooler, longer-lived star, descendants of the human race might persist for yet many more billions of years—that's why degrading the gene pool matters.[18] This was an extraordinary talk—which can only be fully appreciated by reading it in its entirety—especially given his audience of very practical-minded and earth-grounded clinicians. It is a window into an original, unusual and remarkable mind, one of a handful of manifest deep thinkers that I've ever rubbed shoulders with.

Van Praagh was born in London, Ontario in 1930, got his MD from the University of Toronto (1954), trained in pediatrics in Boston and Toronto, and then in pediatric cardiology with Helen Taussig (Fig. 6.2). His postdoctoral training was enriched with yet more advanced study—4 years—with pathologists (John M. Craig, Jesse Edwards, and Maurice Lev), an embryologist, and cardiologists and physiologists at the Mayo Clinic.[19] He joined Boston Children's in 1965 as its cardiac pathologist,

---

[17] Castañeda (2010).

[18] Barratt-Boyes et al. (1973), p. 331–339.

[19] Van Praagh (2012).

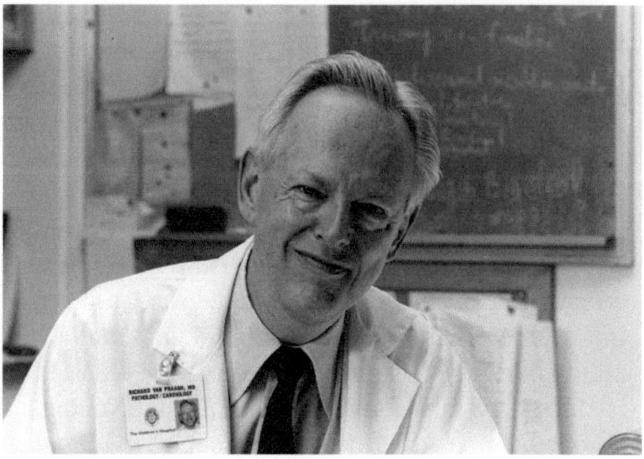

**Fig. 8.1** Richard Van Praggh MD. (With permission from the Bostin Children's Hospital Archives)

staying there until his retirement in 2002. Working with his treasured wife Stella, who made important original contributions of her own, Van Praagh produced as large a shift in the field as any other single contributor since the shape of the heart mattered.[20]

While at the Mayo Clinic (1960–1961), he was given an assignment: Wring as much as you can from the single ventricle heart. The topic was old but unsettled and highly relevant; a single ventricle was sometimes confused with a large ventricular septal defect, with disastrous consequences if repair were undertaken. Pouring over formalin-preserved hearts and other materials, Van Praagh cast fresh eyes on the problem, ultimately producing a work strikingly more advanced than previous efforts.[21] He described four varieties of single ventricles and their embryology, and he detailed the various arrangements of the great vessels and atria. Foreshadowing his subsequent work, Van Praagh produced diagrams concisely displaying the configurations that these malformations can assume. While his approach was not entirely original—Lev had paved the way—he had provided a novel and unprecedentedly deep dive into the nature of the single ventricle. More significantly, he was beginning to rethink *all* cardiac morphology. Van Praagh's seminal "segmental" analysis deals with the heart as three separate but connected segments, as well as two connectors, some or all of which may be abnormal in any given malformation.[22] He used set notation to concisely denote the segments (for example, {S,D,S} for the normal heart) and drafted a table of letters and symbols, lumping and splitting the myriad ways that these segments can go wrong into a condensation so efficient that it will likely never be excelled.[23] Van Praagh also showed how departures from

[20] Van Praagh (2019).

[21] Compare, for example, Van Praagh et al. (1964) with Rogers and Edwards (1951); Abbott (1936), pp. 50–53 and Table.

[22] Van Praagh (1985).

[23] Van Praagh's set is useful for a complex malformation, as it denotes its gross features at a glance (though without providing any details). It's like specifying that a member of the cat family is in the next room; you don't know whether it is a tabby or a tiger, but you know that it is nothing like, say, a wolf or a giraffe.

normal embryologic development account for certain defects (for example, how the aorta can wind up arising from the right, rather than left, ventricle). And, for good measure, he invented two new cardiac operations—performed by colleagues, of course![24] Segmental analysis proved a compelling way of structuring how one thinks about malformed hearts, deeply influencing even his transatlantic sparring partner, as we'll soon see.

Van Praagh operates on a plane rather higher than most. Castañeda—a highly intelligent fellow for whom an acute facility with cardiac anatomy was essential—confessed that "not infrequently, I failed at first to recognize the essence of his arguments and only after further reflection managed to grasp the importance or validity of his ideas."[25] But mental virtuosity only partly accounts for his morphology. Nothing in cardiac structure ineluctably leads to the Van Praaghian system; it owes its structure to its creator's cognitive proclivities. Mathematics is one. The logic of segmental analysis—taking discrete, definable elements and combining them to sum up the general layout of any given heart—is a sort of math, even if exceedingly limited. Van Praagh tumbled to set notation while helping his son do math homework, and years later elaborated it into "equations"; for example, the normal heart became: SNRGA{S,D,S} = 0R + 4 L.[26] His keynote address at *Neoheart: Cardiovascular Management of the Neonate* (2019) was entitled "A Contribution to the Algebra and the Geometry of Normally and Abnormally Related Great Arteries." Van Praagh's hankering to apply math, or something resembling it, to morphological concepts is, to put it mildly, peculiar, even in an era where quantification is king.

And his imagination is as free-ranging as it is numerically inclined. As a fellow, I enjoyed a few weeks as one of Jesse Edwards' (eventual) five hundred trainees. (I can recall hearts reeking of formalin in his one hand, the other wielding a silver probe to push open a flap of tissue or delineate the path of blood flow.) He was a patient and rather solemn man, methodical and attuned to detail, focused and business-like. My take on Van Praagh—which takes almost no time to form—could not be more different. Castañeda put it well: "[Van Praagh's] alert and inquisitive mind often races in various directions simultaneously. His attention, therefore, can be distracted from one moment to the other by ever new ideas, which can at times make it difficult to keep a conversation or teaching session on track."[27] When Van Praagh told me that he is "interested in everything," I thought of his 1972 space-time speech, and his 1985 book, *Survival: A New Approach From the Life Sciences to the Major Problem of Our Time*.[28] In this slim volume, written for "everyone, every-

[24] Van Praagh et al. (1971); Barratt-Boyes et al. (1973), p. 99.

[25] Castañeda (2010).

[26] Steve Sanders (a colleague of Van Praagh's) recalled that Van Praagh developed a case of "physics envy" after attending a physics lecture, inspiring his numerical elaboration of segmental notation. When I asked Van Praagh about this in 2020, he could not recall the lecture, but remembered developing his equations while preparing a paper to follow-up a medical meeting in Cracow, Poland.

[27] Castañeda (2010).

[28] Van Praagh (1985).

where," Van Praagh suggests that a new way of thinking—rational, truth-seeking, and biologically derived—is needed to avoid the ultimate catastrophe of nuclear holocaust. An astonishing range of ideas and history—religion, economics, anthropology, politics, philosophy, and more—are drawn together to fashion his argument. Van Praagh, being drawn to the big picture, hankered to construct a general theory of cardiac malformations, rather than settle for descriptions of individual defects. Grand synthesis, after all, is what his diagrams aim to do: organize and compress the universe of cardiac defects—their segmental arrangement, not every detail—into a concise and elegant summary, something akin to Mendeleev's periodic table. His numerically-enhanced segmental sets reflect both a mathematical bent and an effort to distill; an alpha-numeric shorthand links segments and great vessel connections with his embryological explanation for the latter. Were it not to do grave injustice to this indefatigable and passionate morphologist, one might gloss Van Praagh as a philosopher trapped in the body of someone whose work is describing the shape of a body part.

Van Praagh's opus helps us engage a difficult subject, but it is also pretty abstract, and it could have gotten buried in academic medicine's pulped and processed trees. As Castañeda's footprint exceeded his surgical results, so did Van Praagh's influence flow from more than papers and talks. Richard being Richard, and the pulpit provided by the Boston Children's cardiac program, account for much of his success. Children's was (and is) one of the largest training centers for congenital cardiologists and surgeons, and its trainees flocked to Van Praagh's teaching sessions. These were generally held at the end of the day, with Stella's home-baked treats providing additional inducement and stamina. Morphology melts in Richard's mouth: His extraordinary fluency with his subject and facility for riffing endlessly off a question or idea, articulated with an unusual grimace-tinged smile, is engaging stuff. (At a conference in Auckland, New Zealand, cardiologist Peter Vlad asked Van Praagh a question admitting to a fairly compact answer; the response was so painfully long and statistically elaborate that at its conclusion Vlad replied, "Thank you Mr. Chairman, I am sorry I asked!")[29] As a student, Van Praagh struck me as a fast, deep, and wide river of knowledge, helplessly overflowing its banks, exactly as he still does, decades later. The many fellow travelers passing through Boston have carried Van Praaghian concepts with them throughout congenital cardiology, though many have not stuck.[30]

Indeed, as it turns out, although segmental analysis is now standard stuff, despite his countless pupils, many have little regard for much of Van Praagh's most distinctive work. His set notation is often ignored, and other Van Praaghian ideas—for example, the "connecting segments"—hold little appeal for most.[31] His diagrams, ingenious as they are, have not become standard fare. There has

[29] Barratt-Boyes et al. (1973), p. 193.

[30] Besides teaching sessions at Children's, Van Praagh gave many talks at meetings, visited outside institutions, and produced a 22-lecture video series in 1991.

[31] Freedom (1984).

been a long-running (since the early 1970s) and well-known dispute between Van Praagh and Robert Anderson, even though the domain of pickled hearts would seem the last place one might expect to find public controversy.[32] Lillehei's cross-circulation operations and their risk of 200% mortality, as well as surgery possibly inflicting pointless pain and suffering on HLHS babies, understandably stirred the hornet's nest, but this was a squabble between people describing heart defects. How did it escape the experts' lair, far outlasting the surgical controversies? That its chief protagonists were two of congenital cardiology's most engaging personalities surely had a lot to do with it.

Born (1942) in Wellington, Shropshire, England, Robert H. Anderson got his medical degree (and another in anatomy) from the University of Manchester in 1966. Initially leaning toward ophthalmology, he soon plunged into cardiac anatomy and trained with Anton Becker at the University of Amsterdam in 1973. Anderson worked 25 years at the Royal Brompton, then eight more at Great Ormond Street Hospital Institute of Child Development. An emeritus professor at University College London since 2007, he has been a visiting professor or fellow at several other centers[33] (Fig. 8.2). While Anderson declared that Van Praagh's segmental (sequential is Anderson's term) analysis "revolutionized" the field,[34] his approach contrasts in multiple ways, in part as noted above.[35] He favors precise, systematic description to specify cardiac anatomy while eschewing Van Praagh's set notation, and their terminologies sometimes diverge. Their head-butting "letters to the editor" are highly technical and difficult for even well-informed non-morphologists to adjudicate. A certain amount of pique also shows through, with Anderson complaining—with some justification—that Van Praagh ignores his work, and Van Praagh suggesting that sometimes Anderson just doesn't get the point.[36] They avow respect for and friendship with the other, but both are hard-headed and certain enough of their point of view that neither can understand why the other hasn't long ago cried uncle.

Both men have trained their share of devoted disciples, as the genesis of the *Atlas of Congenital Heart Disease Nomenclature* affirms.[37] The *Atlas,* which compares and contrasts the Van Praaghian and Andersonian systems (and serves as a catalogue raisonné of their ideas), is peculiar; other such tracts discuss one or

[32] Moodie (2015); Goreczny et al. (2018); Ezon et al. (2015); Castañeda (2010).

[33] Moodie (2015); Goreczny et al. (2018).

[34] Moodie (2015).

[35] Tynan et al. (1979); Ezon et al. (2015).

[36] For those interested in the fine grain of the controversy between Van Praagh and other morphologists (not just Anderson), the following citations are for letters from Van Praagh to the editors of various journals, in response to criticism: *Am Heart J* (1977) v.93:810; v. 94:670; 671; *Circ* (1978) v.57:1036; (1980) v.61:1057; *Am J Cardiol* (1982) v.50:929; *Cardiovasc Intervent Radiol* (1984) v.7:320; *Pediatr Cardiol* (1987) v.8:151; *J Thorac Cardiovasc Surg* (1989) v.97:476; *Euro J Cardiothorac Surg* (1990) v.4:213; *Am Heart J* (1995) v.129:123; *Ann Thorac Surg* (1995) v.60:1163; *J Thorac Cardiovasc Surg* (1996) v.111:1107.

[37] Ezon et al. (2015).

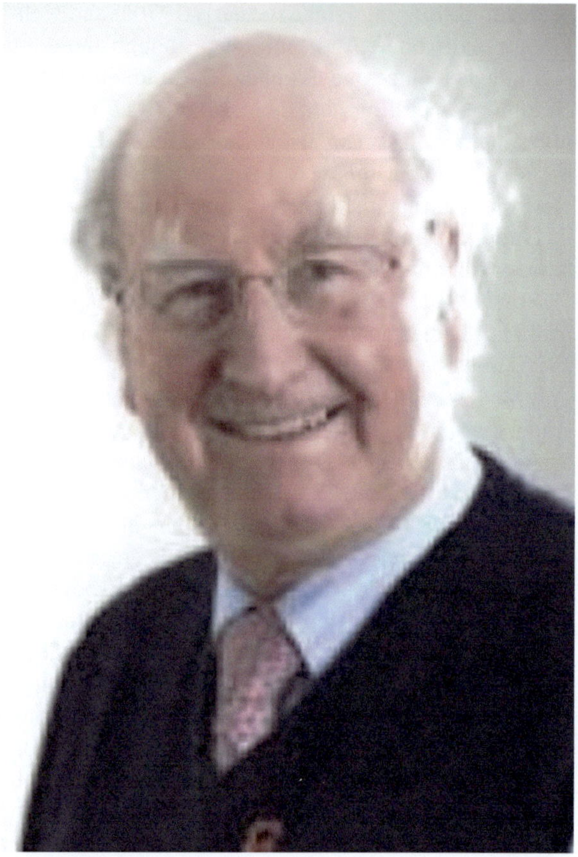

**Fig. 8.2** Robert Anderson MD. (Courtesy of Robert Anderson MD)

the other, or a hybrid, of these two systems.[38] When I asked its first author what inspired this unusual effort, he implicated two influential mentors, one fiercely subscribing to Anderson's view and the other to Van Praagh's, leading him to conclude that facility in *both* systems is required for fluency in congenital cardiology.[39]

I'm not so sure. At Boston Children's, *the* Van Praaghian stronghold, set notation (sans the numbers) is routine, but clinicians don't talk about connecting segments, do use unapproved terminology, and routinely utter "single ventricle" in ways utterly inconsistent with both his and Anderson's lexicons. In Boston—and surely in centers partial to Anderson—descriptive formalism is often shorn from working discourse. And speaking with Boston surgeons, I find a wide range of opinions regarding the utility of both systems. If their terminology is only

[38] Keane et al. (2006).

[39] Personal communication (email) with David S. Ezon, November 2020.

inconsistently applied, and many practitioners' anatomic expertise is not directly derived from Van Praagh and Anderson's systems, how much have they really added to congenital cardiology? To go further, could it be that Jesse Edwards (and others) provided essentially all the maps needed to negotiate the malformed heart, and that later contributors are talking about angels and pins? What is and will be the influence of these two dynamos, the most *present* of the modern morphologists? The stories of the Baltimore trio and Lillehei and Norwood (see Chap. 11) are compelling and durable because they show us that something specific and very special, and hitherto seemingly unlikely or impossible, could be done, and how to do it. They stand out from the rest of their landscape like a lone pine on the tundra. On the other hand, Van Praagh and Anderson's morphological constructs, *viewed strictly through the lens of the tools required for effective therapy*, hardly penetrate the horizon.

But perhaps that is the very nature of their contribution. The language of cardiac defects is like a language: As students, we learn formal elements of sentence structure, but we speak and write long after the meanings of gerund and infinitive have escaped memory, and occasionally hang a participle, yet we communicate more precisely and gracefully thanks to the residua of our formal instruction. So, too, with the heart: Whether we remember or care to adopt either morphologist's dictionary, having been directly or indirectly (via our mentors) so indoctrinated, we are bound to speak and think at least a little more clearly than otherwise. Our understanding of cardiac *structure*—as opposed to the names applied to its features—is also subtly, even unconsciously enriched by exposure to the systematic and penetrating analysis of Van Praagh and Anderson. Their papers and pedantry have diffused into our field and have advanced morphological understanding in ways on which it is hard to draw a steady bead. Richard and Bob will, I predict, merge into the landscape in the way that influencers always have. Congenital cardiology is mostly fashioned from the innumerable incremental advances in knowledge and craft that we apply, unaware of their origins and originators. Van Praagh and Anderson have taught us things whose roots are—or will be—lost to us. In that sense, they stand in for most of what makes congenital cardiology function and inch ahead. Not just the lone pines, but the earth into which their roots are sunk.

The days of sword-crossing over morphological arcana are drawing to a close. The International Society for Nomenclature of Paediatric and Congenital Heart Disease has imposed some terminological order (the International Paediatric and Congenital Cardiac Code).[40] Cardiac morphology taught face-to-face with morphologists and real hearts will remain invaluable, but new methods of teaching, utilizing computerized reconstructions, will substitute for, and maybe even supersede, hands-on experiences.[41] Going forward, the morphologist's deepest achievements may be

[40] Franklin et al. (2017).

[41] Goreczny et al. (2018).

contributions to cellular and molecular investigations of cardiac development. We should hope that the color like that of these four 'Lone Pines"[42] will never leave cardiac morphology, and given its history of dynamic and vivid contributors, my hunch is that it never will.[43]

***

## References


Abbott ME (1936/2006) Atlas of congenital cardiac disease. McGill-Queen's University Press, Montreal

American Association of Clinical Anatomists. Robert Anderson. Accessed 20 Aug 2024. https://clinical-anatomy.org/Robert_Anderson_MD_PhD_FRCPath

Barratt-Boyes BG, Neutze JM, Harris EA (1973) Heart disease in infancy: diagnosis and surgical treatment. Williams & Wilkins, Baltimore

Becker AE, Anderson RH (1982) Atrioventricular septal defects: what's in a name? J Thorac Cardiovasc Surg 83:461–469

Bharati S (1994) Maurice Lev, MD. 1908 to February 4, 1994. Cardiovasc Pathol 3:145–145

Castañeda AR (2010) Richard van Praagh. Thorac Cardiovasc Surg 58:320–321

Desnick SJ, Neal WA, Nicoloff DM, Moller JH (1976) Residual right-to-left shunt following repair of atrial septal defect. Ann Thorac Surg 21(4):291–295

Evans WN, Acherman RJ, Anderson RH (2009) One hundred years of texts describing congenitally malformed hearts from 1814 to 1914. Cardiol Young 19:12–29

Ezon DS, Goldberg JF, Kyle WB (2015) Atlas of congenital heart disease. Ezon Educational Services, Houston

Franklin RCG, Bréland MJ, Colan SD et al (2017) Nomenclature for congenital and pediatric cardiac disease: the International Paediatric and Congenital Cardiac Code (IPCCC) and the eleventh iteration of the International Classification of Diseases (ICD-11). Cardiol Young 27:1872–1938

Freedom RM (1984) The anthropology of the segmental approach to the diagnosis of complex congenital heart disease. Cardiovasc Intervent Radiol 7:121–123

Freedom RM, Yoo S, Mikailian H, Williams WG (2004) The natural and modified history of congenital heart disease. Wiley-Blackwell, New York

French RK (1994) William harvey's natural philosophy. Cambridge University Press

Fye WB (2015) Caring for the heart: Mayo Clinic and the rise of specialization. Oxford University Press, Oxford

Goreczny S, Ivy D, Anderson R (2018) "The person who influenced me most was the person who disagreed most strongly with me": an interview with professor Robert Anderson. Cardiol Young 29:259–262

Keane JF, Lock JE, Fyler DC (2006) Nadas' pediatric cardiology, 2nd edn. Saunders, Philadelphia

Lev M (1966) Some newer concepts of the pathology of congenital heart disease. Med Clin North Am 50:3–14

Moodie DS (2015) Interview with Roberts [sic] Anderson. Cong Heart Dis 10:96–104

Peacock TB (1858) On malformations, &c., of the human heart. John Churchill, London. Reprinted in the classics of medicine library. Gryphon Editions, Ltd., Birmingham, 1981


---

[42] Tom did not quite consider these four "Lone Pines", hence the quotes, but they were darn close. You can make your own decision.

[43] Tom would like to thank Drs. Richard Van Praagh, Stephen P. Sanders, and Robert H. Anderson for discussions relative to this chapter.

Roberts WC (1998) Jesse Efrem Edwards, MD: a conversation with the editor. Am J Cardiol 81:902–911

Rogers HM, Edwards JE (1951) Cor triloculare biatriatum: an analysis of the clinical and pathologic features of nine cases. Am Heart J 41:299–310

Saunders JBC, O'Malley CD (1982) The anatomical drawings of Andreas Vesalius. Bonanza Books, New York, NY

Tynan MJ, Becker AE, Macartney FJ, Jiménez MQ, Shinebourne EA, Anderson RH (1979) Nomenclature and classification of congenital heart disease. Br Heart J 41(5):544–553

Van Praagh R (1985 July) The importance of segmental situs in the diagnosis of congenital heart disease. Semin Roentgenol 20(3):254–271

Van Praagh R (2012) The Farber-landing lecture: pediatric pathology—the clinician's "open sesame" and its importance in pediatric cardiology and cardiovascular surgery. Ped Dev Pathol 15:431–449

Van Praagh R (2019 Jan) The story of Dr Stella (1927–2006). World J Pediatr Congenit Heart Surg 10(1):125–128

Van Praagh R, Ongley PA, Swan HJC (1964) Anatomic types of single or common ventricle in man. Morphologic and geometric aspects of 60 necropsied cases. Am J Cardiol 13:367–386

Van Praagh R, Bernhardt WF, Rosenthal SA, Parisi LF, Fyler DC (1971) Interrupted aortic arch: surgical treatment. Am J Cardiol 27:200–211

Wakai CS, Edwards JE (1958) Pathologic study of persistent common atrioventricular canal. Am Heart J 56:779–794

# Chapter 9
# Strange Operation—Fontan

Nothing is ever—quite—an innovation.
–Stephen Greenblatt, *The Swerve.*[1]

In biology, wild type is the normal type. Doctors strive to purchase it. Heart surgeons close a hole; buttress a leaky valve; widen a narrowed artery. Cardiologists prevent the heart from shuddering to a sudden stop; if weak, increase its squeeze; align an irregular rhythm with the normal metronome. Practitioners don't presume to redesign the human body, but rather to adjust faulty tissues or organs so that they work as such components normally do.

I note in Appendix 4 the limitations of animal models for developing new therapies. But such models were absolutely crucial to creating open-heart surgery. Inventing ways of safely invading and repairing the heart would never have happened—or if so, at stupendous human cost—without using animals to learn the physiology, create new tools, and hone surgical craft. The debt owed our animal friends—mostly dogs and an occasional cat in this case—is truly incalculable.

But to rescue the single ventricle, doctors had to do more than manipulate an idled pump; they had to invent a new physiology. Laboratory work suggested novel and even strange operations, aiming not to convert the patient's circulation to the wild type—that is, to normal—but rather to something Nature had left in the water. The Fontan operation is its ultimate expression, and the final modality of treatment for most single ventricles today. *Strange Operation* tells the story of how this treatment evolved, in the hands of the son of a famous Tour-de-France cyclist, and how this surgery was generalized beyond a tiny fraction of the single ventricle crowd. Fontan operations were initially mostly applied to a rare malformation (tricuspid atresia), leaving many single ventricles stranded. Congenital cardiology's last major surgical development—at least by my lights—was surgery to rescue babies with hypoplastic left heart syndrome, and similar defects, which are far more common than tricuspid atresia. The creation of the iconic Norwood procedure brings us to what in many ways is congenital cardiology's acme (Chap. 11).

---

[1] Greenblatt (2011), p. 286.



T. J. Kulik, M. Dick, *Reimagining a Child's Heart*,
https://doi.org/10.1007/978-3-031-88608-9_9

But first, the cardiovascular reconfiguration crafted by Francis Fontan. As Harvey showed centuries ago, blood pumped by the left ventricle to the body returns to the right ventricle, which propels it through the lungs and into the left ventricle, where the cycle begins afresh. With the "Fontan," evolution is heaved out the window. In it, the solo ventricle pumps to the body but blood traverses the lungs by virtue of the pressure remaining after passing through tiny vessels in muscle and gut and other tissues (Fig. 9.1). This unlikely arrangement only works thanks to the exquisite efficiency of the vascular system: just one watt of power, the amount consumed by a tiny incandescent flashlight bulb, is enough to circulate the blood in a resting adult.[2] Normal physiology isn't *possible* with a single pumping chamber, but that only adds to the *strangeness* of the operation. Medicine aspires to return an ailing body to the wild type, and there are precious few examples of such flagrant violation of this principle as the Fontan. The Blalock-Taussig-Thomas shunt is seemingly another, but even it mimics the (naturally occurring) patent ductus arteriosus—in fact, the ductus was its inspiration. The Fontan is not like anything found in nature—at least not quite.

But as peculiar as it is, the operation that stands at the apogee of solo ventricle palliation had always been out there, waiting to be exploited, like alluvial gold. It could have been invented shortly after open-heart surgery's arrival, yet it hung fire for over ten years, and took nearly ten more before garnering widespread buy-in. Clues suggesting its viability lurked just below the surface. Experiments were performed in the 1940s where the contractile function of a dog's right ventricle was intentionally destroyed, yet trans-pulmonary blood flow proceeded unabated; a 1952 paper describing a baby alive for seven months despite lacking a functional right ventricle suggested that this chamber wasn't so essential after all. (A similar patient, living one year, was described in 1961, and subsequently adults with an "Uhl's heart" have been documented.)[3]

In fact, nature had been dropping hints for five hundred million years that a second ventricle is not *de rigeur*. Fish have only one ventricle, and a circulation something like a reverse Fontan. Blood is pumped first to the organs of gas exchange (the gills), then distributed to the body's tissues, finally returning to the heart. Physician-physiologist Simon Rodbard described this circulation as "primitive,"[4] yet it is anything but. Depending upon the species, fish can burst up to 60 miles an hour—through a medium 800 times as viscous as air and 60 times as dense—and range over thousands of miles, never stopping to rest. Massive great white sharks slink through the brine, dive thousands of feet, and may live for 70 years powered by this "primitive" system. Despite the fact that seawater contains only three percent as much oxygen as air, a tuna's maximum oxygen consumption—a measure of the cardiovascular

---

[2] Williams et al. (2001). The power (watts) needed to circulate the blood = cardiac output (l/min) × mean arterial pressure (mmHg) × $2.22 \times 10^{-3}$. For an adult with a cardiac output of 5 l, and a mean arterial pressure of 100 mmHg, the power = 1.1 watts, though the total amount of power *generated* is higher since the heart is not perfectly efficient.

[3] Uhl (1952, 1996); Arcilla and Gasul (1961).

[4] Rodbard et al. (1949).

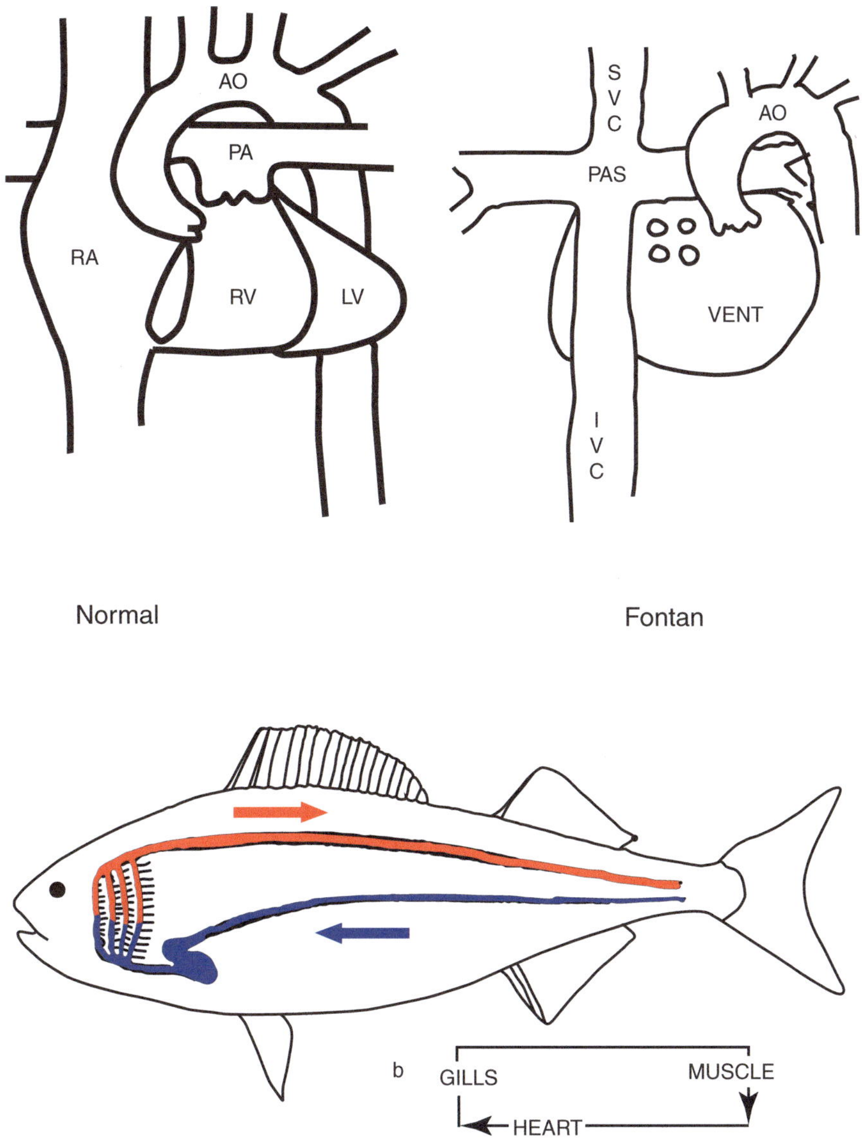


**Fig. 9.1** Top: Left—cartoon of Normal heart. Right—cartoon of Fontan Heart. Bottom: cartoon of fish circulation. See text

system's overall capacity—is is nearly as high as a human's.[5] This is not to say that a person's plumbing can be reconfigured to that of a fish. Indeed, the Fontan circulation isn't quite that of a fish's, since with the former the blood first perfuses the body rather than the lungs[6] (Fig. 9.1). A fish's environment is different and, in some ways, easier, as fish do not walk upright and against gravity. Their gills can operate at higher vascular pressures than our lungs, since any fluid leaking out of their super-thin capillary vessels is into the water, not into the alveoli. And one feature of piscine physiology would prove most inconvenient for even the most restless land-lubber: many fish must unceasingly "fish" for oxygen-containing water to suffuse their gills, lest they suffocate. But the example of fish can make us think differently about the number of pumping chambers needed, even in the human.

The clues were there, but the Fontan's gestation remained halting. The very strangeness of the central idea of this operation—blood eking its way across the lungs without a right ventricle, the second pump—likely fettered the conceptual leap needed for its acceptance, but there were also other reasons. The Fontan's creation story recalls the early use of artificial pumps for organ perfusion; isolated experiments were performed, lacking follow-up, so people didn't capitalize on lessons learned. Animal models, our best friends, and our worst enemies, were confusing and contributed to the muddle. And cardiologists didn't always appreciate just how limited, in vigor and duration, their single ventricle patients' lives were, which moderated any tendency to try radical new treatments. It's perhaps not surprising that the Fontan's development was slow.

Before we engage the Fontan story, we must first take a step back and consider another critical development, first appearing just in advance of open-heart surgery, that helped make modern congenital cardiology modern. The physiological and clinical insights that *cardiac catheterization and angiography* delivered rapidly expanded cardiology's toolbox, enormously increasing the range and power of open-heart surgery, including single ventricle therapy. This immensely useful tool first hit the scene at the provocation of WWII, not in the service of ailing hearts but rather shock victims, and at the hands of pulmonologists rather than cardiologists, though it was soon hijacked by the latter. Its history is one of our familiar themes of persistence and courage, but this time with a different twist. We've seen foundational contributions made only by dint of unusual courage, but here we examine courage as an end unto itself: a brave investigator who is firmly ensconced in cardiology's historical cannon, despite lacking any such culminating achievement. And

[5] Brill and Bushnell in Block and Stevens (2001); Evans et al. (2005); National Maritime Research Institute. The maximum oxygen consumption for an athletically untrained 30-year-old man is roughly 41–48 ml/min/kg, and 34–39 ml/min/kg for a woman (Paap and Takken 2014). For a skipjack tuna, it is at least 32 ml/min/kg (Brill and Bushnell in Block and Stevens 2001, p. 88).

[6] Crustaceans—for example, lobsters and crayfish—have a single ventricle, and their hemolymph (blood equivalent) is pumped to the body's tissues before passing through their gills, reminiscent of Fontan flow. But their circulatory systems are very different—the hemolymph sloshes through the tissues rather than being contained in blood vessels—and crustaceans' repertoire restricted to scuttling across floors of silent seas, as T.S. Eliot put it; any comparison with human single ventricle physiology seems a stretch.

in *Strange Operation* we meditate again on the vagaries of credit in congenital cardiology, but with a fresh slant: Blalock and Taussig initially got all of the recognition for their seminal innovation while an indispensable contributor was neglected. But we soon see that even big cheeses with temporal precedence can lose out on name-fame if they don't play their cards right.

We begin with something else new, though sporting a long and distinguished history: physicians first hazarding new procedures not on their patients, but on themselves.

We've encountered pioneers whose achievements demanded serious courage. Robert Gross's career would have likely exploded on the launching pad had his first ductal ligation gone awry. Walt Lillehei's thrusting to operationalize open-heart surgery provoked critical parries, and the predictable and painful need to break terrible news to families after an operation's failure. Blalock and Taussig exposed themselves to fallout from the inevitable deaths; it would have been easier to apply, while bemoaning, the sorry existing state of the art than a risky new operation. But we remember these people not for their backbone (at least not mainly), but for what they accomplished. Werner Forssmann on the other hand, collected the acme of accolades—the Nobel Prize in Physiology or Medicine—*for* courage. Forssmann was one of three men so honored in 1956, along with Dickinson W. Richards and André F. Cournand for developing cardiac catheterization (Fig. 9.2). The Nobel presentation speech of Göran Liljestrand tells the story.[7] Turning to the awardees, Liljestrand said: "Professor Cournand and Professor Richards. The practical value of cardiac catheterization has been definitely proved by you and your co-workers. This method, combined with those already available before, has *in your hands led*

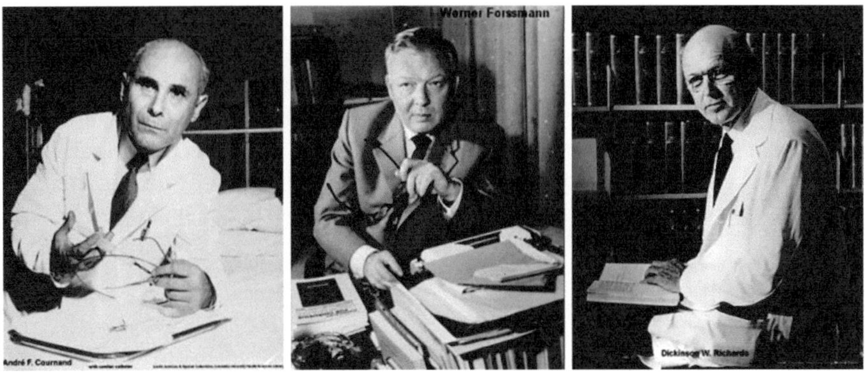


**Fig. 9.2** Andre F. Cournand (left); Werner Forsman (middle); Dickinson W. Richards (right). (Reprinted by permission of Oxford University Press on behalf of the European Society of Cardiology)

[7] Liljestrand (1956).

*to many important new observations, to diagnostic as well as therapeutic advances*" (emphasis mine). But for Forssmann: "Professor Forssmann. As a young doctor you have had the courage to submit yourself to heart catheterization. As a result of this, a new method was born which since that time has proved to be of very great value." The rest of Liljestrand's speech lauds the major contributions that Cournand and Richards made to respiratory physiology, shock, and the physiology of congenital heart disease, while the German was mostly fêted for his "by no means harmless experiments on himself," thereby demonstrating the safety of cardiac catheterization in humans. Forssmann never exploited this technique for basic or therapeutic investigations, partly because he could never gather support from his superiors. But Cournand thought that Forssmann had little scientific bent and wasn't good at working with others, which may be a better explanation.[8]

Self-experimentation, or experimenting on one's family members, has a surprisingly ample pedigree. Physician and medical historian Allen Weisse collected 514 instances of this practice, surely an underestimate.[9] Self-experimenters in the realm of infectious disease, by Weisse's count, are the most numerous. In 1721, for example, Zabdiel Boylston in Brookline, Massachusetts, attempted to immunize his 13-year-old son against smallpox using pus from a pock (he himself was immune, having had the disease).[10] Jonas Salk administered his polio vaccine to himself and his wife and children before commencing field trials, and Albert Sabin did much the same with his vaccine. Cardiac practitioners have been just as brave. In addition to Forssmann, several notable physicians have submitted to heart catheterization in pursuit of their research, including Howard Burchell, Earl Wood, and Andreas Gruentzig.

Weisse identified eight Nobel Prize winners who had self-experimented in areas relevant to their Prize. But when one reviews the scope of their work, Forssmann stands out as the only one who took an existing idea, previously well-developed in animals, and merely showed that it could be safely applied to a human (and only one human, at that). The other self-experimenting laureates executed elaborate lines of discovery culminating in a major discoveries.[11] In fact, exactly how convincing Forssmann's demonstration was is unclear to me; after all, it was an *n* of only one, and the procedure lasted only a few minutes. In his 1944 Harvey Lecture, Richards said that he and Cournand knew of Forssmann's demonstration and other work in

[8] Weisse (2002), pp. 28–30.

[9] Weisse (2012).

[10] Moore (1969).

[11] For example, Barry J. Marshall, an Australian physician who, with Robin Warren, was awarded the 2005 Nobel Prize for Physiology or Medicine for discovering that the bacteria *H. pylori* is often the cause of pyloric ulcers. Marshall, pursing an idea that grew from the work of Warren and others, showed that *H. pylori* is often present in the stomach of patients with gastritis, while absent in normals. Frustrated with the lack of success of establishing an animal model for further studies, he—after undergoing a baseline endoscopy—drank a cocktail with the bacteria. Developing symptoms a few days later, a repeat endoscopy and biopsy showed inflammation and the bacteria in the stomach lining. He also conducted a clinical trial of antibiotics to treat ulcers. Marshall published dozens of papers on the subject. Marshall et al. (1985); Nobel Prize (2005).

Europe, but they were still afraid that it might be dangerous and had "vacillated for eight years," making only "desultory" efforts, mostly in animals, to develop catheterization.[12] Forssmann's volume of work-product paled in comparison with his Nobel littermates. Cournand published 70 papers between 1941 and 1955, and Richards 81 (although not all were related to catheterization, and many of the reports were shared), as contrasted with Forssmann's two. Nils Hansson, a scholar who has published extensively on the Nobel prize, discussed (along with colleagues) Forssmann's award in "*From nobody to Nobel laureate*" (English translation): Archival material from the Nobel Foundation reveals that Gören Liljestrand (secretary of the Nobel Committee), who was primarily responsible for reviewing Forssmann's contribution for consideration for the award, found it insufficient to merit the prize. Hansson concludes that this "highly remarkable" awarding of the Nobel, done despite Liljestrand's skepticism, can be accounted for by the fame of those who nominated Forssmann for the prize, and the fact that Cournand, Richards, and Paul Dudley White (perhaps the most prominent American cardiologist at the time), cited him in their written accounts of the origin of cardiac catheterization, and provided other forms of support.[13]

Whether Forssmann's contribution was of the stuff usually associated with the Nobel or not, cardiac catheterization (introducing a thin tube [catheter] into a peripheral vein or artery and advancing it into the heart using X-ray fluoroscopy) was a major and necessary advance for congenital cardiology. To make sense of a defect's physiology, cardiologists needed to measure pressures and blood oxygen content inside the heart, and flow to the body and lungs. And revealing a malformed heart's architecture is equally key to executing repairs. Much of this information is now obtained using echocardiography, computerized tomography (CT), and cardiac magnetic resonance imaging (cMR), but these technologies were decades off in the 1950s. Doctors had only heart catheterization for hemodynamics, and angiography (injecting a radiopaque liquid through a catheter to outline the interior of the heart and blood vessels using x-rays) for imaging. While physical examinations, X-rays, and electrocardiograms sufficed for the New Dawn of congenital cardiology (but allowing for a significant number of inaccurate diagnoses), its Modern era required vastly better diagnostic information.

Cardiac catheterization in animals anticipated Forssmann by at least two hundred years. The Rev. Stephen Hales ordered a mare, 14 hands high, tied down and introduced a brass pipe, spliced onto a nine feet long glass tube, into its crural artery; blood levitated eight feet and three inches above the heart, thus quantifying its pressure (*Haemastaticks,* 1733).[14] Claude Bernard, arguably history's premiere physiologist, first performed "catheterism" to ascertain where animal heat is generated. Antoine Lavoisier had surmised the lungs, while others though it elsewhere. Passing heat-sensing catheters into a horse's right and left ventricles and finding the

[12] Richards Jr. (1944).

[13] Hansson et al. (2015).

[14] See also Pickering in Fishman and Richards (1964), p. 489.

temperature a bit higher in the right ventricle than the left, Bernard deftly dislodged the site of heat production from the lungs (1844). He measured ventricular pressures in other animals, including a dog named King Charles.[15] Auguste Chauveau and Jules Marey famously catheterized a horse in 1861, which served a pivotal inspiration for Forssmann.[16] Others followed, but until Forssmann, this procedure was considered too dangerous for people. Cournand wrote that the risk lay in blood clots and thrombophlebitis (inflammation or infection of veins),[17] although abnormal heart rhythms and cardiac perforation or damage must have also spooked physicians. Werner Forssmann's great accomplishment was to allay that fear, forcing people to think differently about that procedure.[18]

Forssmann was Berlin-born, in August 1904.[19] He entered Friedrich Wilhelm University in 1922 and was licensed as a physician by February 1929. His internship commenced in Eberswalde, a small Prussian town northwest of Berlin, at the Auguste Viktoria Home, supervised by Dr. Richard Schneider, head of the second surgical department. Bernard, Chauveau, and Marey's research mesmerized Forssmann early in his university days: a diagram of Marey standing in front of a horse, grasping a tube inserted through the horse's jugular vein into his heart, so "excited" Forssmann that "it haunted me day and night." Forssmann and his friend Peter Romeis hashed over the sorry state of cardiac diagnostics for hours, envisioning catheterization's revolutionary potential. In the summer of 1929, "After endless debates of the pros and cons, I resolved upon the action that was to decide my fate." He would open a superficial vein in the arm, insert a ureteral catheter, and advance it into the heart. He presented his plan to Schneider, who despite being generally supportive and sympathetic, answered in the negative; risky ventures of this sort are best launched in a major hospital. Forssmann, "so obsessed with my plans that I would not consider abandoning them," instantly regrouped, proposing to catheterize himself, a proposition no more satisfactory from Schneider's perspective. "Remember your mother," was Schneider's rejoinder, "I am also responsible to her for what you do. Imagine how it would be if I had to inform this lady, who's already lost her husband during the war, that her only son had died in my hospital as a result of an experiment which I had approved."[20]

But Forssmann was implacable. The major hurdle was getting his hands on the sterile instruments, locked away in custody of one Gerda Ditzen, needed to cut down onto and slit his vein. The intern figured that she would not readily surrender these tools, so he "began to prowl around Nurse Gerda Ditzen like a sweet-toothed

[15] Cournand (1980).

[16] Cournand in Fishman and Richards (1964), pp. 49–50.

[17] Cournand and Ranges (1941).

[18] Cournand wrote that Claude Bernard invented cardiac catheterization, but Johan F. Dieffenbach catheterized animals, and possibly a human, in 1832. Ernest Unger introduced a catheter into the arm vein of a colleague, Frtiz Bleichröder, and three other people, in 1905, though reported it only seven years later and did not document that it reached the heart.

[19] Forssmann (1974).

[20] Forssmann (1974), pp. 81–84.

cat around the cream jug."[21] They gossiped around cups of coffee, hashed over books, and when the time was right, he confessed his obsession to Gerda. Sharing his anatomy and physiology books, he made his vision hers. After two weeks of schmoozing, she was all-in, even asking Forssmann to perform the catheterization on her. "Ya," Forssmann replied, and the procedure was perpetrated during the hospital's after-lunch siesta. As described in his autobiography, Forssmann induced Ditzen to allow him to immobilize her on an operating table (he didn't want her to fall off, he said) and applied disinfectant solution to her arm as though preparing to incise her skin. But somehow during this charade he applied local anesthesia to *his* arm, opened a vein, and slid in a ureteral catheter, all out of her line of sight. He was fixing to walk down to the basement X-ray machine, catheter hanging from his arm, before Gerda realized that she had been duped. When an X-ray showed the thin tube shy of the heart, Forssmann pushed it in another foot, where it found the right atrium.[22] The news diffused quickly. Within minutes, Schneider sent for him, and after expressing his disappointment at Forssmann's breach of trust, he congratulated his trainee. They celebrated Forssmann's "heart probe" at Kretschmar's (presumably a restaurant) that evening. Whether to provide richer opportunity for his precocious trainee, or rather to re-locate a loose cannon, Schneider advised Forssmann to decamp to a flagship hospital. (Schneider did allow Forssmann to place a catheter in a patient dying from sepsis [bacteria in the blood] before he left.)

Forssmann soon secured a position at German surgery's Mecca, Berlin's Charité hospital, under Ferdinand Sauerbruch. But he could garner no support for research and soon clashed with this powerful boss, was fired, and found himself back in Eberswalde by January 1930. His vision still unsatisfied, Forssmann now hoped to outline the heart's interior by injecting, through an intracardiac catheter, X-ray-opaque contrast material. While the Auguste Viktoria didn't have suitable X-ray equipment, the Neukölln municipal hospital did. However, it had no animal housing, so Forssmann kenneled study dogs in his mother's apartment. On the day of an experiment, he sedated the dog with morphine, hauled it in an old potato sack to the hospital, did the experiment, and returned the incontinent animal to his mother's bathtub that night. (Apparently the only problem with this arrangement was that his mother and grandmother would get so attached to the dogs that they could hardly let them go.) After satisfying himself that angiography was safe, Forssmann twice injected contrast in his own heart and took X-rays. But the angiograms were of poor quality and of little use.[23] He abandoned cardiac investigations and eventually carved out a career in urology.[24]

Forssmann dispelled unfounded and paralyzing fear of cardiac catheterization, but Cournand and Richards were the first to systematically exploit this tool to break

[21] Forssmann (1974), p. 84.

[22] Forssmann (1974), p. 86. Forssmann couldn't recall the date of this first catheterization, only that it was in early summer 1929.

[23] Forssmann said that he performed a total of nine self-catheterizations, while providing few details.

[24] Forssmann (1974).

new ground in physiology and pathophysiology. These extraordinary men, working at New York's Bellevue Hospital, formed a rare partnership, lasting until Richard's death 41 years later. Cournand reckoned them a "perfect combination,"[25] and their collaboration surely ranks amongst medicine's most notable. Richards hailed from Orange, New Jersey (both he and Cournand were born in 1895), got his BA and MA at Yale, and his MD from Columbia.[26] Cournand described Richards as "a humanist; he was a Hellenist; he was a scientist; he was a superb clinician; and he was an outstanding gentlemen. I have never met another man as remarkable as he."[27] A Hellenist, indeed—Richards had devoured Greek at the Hotchkiss School and copped the highest score ever on the Greek entrance exam at Yale. He studied Hippocrates and had the expertise and self-confidence to offer an alternative to the usual translation of the Greek physician's first aphorism.[28] Richards deeply contemplated medicine and research, putting them into broad historical and societal context,[29] yet transcended the ivory tower. Deeply offended by the decrepit state of Bellevue Hospital, Richards repeatedly complained to its administration and to the press: "I can win the Nobel Prize in medicine, but I can't take care of my patients at Bellevue."[30]

Cournand was a Parisian. He earned his BA from the University of Paris, and then moved to Bellevue in 1930.[31] This "enzymatic" dynamo was described in his 90th year as a man of "probity, culture, wisdom, and charm. He is hard of hearing but easy of understanding. He remembers the past, thinks of the future, and integrates the two with vision and clarity." Both Richards and Cournand were humanists, curious, and sustained in their labors to advance their science.[32]

Their partnership gelled in February of 1932, Richards an assistant attending physician at Columbia Presbyterian and Cournand chief resident on the chest service at Bellevue.[33] Pulmonary, not cardiac physiology, was their chief interest, and they began by pondering their subject, broadly and deeply. They delighted in parsing the various factors which define cardiorespiratory physiology, and how they might be quantified. They envisioned a comprehensive plan for investigating cardiopulmonary dynamics, summarizing it in a figure they returned to often (Fig. 9.3). They explored cardiac catheterization starting in 1936, using animals, and Cournand first catheterized a human in 1940.[34] World War II provoked an acute need to better understand and treat shock, an all-too-common battlefield concomitant; Alfred

---

[25] Cournand in Weisse (2002), p. 38.

[26] Cournand (1989).

[27] Cournand in Weisse (2002), p. 38.

[28] Richards (1970), p. ix.

[29] Richards (1970).

[30] Oshinsky (2016), pp. 244–247.

[31] Weibel (1995).

[32] Merton in *Andre Cournand, 1895–1988* (1988), pp. 16, 22–23.

[33] Weisse (2002), pp. 28–38; Richards Jr. (1944, 1956); Cournand (1989).

[34] Cournand and Ranges (1941).

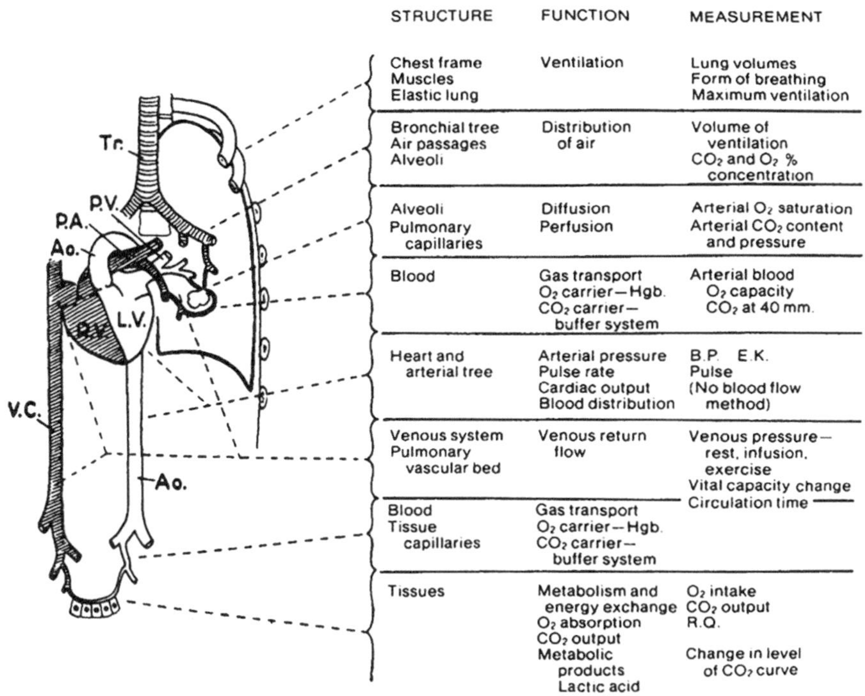


**Fig. 9.3** Richards and Cournand's master plan for investigating Cardiopulmonary Physiology. (J Thoracic and Cardiovascular Surgery (1938))

Blalock had studied shock in dogs (Chap. 6), but it was little explored in humans. Chatting with Blalock, the chair of the government's "shock committee," at a conference just after Pearl Harbor, Cournand described his exciting new catheter work. Impressed, the Baltimore surgeon quickly advanced a grant for the Bellevue group to probe shock in humans,[35] temporarily diverting Cournand and colleagues from cardiopulmonary physiology.

These clinical studies proved a far tougher proposition than investigations using animal models. Unlike a lab scientist, who has the luxury of scheduling experiments, Cournand's team was activated—anytime, day or night—whenever a shock victim rolled through the doors of Bellevue's emergency department. They catheterized gravely ill, sometimes dying people, with all the attached drama and intensity. Stanley Bradley, a trainee working with Cournand, recalled "the large, high, long room—the Emergency Ward at Bellevue—darkened and filled with quiet, purposeful movement, hushed voices and muffled sounds of transport and the coming-and-going of staff. . . . The looming X-ray head, the sudden, total darkness as the course of the catheter was followed fluoroscopically and André's quiet, tight,

[35] Weisse (2002), pp. 34–35; Fye (2015), p. 169.

but high-pitched voice calling the time sequence, calling for breathing rhythms in a sort of ceremonial chant, issuing soft but sharply demanding orders and criticisms."[36] They were responsible for desperately ill people needing therapy even as the investigations continued; Cournand had to juggle scientific exploration and life-saving clinical management.[37]

Their shock work was only the first tranche of many catheter-based studies. Seminal observations were made on many fronts: congestive heart failure; lung disease's impact on the heart; the effects of positive pressure breathing; the physiology of congenital and acquired heart disease; and the results of therapy. Congenital cardiologists and surgeons finally developed a quantitative appreciation of blood flow across holes in the heart, and how malformations impact pulmonary artery pressure. They learned how abnormal blood flow and arterial oxygen are related, and who will benefit from a surgical shunt, and who will not. Surgeons landed upon the shore of a new world thanks to angiography: Unimaginable procedures became routine, and others (such as the Blalock-Taussig-Thomas shunt) became much safer as anatomical information provided more reliable diagnoses.[38]

As people peeled back layers of normal and abnormal cardiovascular function, they began to explore *unnatural* physiology. In 1943, physicians at the University of Pennsylvania, studying congestive heart failure, asked: What happens to venous pressure if the right ventricle can no longer contract? In anesthetized, open-chest dogs, they devitalized the right ventricle using cautery and measured systemic and venous pressures. Killing the right ventricle only mildly reduced systemic blood pressure, and little increased venous pressure, suggesting that—at least under those conditions—that ventricle is not essential for blood flow to cross the lungs.[39] Similar experiments and observations from others followed.[40] But what had been discovered—that the right ventricle is dispensable[41]—was of questionable clinical utility; the experiments mostly involved dogs under anesthesia, with scarce observations made in awake, exercising animals. And it seemed that the left ventricle might be interacting with the devitalized right ventricle to help propel blood,[42] implying that surgically re-arranging a single ventricle circulation to send venous blood directly to the lungs might not be feasible. But even if these experiments offered only feeble proof of concept for the Fontan circulation, they did induce people to think differently: Perhaps a single pumping chamber would be quite enough, if the circulation were appropriately reconfigured.

---

[36] Bradley in *Andre Cournand, 1895–1988* (1988), p. 7.

[37] Richards Jr. (1944).

[38] In addition to Cournand and associates (especially Janet Baldwin and Aaron Himmelstein), Richard Bing (Johns Hopkins), Lewis Dexter (Harvard), and Earl Wood (Mayo Clinic) used cardiac catheterization to study hemodynamics in congenital heart disease.

[39] Starr et al. (1943).

[40] Landis et al. (1946); Rodbard and Wagner (1949); Bakos (1950); Kagan (1952); Donald and Essex (1954).

[41] Sade and Castañeda (1975).

[42] Kagan (1952).

In 1950, a fledgling northern Italian surgeon showed much more—that venous pressure alone could push superior vena caval blood through the right lung in long-surviving dogs, not merely during an hours-long experiment. Born in 1919 in Nola, near Naples, and raised in Venice, Carlo Carlon earned his MD at the University of Padova. Drafted into the Italian navy and serving as a medical ensign until the end of WWII, he began his general surgery residency shortly after discharge and got interested in thoracic and cardiovascular surgery. Italian heart surgery being even less mature than in the States, Carlon figured that he best look for training opportunities abroad. So between 1946 and 1950, he was on the road, with Blalock in Baltimore, Holman in New York, at the Karolinska Institute in Stockholm, and in London. Soon after returning to Padova, he aspired to create a better shunt than Blalock's, more physiologically efficient and easier to craft.

What Carlon had in mind was utterly new. Blalock's shunt was tough to execute in babies. Surgeons—Willis Potts, Denton Cooley, and David Waterston—had invented technically-easier alternatives, but these operated on the Blalock-Taussig-Thomas principle—arterial blood directed through the lungs. Thinking differently, Carlon imagined a truly novel shunt, where venous blood, rather than arterial, increases pulmonary blood flow.[43] He laid out a detailed argument for his idea, including noting physiological precedent: the venous pressure needed for transpulmonary flow, while higher than normal, is seen in people with chronic constrictive pericarditis.[44] Venturing into the dog lab, he connected the superior vena cava (using the azygous vein) to the right pulmonary artery, so that its flow crossed the lung by virtue of venous pressure only. Three animals not only survived the procedure, but showed no symptoms, were "lively and strong," and just as smart and affectionate as any other dogs.[45] While Simon Rodbard is generally credited with first suggesting the feasibility of right-heart bypass,[46] Carlon was the first to actually show that a substantial amount of venous return can bypass the heart in an awake and apparently normally-functioning animal. And his data intimated that an even more radical and useful operation might be possible: If one lung could accept the superior caval blood, might both lungs accept both caval flows?

But Carlon's contribution suffered the same fate as the insights of Ibn al-Nafis and Michael Servetus: limited dissemination (Chap. 1). His 1950 paper was in Italian and published in a barely-read—outside the country—Italian journal, and his 1951 report appeared in an organ only a little less obscure. The hotbed of cardiac innovation was the US and a few centers in Europe and Canada, whose cardiac surgeons were largely unaware of Carlon's shunt. His breakthrough was widely appreciated only decades later, long after credit for this type of shunt fell to William

[43] With Blalock's and other aortopulmonary shunts, the ventricle pumps blood to the lungs, as well as to the body. With Carlon's, blood perfuses the right lung via residual pressure in the venous circuit, hence the total amount of blood the heart needs to pump is less than with the Blalock-Taussig-Thomas shunt, all other things being equal.

[44] Carlon et al. (1950, 1951).

[45] Robiseck et al. (1969); Robiseck (1981).

[46] Rodbard et al. (1949); Sade and Castañeda (1975); Robiseck (1992); de Laval (2005).

Glenn (later discussed).[47] Although Carlon's international reputation lagged his imagination, he was highly regarded at home. Appointed Chairman of Surgery in Udine in 1959, he returned to Padova as the same in 1963, remaining chair until retiring in 1990.[48] He died the following year.

Lack of persistence and follow-through also explain Carlon's incomplete impact. With only rare exceptions, the most influential surgeon-innovators have been those who exported laboratory insights into the hospital's operating theater.[49] William Glenn, Chief of Cardiovascular Surgery at Yale, had the same idea as the Italian surgeon, but was more persistent. Over the course of many experiments, he connected one or both 'cava to canine pulmonary arteries, first reporting his results in 1954.[50] Three additional papers were published subsequently, including one first-authored by Sherwin Nuland, then a research fellow at Yale and subsequently a surgeon and an award-winning author.[51] Glenn concluded that, while the superior 'cava could be connected to the right pulmonary artery, serving as its sole source of blood flow, the inferior 'cava could not be so diverted without unacceptable side effects. In February 1958, Glenn anastomosed the superior vena cava to the right pulmonary artery in a deeply cyanotic and exercise-strapped seven-year-old boy with a solo ventricle. The lad left the hospital wearing only the faintest tinge of blue and fit to "walk up the hill." Glenn's single case report in the *New England Journal of Medicine* (1958) forever affixed his name to that procedure, even though its first successful clinical application was actually in Russia and anticipated Glenn's by nearly two years.[52] Evgenii Meshalkin's maiden successful clinical case (following extensive experimentation) was in April of 1956, and he reported 24 patients in the Russian literature later that year; two other Russian surgeons, Alexander Vishnevsky and Nikolai Galankin, also had also done similar operations in 1956.[53] Neither publication in Russian surgical journals, nor presentation at Russian meetings, got the word out, and the Meshalkin—like the Carlon—shunt was never to be.

There's a pattern here, and a lesson—being second or third, with better publicity, can beat being first. Italian cardiac surgeons, highly imaginative but never missing

[47] Robiseck et al. (1969); Robiseck (1981).

[48] I am grateful to Carlon's daughter Barbara, for discussion and email correspondence; his son Graziano, for email correspondence in April 2004; and colleague Giovani Stellin for discussion and correspondence.

[49] Only one such exception comes to mind. Giancarlo Rastelli, a research surgeon in an animal laboratory at the Mayo Clinic, developed a novel surgical procedure named for him; it was colleagues rather than Rastelli who applied this operation clinically (Squarcia and Squarcia 2007; Konstantinov et al. 2005; Rastelli et al. 1969).

[50] Glenn and Patino (1954).

[51] Patino et al. (1955); Nuland et al. (1958). Nuland's graceful style suffused many lay articles and books, including *Doctors: The Biography of Medicine* (1989) and *How We Die: Reflections on Life's Final Chapter* (1995).

[52] Glenn (1989). In a 1989 article, Glenn confessed that "because of our lack of scholarship" he was unaware of Carlon's work until he first applied the shunt clinically.

[53] Konstantinov and Alexi-Meskishvili (1999).

an opportunity to miss an opportunity, have been exemplars.[54] Glenn's shunt has been almost entirely superseded by the bidirectional cavopulmonary shunt (aka the "bidirectional-Glenn," where the superior vena cava is connected to *both* pulmonary arteries. The first such shunt was crafted by Archille Dogliotti in Torino in a five-year-old girl with tetralogy of Fallot and reported in 1961.[55] And Gaetano Azzolina, in Massa (Italy), operated upon nine patients between 1968 and 1970, most of whom received a complete (in several it was incomplete) bidirectional shunt.[56] As was true for for Carlon's report, Dogliotti's paper was in Italian in a minor journal, although Azzolina's was in English and in a more widely circulated one. When this operation fully emerged in the 1980s, Azzolina's priority was acknowledged—Dogliotti's recognition came later—but the connection was too distant for either to become eponyms.[57]

Perhaps not every new procedure merits the innovator's name, but the congenital cardiac community has not been stingy with these honors: By my count (probably missing a few), 32 names have clung to a procedure often or exclusively used in congenital heart surgery.[58] But also fickle. Some of the greatest pioneers—Gross, Lewis, and Lillehei come to mind—remain without such recognition. And highly impactful procedures have escaped concise identification via having a person's name attached. For example, Marc de Leval's brilliant and highly-influential evolution of the Fontan procedure remains the "total cavopulmonary connection" or "lateral tunnel Fontan"—try letting those roll off your tongue—rather than "the de Leval.".[59]

Glenn and others had established a trailhead, but efforts to hack out a path to the Fontan were desultory and dead-end. Part of the problem was that would-be trailblazers had a map—animal research—which proved unreliable. Results from dogs were inconsistent and often misleading, for reasons sometimes obvious, usually not. John Rose[60] at Georgetown found that complete right ventricular bypass in dogs was not tolerated, but inspection of his data reveals that an unappreciated technical problem[61] could explain the unsatisfactory results. But, as noted above, Glenn's excellent work also suggested that complete right heart bypass was problematic

[54] Abba Eban used "never miss an opportunity to miss an opportunity" in a different context.

[55] Konstantinov and Alexi-Meskishvili (2000).

[56] Azzolina et al. (1972).

[57] Hopkins et al. (1985); Konstantinov and Alexi-Meskishvili (2000).

[58] Baffes, Bentall, Blalock, Brock, Brockenbrough, Cooley, Damus, De Vega, Fontan, Glenn, Hanlon, Jatene, Kawashima, Kaye, Kreutzer, Mee, Mustard, Nikaidoh, Norwood, Ozaki, Potts, Rashkind, Rastelli, Ross, Sano, Senning, Stanzel, Starnes, Taussig, Thomas, Waldhausen, Waterston, and Yasui are the names; not all are surgeons.

[59] de Laval et al. (1988).

[60] Rose et al. (1955).

[61] A tube graft was used to convey blood from the proximal inferior vena cava to the pulmonary artery; their data (Table II) reveals significant obstruction between the vena cava and the pulmonary artery, which could account for their negative results.

in dogs, and others observed the same.[62] One surgeon labored for years for complete experimental bypass of the right heart, but achieved little of clinical value since his operation—which routed inferior vena cava blood into the left atrium—would have left many patients as blue or bluer than they were before the surgery.[63]

There were at least two reports suggesting complete bypass of the heart *might be* well-tolerated in dogs, but this work was apparently never further developed. Herb Warden and colleagues at the University of Minnesota created the equivalent of canine tricuspid atresia (complete under development and closure of the tricuspid valve, resulting in a markedly hypoplastic right ventricle) that bypassed the right ventricle; three animals survived at least three months.[64] But they did not prove that the tricuspid valve was completely closed and pursued no follow-up of these promising results. (At least none that were published.). Alex Haller and associates did much the same in a canine model, with three survivors, although the length of survival was not given, nor how healthy the dogs were. Haller, too, published no subsequent studies.[65] One senses that these surgeons' hearts weren't really into tossing out the right ventricle, perhaps related to the sheer audacity of the idea.

There were also sporadic *clinical* attempts at venous bypass. Elliott Hurwitt did so in a four-month-old baby thought to have tricuspid atresia, who died at the operation's end. The diagnosis was revealed to be incorrect on post-mortem, and the operation was doomed to failure given the cardiac anatomy.[66] At conferences, a few surgeons shared brief anecdotes of unsuccessful attempts at complete exclusion, but these contributed little to the craft, as minimal information was presented, or—as was the case for Hurwitt's patient—it seems clear, at least from this distance, that the patients' malformations were simply not amenable to such surgery.[67] Throughout the 1950s and 1960s, surgeons lacked a trail that led them to complete venous bypass. Bushwhacking was required.

The adjective *data-driven* means that progress in an activity is compelled by data, rather than by intuition or by personal experience.[68]

Victor Fontan was a professional cyclist[69] of substantial success. Competing from 1913 to 1930 and logging a respectable 20 victories along the way, he is perhaps best known for his heartbreaking 1929 Tour de France. Fontan was hammering from Luchon to Perpignan, in the lead, when his front forks collapsed. Today, team and neutral service cars roll ready to assist riders with flats and broken bikes, but in the ancient Tour days you were pretty much on your own. Victor eventually begged

---

[62] Puga and McGoon (1973); Robiseck et al. (1966).

[63] Robiseck et al. (1956, 1966).

[64] Warden et al. (1954).

[65] Haller et al. (1966).

[66] Hurwitt et al. (1955). The patient had a single ventricle, two atria (with a patent foramen ovale), and both atria communicated with the ventricle via the atrioventricular valve.

[67] Hurwitt et al. (1955); Bopp et al. (1961).

[68] Wikipedia, July 22, 2020.

[69] Tom, not incidentally, was an ardent amateur cyclist; he followed the Tour de France closely each year.

a replacement bike, but the additional time lost from a punctured tire dragged him from the fray. He wound up in the bushes, dropped-out of the Tour and crying.[70] If 1929 was miserable relative to Victor's Tour de France aspirations, it was marvelous for his family and for congenital cardiology: His son Francis was born on July 2, drawing his first breath in Nay, a tiny commune adjacent to the French Pyrenean foothills.[71] Francis entered the Faculté des Medicines at the University of Bordeaux at age 17 and commenced his residency as an Interne des Hopitaux at the University Hospitals six years later. The Department of Cardiac Surgery was his selection for his third year of internship, where he completed his doctoral thesis on cardiopulmonary bypass in 1959. Fontan was appointed the Chef de Clinique in the Medical Department of Cardiology, and by 1960, he had the same title in the Surgical Department of Cardiac Diseases. He was appointed head of that department at the University of Bordeaux, at the Hôpital du Tondu, in 1968.

Fontan's interest in tricuspid atresia was piqued by a teenager with this malformation who had died while he was an intern. Influenced by the Russian surgeons and William Glenn, Fontan created a canine model of tricuspid atresia and directed venous blood straight into the lungs (1964–66) and, like others before him, had no survivors. But dogs have a thin-walled right atrium—unlike patients with tricuspid atresia, who have more muscular atria—which Fontan figured was ill-equipped to push blood through the lungs. This notion gave him permission, he decided, to shrug off his and others' discouraging laboratory results and hazard the definitive test in a patient. When Fontan was approached in 1968 by Pierre Broustet, a well-known French cardiologist, with a plea to rescue a deeply cyanotic twelve-year-old girl with tricuspid atresia, he was ready to make his wager. Fontan didn't have to chance complete venous bypass—a Blalock-Taussig-Thomas type of shunt, or even a Glenn, would have been standard at the time. But he did.

Fontan's justification for risking his operation differed from that of Gross, Blalock, and Lillehei, who had provided reasonably strong proof-of-principle of the proposed surgery in the animal lab and the morgue. (Blalock wasn't certain that his shunt would pink-up his patients, but Taussig's anecdotal experience strongly suggested as much.) And as for abnormal cardiac communications, Gross and Lillehei had cogent reasons to believe that their operation was likely to be beneficial, and laboratory trials indicated that they could safely do so. (Of our foundational clinical innovators, only Bailey [Chap. 4] had no preclinical confirmation that his experimental operation for relieving mitral stenosis was sound.) In fact, information available to the French surgeon indicated that total venous bypass would *not* work, save for the flawed Warden and Haller papers. (And they go unmentioned in his report, so we do not know if he was even aware of them.) Fontan's intuition didn't let him down—complete heart bypass could work and did. But it *was* intuition, at the bottom, not evidence, that green-lighted his operation. His notion that a hypertrophied

[70] *Velo Archive.* Tour, 1929.

[71] Anderson (1999, 2018); Watts (2018).

right atrium was required to make the difference between a failed and a successful operation was merely a hunch, and one we now know to be incorrect.[72]

Fontan's first Fontan was performed on April 25, 1968. A somewhat rocky post-operative course preceded hospital discharge, but the young lady went on to do well for many years.[73] Unlike Glenn, who hurried to publish his single case of a less remarkable innovation, Fontan reported nothing at the time. A second patient (January 1970), 36 years old and with a similar diagnosis, also enjoyed considerable improvement after surgery. His third case (March 1970) died after operation, which Fontan attributed to mitral valve leakage.[74] Argentina's Guillermo Kreutzer effected a similar procedure in two patients shortly thereafter (July and December 1971); both survived to hospital discharge, although one died six months later.[75] Kreutzer was unaware of Fontan's paper.[76] (The operation is sometimes referred to as the Fontan-Kreutzer procedure) (Fig. 9.4). Fontan soon attracted adherents outside Bordeaux, and he and surgeons in Leiden, the Netherlands, operated upon 100 patients with tricuspid atresia between 1968 and 1981.[77] The procedure evolved in configuration, and people quickly learned that patients with certain characteristics—such as increased resistance to blood flow through the lungs, poor

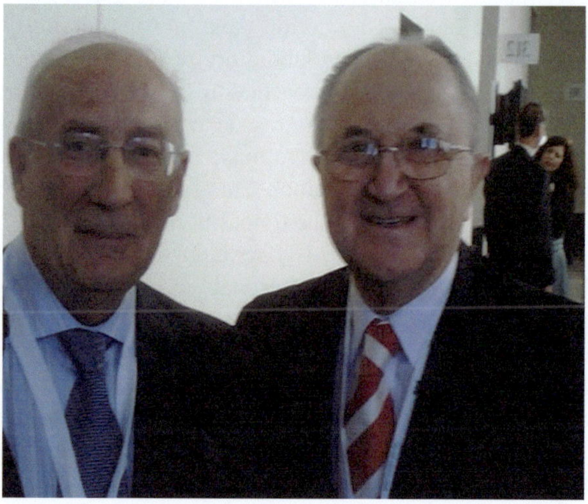

**Fig. 9.4** Francis Fontan MD (left) and Guillermo O. Kreutzer MD

[72] de Laval and Deanfield (2010).

[73] Anderson (1999).

[74] Fontan and Baudet (1971).

[75] Kreutzer et al. (1973).

[76] August 2010 interview with Guillermo Kreutzer, World Society for Pediatric and Congenital Heart Surgery, https://www.wspchs.org/, accessed Aug. 25, 2020.

[77] Fontan et al. (1983).

ventricular function, and mitral valve leakage—often did poorly after the procedure. Fontan and associates elaborated their hard-won observations into a book chapter including "ten commandments"[78] regarding patient selection for successful Fontan palliation, probably the single most famous piece of solo ventricle pontification.[79] While people eventually learned which of these rules were firm and which were fragile, the commandments served as a rough framework for selecting the correct patients for surgery, and they were essential for improving survival.

No one-trick pony, Fontan was an excellent general congenital heart man, active in adult cardiac surgery and transplantation, and a driving force in the formation of the European Association for Cardio-Thoracic Surgery. Like the wine he so savored, he was the product of his terroir, familial and regional. It's perhaps no surprise that Fontan was a mean skier, given that his father was a professional cyclist. And while many relish fine food and wine, precious few take it to Fontan's level. He, his wife Maryse, son Edouard, and a friend raised Chateau l'Ermitage, a vineyard flanking the Ciron River near Preignac, from dereliction to an award-winning producer of Sauternes. Traveling and golf occupied what little spare time Fontan must have had. Francis Fontan died in 2018 with one of the two most uttered names in single ventricle history, if not congenital cardiology (we meet the other in our Chap. 11).

> It seemed to me possible that democratic faith might be imparted better by contagion than by argument.
> –Dean Acheson, *Present at the Creation.*[80]

The Fontan stands at the apogee of single ventricle surgical palliation, the preferred destination for the vast majority of single ventricle souls, even over a half century after its creation.[81] *Why* this is so explains how most new ideas become therapy. The physiologist's reason for the Fontan's preeminence, concisely put, is that this surgical reconfiguration offers the most arterial oxygen content for a given quantity of blood pumped. With the Blalock-Taussig-Thomas and other aortopulmonary shunts, the price paid for pink is increased volume work, since the solo ventricle re-pumps blood to the lungs which had previously so circulated. The extra work eventually weakens cardiac muscle and provokes other problems. And you don't get as much pink as desired, since the arterial oxygen content is invariably less than normal. The Glenn and bidirectional cavopulmonary shunts do not increase volume load, but neither do they normalize arterial oxygen content, which limits exercise capacity and causes long-term complications. The Fontan is the most efficient configuration, relative to oxygen delivery, that has yet been invented.

But I'm reminded of a cartoon I saw a number of years ago. A professorial type was chatting with a young woman at a cocktail party: "In theory, Mrs. Brown, yes," he intoned, "But also in theory, no." This Fontan is a compromise, not a miracle. Its efficiency at delivering oxygen comes at a price—high systemic venous pressure.

---

[78] Choussat et al. in Anderson and Shinebourne (1978).

[79] Anderson and Shinebourne (1978), pp. 559–566.

[80] Acheson (1969), p. 461.

[81] Some single ventricle patients, a minority, are not candidates for Fontan palliation because their physiological characteristics—for example, poor ventricular function or high resistance to blood flow through the lungs—or non-cardiac factors make a favorable response to surgery unlikely.

Though healthy lungs present surprisingly little resistance to flow, the pressure needed to urge blood through them is still considerably higher than normal. Venous pressure is normally about 6 mmHg, but it is roughly 12 to 15 mmHg in a "good" Fontan circulation. While venous hypertension goes unnoticed in many patients, in others it causes fluid collection in body cavities or tissues. Over a period of time, the bowel, liver, and other organs can also be adversely affected by venous congestion. Furthermore, without a ventricle to propel blood through the lungs, exercise capacity is blunted relative to the wild type. The Fontan procedure's superior mode of oxygen delivery is, depending upon the patient, to a greater or lesser extent counterbalanced by its unfavorable effect on venous pressure. As it turns out, for most patients its efficiency outweighs the liability of venous hypertension, but the calculus didn't have to work out that way.

Fontan's invention remains at the top of palliation's heap not because of any theoretical advantage, but because with it, people live longer than they otherwise would. When cardiologists at Boston Children's Hospital reviewed their experience with tricuspid atresia before the Fontan, they discovered that only about one-third of their patients, most of whom were shunted, were alive at 20 years of age[82] (Fig. 9.5). Contrast that with the Fontan: Survival 20 years after the operation is at least double that (after first surviving the early postoperative period), and perhaps as high as 85%

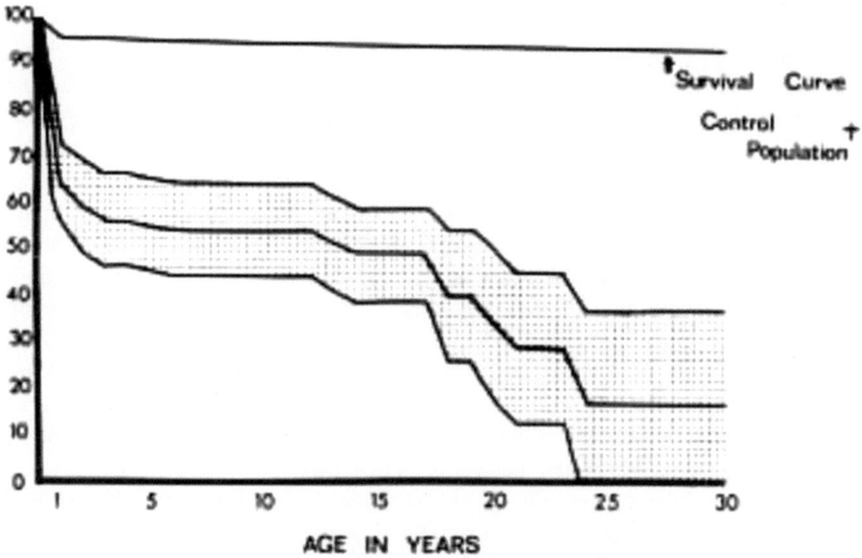


**Fig. 9.5** Survival, tricuspid atresia patients, Boston Children's Hospital; less than 30% were alive at 20 years of age. (Dick, 1975) With permission from the American Journal of Cardiology

[82] Dick et al. (1975).

at 30 years for those who recently had this procedure.[83] Exercise capacity is also better than with a shunt.[84]

Despite the signal advance it heralded, Fontan's paper got a mixed reception. There were enthusiastic early adopters, such as the French surgeons' circle and the Mayo Clinic, while other congenital cardiac practitioners, especially cardiologists, were wary. Up until 1980, thirteen centers (aside from Fontan's and Kreutzer's) had published their experience with the Fontan procedure, but only three had more than five patients. (Although there were surely unreported patients.) Interestingly, the first full report of the operation after Fontan and Kreutzer's papers was from Wilford Hall USAF Medical Center at Lackland Air Force Base in San Antonio, Texas, far off congenital cardiology's beaten path.[85] Compare the reaction, as indicated by papers subsequently published, to Fontan's first report with Walt Lillehei's cross-circulation open-heart breakthrough (Chap. 7). News of the Minnesota surgeon's quantum advance soon spurred a sharp uptick in publications pertaining to open-heart surgery, but Fontan procedure papers lagged noticeably (Fig. 9.6). This was partly due to there being far fewer available patients for the Fontan operation than open-heart surgery. But some of this tepid response can be explained by skepticism related to the fundamental nature—actually, *anti*-nature—of this operation; some people just didn't see it working very well for very long.[86] Some was occasioned by practitioners resorting to the Fontan in patients who were very decompensated and poor candidates; the resulting deaths were devastating for all involved. (Learning who should be offered this operation, and who should not, was crucial to its ultimate adoption.) Another factor was not appreciating how unsatisfactory the current therapy was. At Boston Children's Hospital, it was only after cardiologists reviewed their experience that they appreciated how poor their patients' prospects were. It was an epiphany for the Boston group, compelling them to think differently, and Fontan surgeries soon took off at that hospital (Fig. 9.7).[87]

As Acheson deduced regarding spreading democracy, disseminating this strange operation was a matter of contagion rather than disquisition. Influential centers published mortality figures that were uncomfortably high early on, but rapidly improved. The Mayo Clinic experience was typical: operative mortality fell from 21% for

---

[83] Rychik et al. (2019).

[84] Zellers et al. (1989).

[85] Stanford et al. (1973).

[86] In fact, Alex Nadas—an early leader in the field and head of cardiology at Boston Children's Hospital—directed the first author of the paper to not let the Children's cardiac surgeons get their hands on the list of tricuspid atresia patients collected for their study, lest they set about trying to recruit them for a Fontan procedure. Nadas believed that the patient's cardiologist was responsible for and had the prerogative to make the difficult decision of submitting a patient for this unproven operation (personal communication, Macdonald Dick, II, July 24, 2020).

[87] Conversations and communications with Michael Freed, Macdonald Dick, Peter Lang, and Stephen P. Sanders, cardiologists at Boston Children's Hospital, regarding factors inhibiting adoption of the Fontan at that institution.

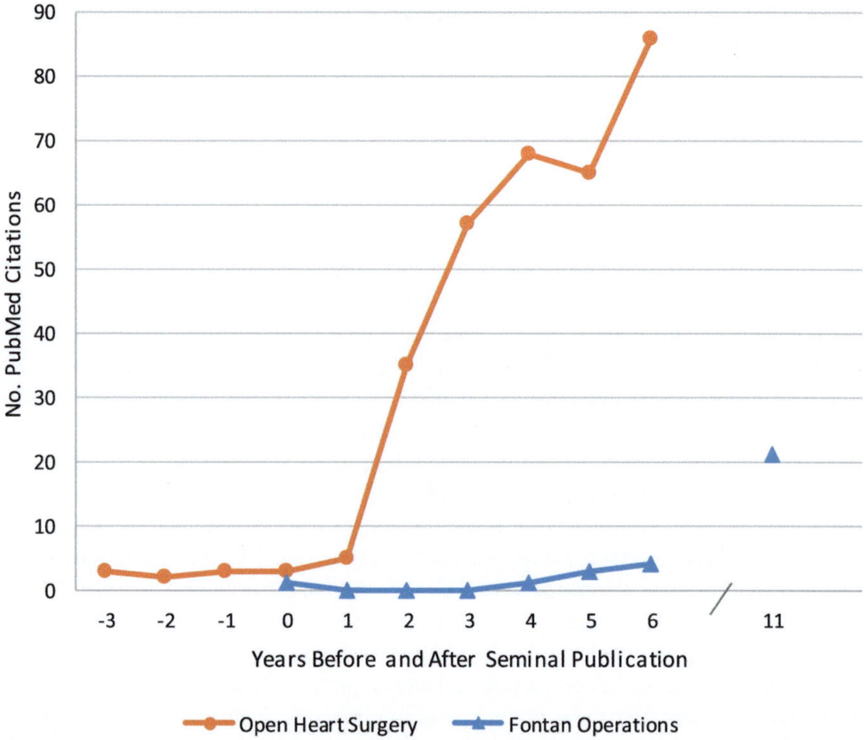


**Fig. 9.6** Number of publications, as cited in PubMed (June 9, 2020), for the search terms "open heart surgery" [red] and "Fontan procedure" [blue]. The seminal publication for open heart surgery is Lillehei's 1954 cross-circulation paper; for the Fontan procedure, his 1971 paper. (Figure by Thomas J. Kulik MD)

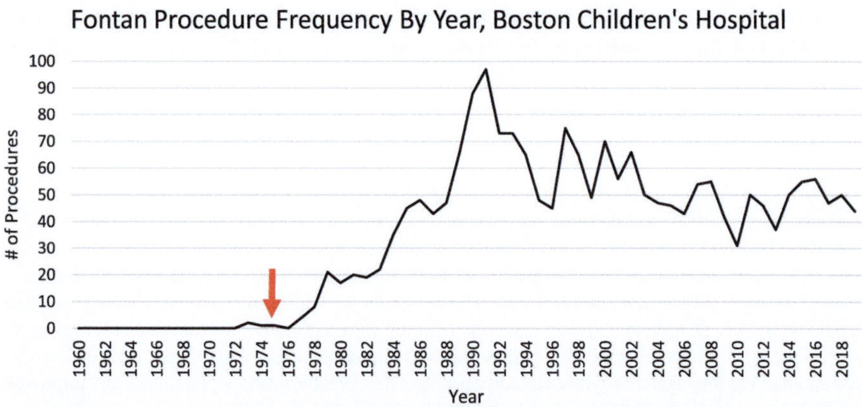


**Fig. 9.7** Fontan's first paper describing his operation was in 1971; a marked uptick in the number of these operations performed occurred only after publication of Macdonald Dick's paper (1975, red arrow) showing poor outcomes of patients with tricuspid atresia treated conventionally. (Figure by Thomas J. Kulik MD)

patients operated upon between 1974 and 1980 to 9% between 1981 and 1989.[88] Other centers had equivalent survival. Fontan's original design was improved and selecting candidates according to the ten commandments also enhanced outcomes. While cardiologists and surgeons still had reservations about the Fontan's long-term durability, by the 1980s results from multiple institutions—disseminated by lectures and articles—compelled the field to follow suit.[89]

I hope I've made the case that, while the Fontan is not perfectly *sui generis* (fish have one ventricle and a series circulation), it's close, and that its utter remoteness from mammalian wild type likely hindered its invention and even adoption. Because precedent facilitates imagination and acceptance, the lack of a precedent for this operation—the example of fish doesn't seem to have entered anybody's mind—got in its way on both accounts. And the vexation of animal models surfaced again in the Fontan story. Without the Glenn shunt, for which experimental work was indispensable, the leap into the Fontan would surely have been at least delayed. In that sense, the penultimate single ventricle palliation was the product of the dog lab. But animal models proved an unreliable compass for a model for the Fontan—one might even argue that it was invented as much *in spite of*, rather than because of, laboratory work. Fontan took a chance with his unproven therapy the same way that all medical innovators must: Because all models are imperfect, any first use of a treatment—even when animal studies have been positive—is a roll of the dice.

We've also seen resolute investigators—Richards and Cournand—add granularity to William Harvey's circulation, setting the table for others to tackle formerly intractable heart disease. Forssmann's self-catheterization and his personal description of it, while a romantic chapter in cardiac history, seems to me at best a distraction, at worst a bad lesson. The brand of courage most tightly cemented to medical advances is that of persistent, different-thinking Lone Pines breaking tedious, exhausting, and at times discouraging trails. The Bellevue physicians are truer examples of how people labor, sometimes over many years, to extract new knowledge and therapies.

In *Collaboration* (Chap. 6) we saw that credit for an innovation rarely extends to all who were vital for its creation. Forssmann's Nobel Prize, contrasted with noteworthy innovators fated to remain only "inside baseball" luminaries, confirms that acclaim is a contingent thing. Publicity is important, but surely other obscure factors are also afoot. That so many people have added so much to congenital cardiology, while accruing so little esteem outside the relatively small circle of their peers, reinforces the idea (Chaps. 7 and 8) that doctors are largely driven by the desire of

---

[88] Mair et al. (1991).

[89] For very young patients—those under roughly one year of age—the risk of dying or a difficult postoperative course after the Fontan is higher than for older children. Most single ventricle neonates require a non-Fontan initial procedure (usually an aortopulmonary shunt, or more complex surgery, Chap. 11), usually followed by a bidirectional cavopulmonary shunt several months later. The Fontan is the third stage in the sequence, usually performed—depending upon the center—between about two and four years of age.

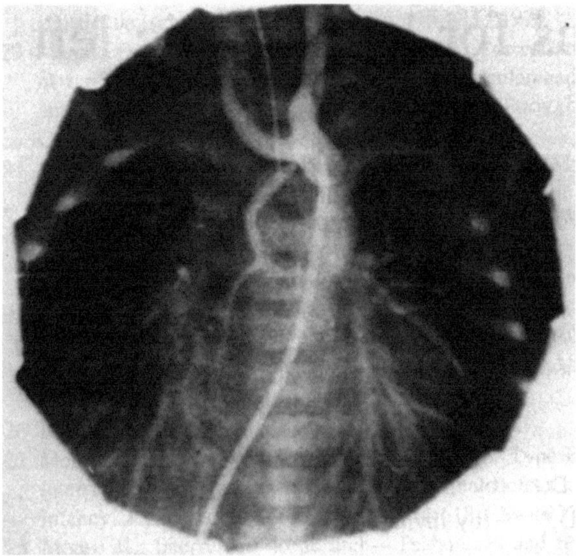

**Fig. 9.8** Hypoplastic Left Heart Syndrome. Angiogram via catheter through inferior vena cava, right atrium, right ventricle, pulmonary artery and patent ductus arteriosus into the thoracic aorta, backfilling with radio-opaque dye into the hypoplastic ascending aorta [AAo], the right coronary artery [CA] and pulmonary arteries [PA]. The hypoplastic left ventricle is not shown but sits immediately under the Hypoplastic AAo

improving their patients, while real fame and fortune, for the vast majority, are absent or at most secondary motivations. That is not to say that ambition is never fueled by a hunger for peer recognition—it surely is—but it seems to me that this is usually only a secondary motivation, and that people tend to be suspicious of those for whom it appears to be the primary driver.

We've arrived at the last two chapters of our story: extending single ventricle rescue to souls formerly stranded. Shunts work for patients with anatomic restriction of pulmonary flow *if* the ventricle's aortic connection, and the aorta itself, are fine. But with many malformations they are not, posing a much tougher problem for the practitioner. Hypoplastic left heart syndrome (HLHS) is the classic example (Fig. 9.8), and it is of special import, since the majority of solo ventricles are this or a variation on the theme.[90] Indeed, even for babies with two ventricles and weighing only a few pounds, repairing the heart and adjacent blood vessels was too much for early open-heart surgeons. Exploring how the craft advanced to manipulating tissue in tiny hearts, and then inventing operations for neonates with complex single ventricles—the Norwood operation -, is the "heart" of Chap. 11. But first we cast the

[90] Hoffman and Kaplan (2002).

single ventricle net more widely and land on a basic biological discovery, made by an Italian biologist and a Canadian physician-scientist working together in Toronto and scarcely known beyond congenital heart aficionados. Their discovery opened the door for babies with hypoplastic left heart syndrome.

## References


Acheson D (1969) Present at the creation: my years in the state department. W.W. Norton & Co., New York

Anderson RA (1999) Francis Fontan. Cardiol Young 9:592–600

Anderson RA (2018) Francis Fontan 1929–2018. Cong Heart Dis 13:161–162

Anderson RH, Shinebourne EA (eds) (1978) Paediatric cardiology. Churchill Livingstone, Edinburgh, UK. dated 1977, published 1978

Arcilla RA, Gasul BM (1961) Congenital aplasia or marked hypoplasia of the myocardium of the right ventricle (Uhl's anomaly). Clinical, angiocardiographic, and hemodynamic findings. J Pediatrics 58:381–8

Azzolina G, Eufrate S, Pensa P (1972) Tricuspid atresia: experience in surgical management with a modified cavopulmonary anastomosis. Thorax 27:111–115

Bakos ACP (1950) The question of the function of the right ventricular myocardium: an experimental study. Circulation 1:724–732

Block BA, Stevens ED (2001) Tuna: physiology, ecology, and evolution. Academic, San Diego

Bopp RK, Larsen PB, Patrick JR et al (1961) Surgical considerations for treatment of congenital tricuspid atresia and stenosis: with particular reference to vena cava-pulmonary artery stenosis. J Thorac Cardiovasc Surg 43:97–113

Bushnell PG, Brill RW (1991) Responses of swimming skipjack (Katsuwonus pelamis) and yellowfin (Thunnus albacares) tunas to acute hypoxia, and a model of their cardiorespiratory function. Physiol Zool 64:887–911

Bushnell PG Brill RW (1992) Oxygen transport and cardiovascular responses in skipjack tuna (Katsuwonus pelamis) and yellowfin tuna (Thunnus albacares) exposed to acute hypoxia. J Comp Physiol 162B:131–143

Carlon CA, Mondini PG, de Marchi R (1950) Su una nuova anastomosi vasale per la terapia chirurgica di alcuni vizi cardiovasculari. Giorn It Chir 6:760–764

Carlon CA, Mondini PG, de Marchi R (1951) Surgical treatment of some cardiovascular diseases. J Intl Coll Surg 16:1–11

Cournand A (1980) Historical details of Claude Bernard's invention of a technique for measuring the temperature and pressure of the blood within the cavities of the heart. Trans NY Acad Sci 39:1–14

Cournand AF (1989) Dickinson Woodruff Richards. October 30, 1896 – February 23, 1973. National Academy of Sciences. Biograp Mem 58:459–467. Washington, DC: The National Academies Press

Cournand A, Ranges HA (1941) Catheterization of the right auricle in man. Pro Soc Exptl Biol Med 46:462–466

de Laval MR (2005) The Fontan circulation: a challenge to William Harvey? Nat Clin Prac Cardiovasc Med 2:202–208

de Laval MR, Deanfield JE (2010) Four decades of Fontal palliation. Nat Rev Cardiol 7(9):520–527

de Laval M, Kilner P, Gewillig M, Bull C (1988) Total cavopulmonary connection: a logical alternative to atriopulmonary connection for complex Fontan operations. J Thorac Cardiovasc Surg 96:682–695

Dick M, Fyler DC, Nadas AA (1975) Tricuspid atresia: clinical course on 101 patients. Am J Cardiol 36:327–337

Donald DE, Essex HE (1954) Pressure studies after inactivation of the major portion of the canine right ventricle. Am J Phys 176:155–161

Evans DH, Piermarini PM, Choe KP (2005) The multifunctional fish gill: dominant site of gas exchange, osmoregulation, acid-base regulation, and excretion of nitrogenous waste. Physiol Rev 85:97–177

Fishman AP, Richards DW (1964) Circulation of the blood. Men and ideas. Oxford University Press, New York

Fontan F, Baudet E (1971) Surgical repair of tricuspid atresia. Thorax 26(3):240–248

Fontan F, Deville C, Quaegebeur J, Ottenkamp J, Sourdille N, Choussat A, Brom GA (1983) Repair of tricuspid atresia in 100 patients. J Thoracic Cardiovasc Surg 85:647–660

Forssmann W (1974) Experiments on Myself: Memoirs of a Surgeon in Germany. Davies H (trans). St. Martin's Press, New York

Fye WB (2015) Caring for the heart: mayo clinic and the rise of specialization. Oxford University Press, Oxford, UK

Glenn WWL (1989) Superior vena cava-pulmonary artery shunt. Ann Thorac Surg 47:62–64

Glenn WWL, Patino JF (1954) Circulatory by-pass of the right heart, I: preliminary observations on the direct delivery of vena caval blood into the pulmonary arterial circulation. Yale J Bio Med 27:147–151

Greenblatt S (2011) The swerve: how the world became modern. W.W. Norton & Company, New York

Haller JA, Adkins JC, Worthington M, Rauenhorst J (1966) Experimental studies on permanent bypass of the right heart. Surgery 59:1128–1132

Hansson N, Packy LM, Halling T, Gross D, Fangerau H (2015) From nobody to Nobel laureate? The case of Werner Forssmann. Urologe A 54(3):412–419

Hoffman JIE, Kaplan S (2002) The incidence of congenital heart disease. J Am Coll Cardiol 39:1890–1900

Hopkins RA, Armstrong BE, Serwer GA, Peterson RJ, Oldham HN Jr (1985) Physiological rationale for a bidirectional cavopulmonary shunt. J Thorac Cardiovasc Surg 90:319–398

Hurwitt ES, Young D, Escher DJW (1955) The rationale of the anastomosis of the right auricular appendage to the pulmonary artery in the treatment of tricuspid atresia. J Thoracic Surg 30:503–512

Kagan A (1952) Dynamic responses of the right ventricle following extensive damage by cauterization. Circulation 5:816–823

Konstantinov IE, Alexi-Meskishvili VV (1999) Cavo-pulmonary shunt: from the first experiments to clinical practice. Ann Thorac Surg 68:1100–1106

Konstantinov IE, Alexi-Meskishvili VV (2000) Early Italian contributions to cavopulmonary shunt procedures [letter to the editor]. Ann Thorac Surg 69:311–320

Konstantinov IE, Rosapepe F, Dearani JA, Alexi-Meskishvili VV, Li J (2005) A tribute to Giancarlo Rastelli. Ann Thorac Surg 79:1819–1823

Kreutzer G, Galindez E, Bobo H, de Palma C, Laura JP (1973) An operation for correction of tricuspid atresia. J Thorac Cardiovasc Surg 66:613–621

Landis EM, Brown E, Fauteux M, Wise C. Central venous pressure in relation to cardiac "competence," blood volume and exercise. J Clin Invest 1946;25(2):237–255

Liljestrand G (1956) Award ceremony speech. NobelPrize.org. Accessed May 18, 2025. https://www.nobelprize.org/prizes/medicine/1956/ceremony-speech/

Mair DD, Hagler DJ, Julsrud PR, Puga FJ, Schaff HV, Danielson GK (1991) Early and late results of the modified Fontan procedure for double-inlet left ventricle: the Mayo Clinic experience. J Am Coll Cardiol 18:1727–1732

Marshall NJ, Armstrong JA, McGechie DB, Glancy RJ (1985) Attempt to fulfil Koch's postulates for pyloric campylobacter. Med J Aust 142:436–439

Moore FD (1969) Therapeutic innovation: ethical boundaries in the initial clinical trials of new drugs and surgical procedures. Daedalus 98:502–522

Nobel Prize. Barry J. Marshall 2005. Accessed August 20, 2024. https://www.nobelprize.org/prizes/medicine/2005/marshall/biographical/

Nuland SB (1989) Doctors: the biography of medicine. Knopf, New York

Nuland SB (1995) How we die: reflections on life's final chapter. Vintage, New York

Nuland SB, Glenn WWL, Guilfoil PH (1958) Circulatory bypass of the right heart, III: some observations of long-term survivors. Surgery 43:184–201

Oshinsky D (2016) Bellevue: three centuries of medicine and mayhem at America's most storied hospital. Anchor Books, New York

Paap D, Takken T (2014) Reference values of cardiopulmonary exercise testing in healthy adults: a systematic review. Exp Rev of Cardiovasc Ther 12:1439–1453

Patino JF, Glenn WWL, Guilfoil PH, Hume M, Fenn JE (1955) Circulatory bypass of the right heart, II: further observations on vena caval-pulmonary artery shunts. Surg Forum 6:189–193

Puga FJ, McGoon DC (1973) Exclusion of the right ventricle from the circulation: hemodynamic observations. Surgery 73:607–613

Rastelli G, Wallace RB, Ongley PA (1969) Complete repair of transposition of the great arteries with pulmonary stenosis: a review and report of a case corrected by using a new surgical technique. Circulation 39:83–95

Richards DW (1970) Medical priesthoods and other essays. Connecticut Printers, Inc, Hartford, CT

Richards DW. The contributions of right heart catheterization to physiology and medicine, with some observations on the physiopathology of pulmonary heart disease. 1956 Nobel lecture. Accessed August 20, 2024. https://www.nobelprize.org/prizes/medicine/1956/richards/lecture/

Richards DW Jr (1944) The circulation in traumatic shock in man: the Harvey lecture. Bull NY Acad Med 20:363–393

Robiseck F (1981) An epitaph for cavopulmonary anastomosis. Ann Thorac Surg 34:200–220

Robiseck F (1992) The history of right heart bypass before Fontan. Herz 17:199–212

Robiseck F, Temesvari A, Kadar RL (1956) A new method for the treatment of congenital heart disease associated with impaired pulmonary circulation: an experimental study. Acta Med Scand 54:151–161

Robiseck F, Sanger PEW, Gallucci V (1966) Long term complete circulatory exclusion of the right side of the heart. Am J Cardiol 18:867–875

Robiseck F, Sanger PW, Moore M, Daugherty HK, Robiseck LK, Bagby E (1969) Observations following four years of complete circulatory exclusion of the right heart. Ann Thorac Surg 8:530–536

Rodbard S, Wagner D (1949) By-passing the right ventricle. Proc Soc Exptl Biol Med 71:69–70

Rodbard S, Brown MD, Katz N (1949) The pulmonary artery pressure. Am Heart J 38:863–71

Rose JC, Cosimano SJ Jr, Hufnagel CA, Massullo EA (1955) The effects of exclusion of the right ventricle from the circulation in dogs. J Clin Invest 34:1625–1631

Rychik J, Atz A, Celermajer DS et al (2019) Evaluation and management of the child and adult with Fontan circulation. Circulation 140:e234–e284

Sade RM, Castañeda AR (1975) The dispensable right ventricle. Surgery 77:624–631

Squarcia U, Squarcia A (2007) Giancarlo Rastelli: the scientist, the man. Clin Cardiol 30:485–487

Stanford W, Armstrong RG, Cline RE, King TD (1973) Right atrium-pulmonary artery allograft for correction of tricuspid atresia. J Thorac Cardiovasc Surg 66:105–111

Starr I, Jeffers WA, Meade RH Jr (1943) The absence of conspicuous increments of venous pressure after severe damage to the right ventricle of the dog, with a discussion of the relation between clinical congestive heart failure and heart disease. Am Heart J 26:291–301

Uhl HS (1952) A previously undescribed congenital malformation of the heart: almost total absence of the myocardium of the right ventricle. Bull Johns Hopkins Hosp 91:197–209

Uhl HS (1996) Uhl's anomaly revisited. Circulation 93:483–484

Velo Archive. Tour, 1929. Accessed August 20, 2024. http://www.veloarchive.com/races/tour/1929.php

Warden HE, De Wall RA, Varco RL (1954) Use of the right auricle as a pump for the pulmonary circuit. Surg Forum 51:16–22

Watts G (2018) Francis Fontan. Lancet 391:932

Weibel ER (1995) Andre Frederic Cournand, 1895–1988: a biographic memoire. National Academy of Sciences. National Academies Press, Washington, DC

Weisse AB (2002) Heart to heart: the twentieth century battle against cardiac disease—an oral history. Rutgers University Press, New Brunswick

Weisse AB (2012) Self-experimentation and its role in medical research. Tex Heart Inst J 39:51–54

Williams SG, Cooke GA, Wright DJ et al (2001) Peak exercise cardiac power output: a direct indicator of cardiac function strongly predictive of prognosis in chronic heart failure. Euro Heart J 22:1496–1503

Zellers TM, Driscoll DJ, Mottram CD, Puga FJ, Schaff HV, Danielson GK (1989) Exercise tolerance and cardiorespiratory response to exercise before and after the Fontan operation. Mayo Clin Proc 64:1489–1497

# Chapter 10
# Bench to Bedside—Prostaglandins

In Chap. 5 about Maude Abbott, I remarked that Big Data is currently all the rage. So too is *translational medicine*. First scuttling onto the scene at the start of this century, this term (AKA, "bench-to-bedside") refers to the process of efficiently and quickly (and hopefully) transforming basic science discoveries into disease prevention, diagnosis, or therapy.[1] It infers a close adjacency of basic biological discovery and its clinical application.[2] Harvey's elucidation of the circulation, for example, ineffably impacted congenital cardiology, but not in a translational way—its practical application was far removed from *De Motu*'s publication. Basic researchers with a foot in the clinic, clinicians closely connected to the lab, or a close working relationship between the two greatly facilitate the process. Translational medicine flourished well before the term was invented, but there is no better exemplar than Flavio Coceani and Peter Olley's urging the fruits of their studies of prostaglandins into the clinical arena. This was and is a critical piece of bench-to-bedside for congenital cardiology: Neonatal cardiac surgery as we know it today would be impossible without prostaglandin $E_1$.

Gas exchange—oxygen in the airways moving into the blood and carbon dioxide in the blood escaping into the air—is primarily what the lungs do. But since this is impossible until the baby's first breath, nature has arranged for right ventricular blood to bypass the lungs via a patent ductus arteriosus (PDA) into the aorta during fetal gestation. This is of considerable advantage, since *both* ventricles—not just the left—can pump to the body and the placenta, where gas exchange occurs in utero. It's also a lifesaver for babies with obstruction of flow from the heart to the body or lungs, allowing for something like normal development in utero and, after birth, survival until ductal closure. Indeed, the vast majority of malformations which render a newborn critically ill—including those with two ventricles—temporarily

[1] Woolf (2008).

[2] Translational research can also refer to assessing how well-established treatments are actually applied to potential beneficiaries.



T. J. Kulik, M. Dick, *Reimagining a Child's Heart*,
https://doi.org/10.1007/978-3-031-88608-9_10

benefit from an open duct. But Nature didn't have cardiac defects in mind when she designed this structure, which normally closes shortly after birth. With closure, the baby may die of a congenital heart defect before being diagnosed or may become too sick to survive an operation. Opening the duct brings improvement (if done soon enough), greatly enhancing the likelihood of a good postoperative outcome. It also means that hurried procedures, undertaken in desperately blue babies in the middle of the night, can be postponed until the light of day. Today, this is routine, but before $E_1$ prostaglandin, practitioners didn't think about it in this way; no neo-Manhattan Project searched for a way to keep the duct open, nor was there much speculation about how great it would be if possible.[3] In fact, Coceani and Olley weren't looking for a way to open the ductus when they started their experiments; in fact, they expected quite the opposite from $E_1$.

The prostaglandin story sprouted in 1933–1934, when a biologically active substance was isolated from human seminal fluid and sheep vesicular glands and named "prostaglandin."[4] It turns out that this is a family of molecules, ubiquitously distributed throughout the body and key players in a variety of processes. (Especially inflammation: History's most important medicine, aspirin, works by inhibiting prostaglandin synthesis.) Their importance is such that the 1982 Nobel Prize in Physiology or Medicine was awarded to three scientists who greatly advanced prostaglandin chemistry and biology.[5] The pages of this story that interest us were composed at Toronto's Hospital for Sick Children (now SickKids). Founded in 1875 and long a flagship pediatric hospital, SickKids has hosted a raft of outstanding cardiologists and surgeons, none having greater impact than Coceani and Olley[6] (Fig. 10.1). The former, a basic scientist—and the latter, primarily a clinician—were born in 1937, Coceani in Trieste, Italy, and Olley in Manchester, England. Coceani earned his MD at the University of Bologna and following postgraduate work in physiology there and in Montreal, he then moved to Toronto in 1968. Olley earned his medical degree at the University of London and arrived at SickKids a year before the Italian.[7]

Coceani was interested in the biology of ductal closure.[8] Increased blood oxygen content after birth stimulates its constriction, that was known; what was not is *how*

---

[3] Email correspondence (October 2020) with Michael Freed and Roberta Williams, practicing pediatric cardiologists at the time. What may seem like a lack of imagination was partly due to the current state of neonatal open-heart surgery: Though advancing, it yet still tenuous, so stabilizing a newborn with poor prospects for successful surgery was of limited use at the time. But this does not explain why an open duct would not have been useful for a baby needing a shunt, which was a standard procedure.

[4] Bergström and Samuelsson (1965).

[5] Sune Bergström, Bengt Samulesson, and John Vane received the Prize.

[6] Hospital for Sick Children, "Our History." I could cite a dozen of the field's biggest names who were there, but I refrain for fear of leaving some out.

[7] Sant'Anna School of Advanced Studies, "Flavio Coceani"; *Globe and Mail*, "Peter Olley Obituary."

[8] Email correspondence from Dr. Flavio Coceani (September and October 2020).

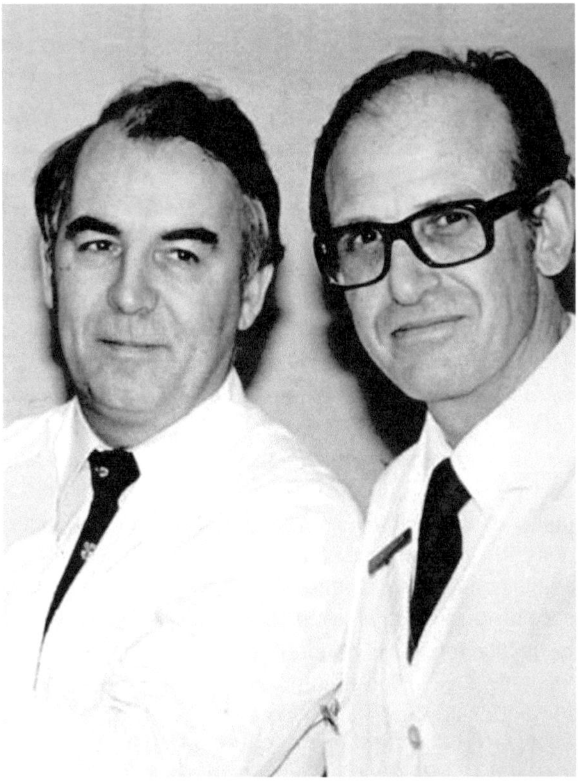

**Fig. 10.1** Peter Olley (left) and Flavio Coceani. (Courtesy of Flavio Coceani)

the oxygen works. But there were clues: Prostaglandin synthesis requires oxygen, and prostaglandin $E_1$ contracts stomach smooth muscle in its presence—might oxygen trigger prostaglandin production, which then closes the ductus? Coceani and Olley's experimental model was simple: They cut a lamb's duct into strips, suspended them in a "physiological" solution, exposed the strips to prostaglandins $E_1$ and $E_2$, and measured the force generated.[9] Anticipating that the E-type prostaglandins would cause contraction, they were surprised to find that the strips *relaxed* instead. Subsequent experiments showed that indomethacin, a prostaglandin synthesis inhibitor, blocked production of prostaglandins—ruling out prostaglandins as mediators of ductal closure—yet the ductus *closed* instead.[10] Their experiments had thus denied their initial notion of prostaglandins as ductal constrictors, but made a strong case that E-type prostaglandins normally *maintain* ductal patency (opening). In fact, all three components that scientists used to determine whether a substance may be a mediator of a particular effect had fallen into place: the presence of the substance in biologically relevant amounts within or in the vicinity of the tissue; the

[9] Coceani and Olley (1973).

[10] Coceani and Olley (1973); Coceani et al. (1976); Olley et al. (1975).

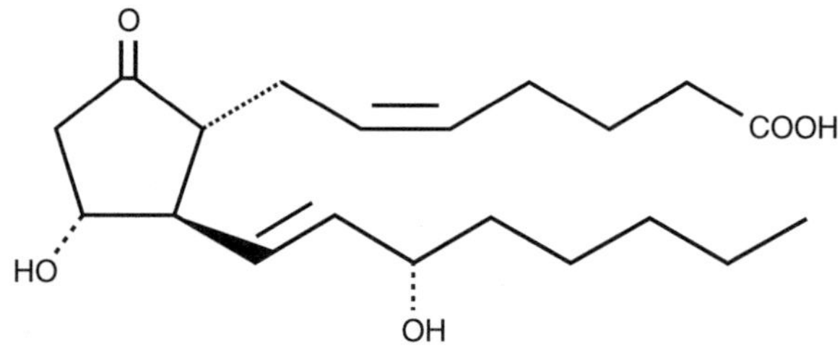


**Fig. 10.2** Prostaglandins $E_2$. In the public domain

substance, in relevant concentrations, having the effect of interest; and selectively blocking the production of, or receptors for, the substance abolishing the effect. Thus, the laboratory data needed to justify trying $E_2$ in babies with cardiac defects were well in hand, and by late 1974, Olley and Coceani were preparing for a clinical trial.

The Toronto investigators had assembled evidence that E-type prostaglandins are ductal dilators,[11] but that was only translation's first step; safety is equally important. For $E_2$, this was relatively straightforward, since prostaglandins are endogenous substances rather than synthetic agents, and $E_1$ had been safely infused into adults and had even found clinical use in obstetrics and elsewhere. Previous experience also provided an estimate of an appropriate dose.[12] Olley's plan was to first try $E_2$ in the intensively monitored environment of the cardiac catheterization lab, knowing that, given its rapid metabolism, any untoward effect(s) would be short-lived after stopping its infusion. For the drug itself, the investigators enjoyed a close working relationship with the supplier of $E_2$, the Upjohn Company. Coceani helped design the clinical protocol, and Olley administered the medication and assessed its effects (Fig. 10.2).

As it turned out, $E_1$ (Fig. 10.3) was first used in babies in late 1974 or early 1975 at Green Lane Hospital in Auckland, New Zealand. M.B. Starling and R.B. Elliott, hard on the heels of the Toronto investigators, had performed experiments in Auckland similar to those at SickKids, and wound up beating them to the punch[13] in

[11] I asked Coceani why $E_1$ or $E_2$ had not been infused into newborn animals to confirm its effect on the ductus *in situ*, prior to human use. He reminded me that their *in vitro* work suggested that $E_1$ was most effective in a hypoxic environment; experiments with hypoxic lambs—as I can attest from my own experience—would have been difficult to conduct. Sharpe and Larsson (1975) confirmed that $E_1$ maintains ductal patency in newborn rats and rabbits, using a whole-body freezing technique, but this was published *after* the first clinical use of $E_1$. But even after $E_1$ was found to be well-tolerated in human newborns, the US Food and Drug Administration required additional studies in fetal lambs before approving its use in babies (Abraham Rudolph, email communication, August, 2017).

[12] Bergström and Samuelsson (1965); Karim et al. (1971); Carlson et al. (1969); Carlson and Eriksson (1973).

[13] The New Zealand group gave $E_1$ to two newborns, one with an inoperable cardiac defect, and the other with fatal heart disease for which the parents had declined an operation. The $E_1$ was apparently given solely to determine its effect on the ductus; this strictly experimental use would be impermissible today, at least in the US.

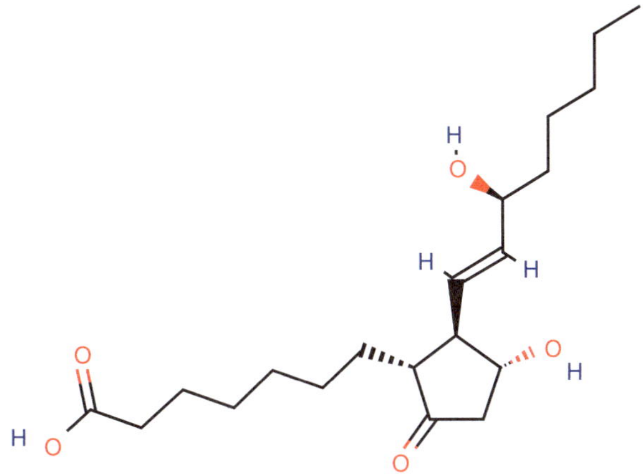

**Fig. 10.3** Prostaglandins $E_1$. In the public domain

its clinical application.[14] In early 1975, Olley and Coceani infused $E_2$[15] into three newborns (reported in the May prostaglandin conference in Florence), and a fourth was enrolled by September. Two had fever and one stopped breathing with $E_2$, which are typical but easily manageable side-effects. All four were rescued from severe hypoxemia, had shunts, and survived to hospital discharge.[16] Other cardiac groups soon followed.[17]

Coceani and Olley's collaboration—like that of Cournand and Richards (Chap. 9)—was attended with splendid mutual regard. (Olley once said that the only disagreement they ever had was with respect to using commas in their manuscripts.) Unlike the Bellevue pulmonologists, whose work was recognized by the Nobel prize, the SickKids pioneers have been afforded only narrow recognition. But they (and the New Zealanders) deserve much better. Neonatal cardiac surgery would be a fraction of what it is today without $E_1$ at the bedside. $E_2$ prostaglandin became the initial treatment—and life saver—for babies with HLHS, as well as other babies with cyanotic heart disease (Fig. 10.2).

Thus, the door was blown wide opened for the development of the Norwood operation, the subject of our final chapter.

---

[14] Starling and Elliott (1974); Elliott et al. (1975).

[15] $E_2$ was used, as it was naturally present in the ductus and therefore presumably optimally selective and efficacious. $E_1$ was later used, as this was what Upjohn had released for other clinical applications.

[16] Olley et al. (1975); Olley and Coceani (1976).

[17] Christensen and Fabricus (1975); Lang et al. (1977); Heymann et al. (1979); Freed et al. (1981).

## References

Bergström S, Samuelsson B (1965) Prostaglandins. Ann Rev Biochemist 34:101–108

Carlson LA, Eriksson I (1973) Femoral artery infusion of prostaglandin $E_1$ in severe peripheral vascular disease. Lancet 1(7795):155–156

Carlson LA, Ekelund LG, Orö L (1969) Circulatory and respiratory effects of different doses of prostaglandin E1 in man. Acta Physiol Scand 75:161–169

Christensen NC, Fabricus J (1975) Letter: medical manipulation of the ductus arteriosus. Lancet 2(7931):406–407

Coceani F, Olley PM (1973) The response of the ductus arteriosus to prostaglandins. Can J Physiol Pharmacol 51:220–225

Coceani F, Olley PM, Bodach E (1976) Prostaglandins: a possible regulator of muscle tone in the ductus arteriosus. Adv Prostaglandin Res 1:417–424

Elliott RB, Starling MB, Neutze JM (1975) Medical manipulation of the ductus arteriosus. Lancet 1(7899):140–142

Freed MD, Heymann MA, Lewis AB, Roehl SL, Kensey RC (1981) Prostaglandin $E_2$ in infants with ductus arteriosus-dependent congenital heart disease. Circ 64:899–905

Heymann MA, Berman W Jr, Rudolph AM, Whitman V (1979) Dilation of the ductus arteriosus by prostaglandin $E_1$ in aortic arch abnormalities. Circulation 59:169–173

Karim SMM, Hillier K, Somers K (1971) The effects of prostaglandins $E_2$ and $F_2\alpha$ administered by different routes on uterine activity and the cardiovascular system in pregnant and non-pregnant women. J Obst Gynecol Brit Commonwealth 78:172–179

Lang P, Freed MD, Rosenthal A, Castañeda AR, Nadas AS (1977) The use of prostaglandin $E_1$ in an infant with interruption of the aortic arch. J Pediatr 91:805–807

Olley PM, Coceani F (1976) E-type prostaglandins: a new emergency therapy for certain cyanotic congenital heart malformations. Circulation 53:728–731

Olley PM, Bodach E, Heaton J, Coceani F (1975) Further evidence implicating E-type prostaglandins in the patency of the lamb ductus arteriosus. Eur J Pharmacol 34:247–250

Sharpe GL, Larsson KS (1975) Studies on the closure of the ductus arteriosus X: in vivo effect of prostaglandin. Prostaglandins 9:703–719

Starling MB, Elliott RB (1974) The effects of prostaglandins, prostaglandin inhibitors, and oxygen on the closure of the ductus arteriosus, pulmonary arteries and umbilical vessels in vitro. Prostaglandins 8:187–203

Woolf SH (2008) The meaning of translational research and why it matters. JAMA 299:211–213

# Chapter 11
# Rescue—Norwood and Others

Classics are embedded in the way we think about ourselves, and our own history, in a more complex way than we usually allow.
—Mary Beard, *Confronting the Classics.*[1]

Case reports are bottom-rungers with respect to academic cachet; "big" papers are usually generated from far more clinical material. But the January 6, 1983, issue of the world's premiere medical journal included just such a report which, though numerically frail, proved to be a landmark for congenital cardiology and especially for solo ventricle therapy. Three physicians—a cardiac surgeon, a pediatric cardiologist, and an anesthesiologist—described a single patient, but a special one: At long last, a newborn with hypoplastic left heart syndrome (HLHS) had been surgically rescued and subsequently palliated with the Fontan. The paper's title, *Physiologic Repair of Aortic Atresia—Hypoplastic Left Heart Syndrome*, (see Fig 9.6 in Chapter) is false advertising. As I've stressed, the Fontan is no repair, and its increased venous pressure is hardly "physiologic." But this was less apparent at the time, and the Boston trio was admirably restrained in their conclusion: "Obviously, determination of the efficacy of such management must await long-term follow-up of a substantial group of patients. However, this child's gratifying postoperative course and current well-being serve to document the feasibility of surgically altering the prognosis of newborns with aortic atresia (completely undeveloped and blocked aortic valve) and other forms of hypoplastic left heart syndrome."[2]

Only a minority of single ventricle neonates can be treated with just a shunt, and those with HLHS or similar defects almost always die in the first few weeks absent an operation. Neonatal surgery, to rescue the baby with HLHS until a cavopulmonary shunt and the Fontan are feasible, requires enlarging the aorta, connecting it with the ventricle, arranging for the correct amount of pulmonary blood flow, and

[1] Beard (2013), p. 8.

[2] Norwood et al. (1983).



T. J. Kulik, M. Dick, *Reimagining a Child's Heart*,
https://doi.org/10.1007/978-3-031-88608-9_11

opening a hole between the two atria—all with a heart weighing two-thirds of an ounce and a key blood vessel the diameter of spaghetti. Inventing neonatal palliation proved elusive for many years after shunts were reasonably reliable for simpler (and less common) malformations.

Bill Norwood (Fig. 11.1) and collaborators were, in a sense, the Henry Ford of single ventricle therapy. Though Ford eventually morphed into a calamitous manager, he did have a big idea: Build cars cheap enough for the working class and pay your employees enough to buy them. Automobile manufacturers had sprouted like mushrooms at the turn of the twentieth century, but their machines were mostly for the well-to-do. Ford rippled ownership out to the working man, thus immeasurably magnifying the auto's utility and impact. The Norwood did the same for babies with HLHS, offering hope for a world of patients previously left stranded and profoundly impacting congenital cardiology to boot. The Norwood procedure accounts for only about three percent of all cardiac surgeries at Boston Children's Hospital, but it is only the first step down the therapeutic pathway; subsequent cardiac catheterizations and operations soon follow, as will hospitalizations unrelated to procedures.

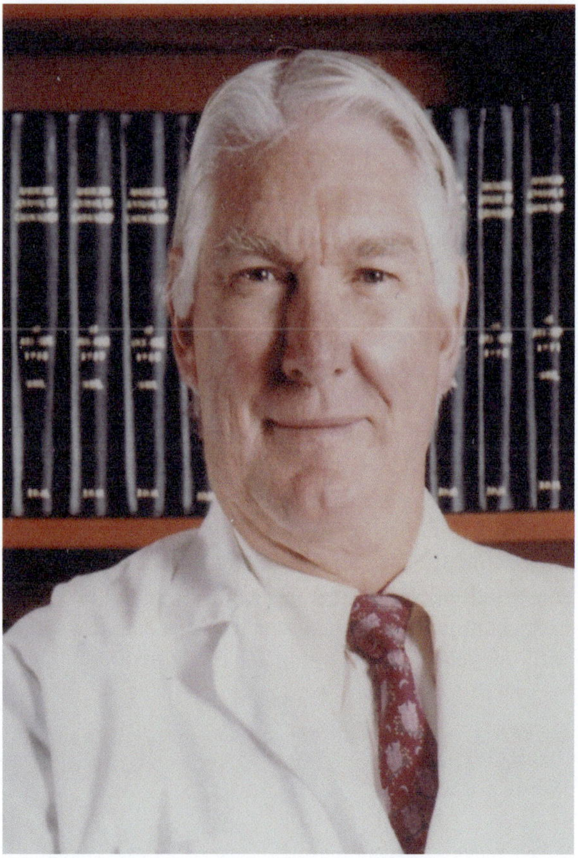

**Fig. 11.1** William Norwood MD PhD with permission of the Boston Children's Hospital Archives

Twenty-nine percent of bedded days in Boston Children's cardiac intensive care unit are currently occupied by patients with single ventricles, most of whom have had a Norwood (or variant) at some point in their life, and this doesn't include hospital days outside the intensive care unit or outpatient visits.[3] The ramifications of this expansion in congenital cardiology's patient base will magnify as the ranks of these folks grow and grow older.

Athena sprang from the brow of Zeus, but "the Norwood" didn't spring from the brow of Norwood—HLHS palliation had long been a grail for surgeons and cardiologists. The earliest operative attempt was innocent of an appreciation of relevant physiology and failed miserably. But people quickly deduced the fundamental requirements of a successful procedure, and by no later than 1968 (before Norwood was even a surgeon), the critical need to control pulmonary blood flow had been recognized. Ways to connect the right ventricle with the aorta were imagined a few years later. But executing this demanding architectural rearrangement, and taming the gnarly postoperative physiology, proved elusive until Norwood and colleagues evolved their operation. They advanced the craft by iterating and failing and learning, using the operating room and intensive care unit as their laboratory. Vivien Thomas perfected the Blalock-Taussig-Thomas shunt in dogs so that his boss was ready to run with his first human. Bigelow and Lewis sweated long hours in the lab to bring hypothermia with circulatory arrest to sufficient perfection so that it worked passably well when first applied to a child; Lillehei did the same for cross-circulation. The animal laboratory was their wind tunnel, their finite element analysis, their proving ground. Human patients were spared many—even if not all—early teething difficulties. Though clinical experience improved new procedures, they were mostly invented *before* their human application. Norwood, on the other hand, couldn't so develop his operation. Animal models didn't exist, and even if one had, he could not have provided the labor-intensive postoperative management needed to nurse an operated animal to recovery. For Norwood and fellow travelers, the clinical crucible was their only lab.

Before we discuss Norwood's project, we need to think small. The earliest HLHS pioneers had, in a sense, gotten ahead of themselves: Open-heart surgery was initially successful mostly in patients at least several months old,[4] yet rescuing a newborn with HLHS couldn't be delayed.[5] Learning how to work inside the neonatal heart was a necessary prelude to the Norwood, and a major challenge on its own. As we will see, to open tiny hearts, surgeons pressed hypothermia, the modality that kicked off intracardiac surgery, back into service, albeit in a more radical way than Lewis and Swan. And technical advances alone couldn't open up neonatal surgery, or at least not very much; treating newborns with critical heart disease *precedes*

[3] Data from Boston Children's Hospital, 2015–2019.

[4] Lillehei et al. (1955); Kirklin et al. (1956); Kirklin and DuShane (1961).

[5] Lillehei's first ten cross-circulation cases ranged in weight from 7.7 to 38.6 kg, the youngest being 18 months old. Kirklin reported 40 open-hearts in 1956, only six of whom weighed as little as 3.6 to 9.0 kg. By 1961, Kirklin had operated upon 34 patients, two to twelve months old, for repair of ventricular septal defect.

their rolling into the operating room. A single ventricle works well enough with an open ductus, but when this vessel constricts, blood flow to the lungs or body is interrupted, and the circulation falls apart. The ability to medically pry open the ductus—developed just as neonatal open-heart surgery was gathering steam—thus stabilizing the circulation, has rescued countless one *and* two ventricle neonates, as highlighted in Chap. 10. In addition, the cardiac morphologists must be praised in the sense that hearts from failed operations often fall into the hands of a pathologist (or cardiac morphologist), who uncovers the surgical misstep(s). Given today's sophisticated imaging techniques, the pathologist is often not the first to discover what went wrong, but in cardiac surgery's earliest days postmortem examinations were indispensable for surgeons to advance their craft (see Chap. 8).

Let's get small.[6]

I'd gotten bitten by the heart bug in college, developed something like an esthetic absorption with it in medical school, and was soon looking for a richer encounter with congenital cardiac surgery than available at my institution. A paper in the *Journal of Thoracic and Cardiovascular Surgery*—I can still recall scouring it in the medical library—suggested that I might find such an experience in Boston. The article, which displayed Aldo R. Castañeda's enviable results repairing heart defects in infants, wasn't the only such report, but Boston seemed exotic yet accessible, and the surgeon's name implied, to me anyway, a certain Latin panache. Perhaps here was a chance to observe not merely cardiac surgery, but a charismatic artist-surgeon at work. July 1976 found me aiming a Chevy down Interstate 80 for the east coast, rolling through lush Iowa and Illinois farmland, the highway hugged by endless rows of towering corn. My previous farmland reconnoitering had been in comparatively hardscrabble eastern Colorado and Nebraska, and I was not a little impressed. Tiny heart surgery in my mind, I was struck with the idea of a surgeons' hands, wielding finely wrought instruments, moving across a few square centimeters of a baby's open chest, while the farmer's métier is expressed in territory too vast for the eye to take in at ground level. This image has stuck with me, poignantly shorthanding the tremendous range in scale of human craft, and how formidable a project usefully manipulating structures refined by eons of evolution really is. During my six weeks in Boston, I saw many surgical masterpieces, where a handful of well-placed incisions and a few centimeters of suture line took an entire morning's work but was repaid with a life rescued. As it turned out, my sojourn proved even more interesting than I had hoped, but that is not where we pick up the trail of neonatal heart surgery.

Half a world away from Boston and a decade before Castañeda had arrived there, Togo Horiuchi and colleagues, in Sendai, Japan, published *Radical Operation for Ventricular Septal Defect in Infancy* (1962).[7] *Radical* referred to the age of their patients. Heart-lung bypass, especially for extended periods, was poorly tolerated in the very young, partly because bypass equipment was insufficiently refined for

[6] Acknowledging Steve Martin's classic 1977 album.

[7] Horiuchi et al. (1963).

diminutive patients. By 1960, John Kirklin's infant ventricular septal defect repairs, conducted on bypass, had reasonably good results, although only a few patients had been operated upon by then.[8] Repair was typically deferred for an older age, or pulmonary artery banding[9] was performed to manage the defect until it could be closed later.[10] The Sendai group cut across the grain in operating on infants, their key to success being hypothermic circulatory arrest. Infants were cooled to 24–27 °C, and repairs were effected in six to twelve minutes.[11] They employed a similar technique used for the first successful open-heart operation (Chap. 7), now largely abandoned to the heart-lung machine, but hadn't pushed it far enough for lengthier repairs. A few years later, another Japanese surgeon, Yorinori Hikasa, dared more: Patients as young as four months, and weighing only four kilograms (about nine pounds), were cooled to as low as 17 °C, with circulatory arrest of up to 75 minutes.[12] Surgeons at the University of Washington in Seattle were doing much the same, and others followed quickly.[13]

Deep (aka "profound") hypothermic circulatory arrest substituted for bypass and offered other advantages besides. The cannulas (tubes) used to conduct blood to and from the heart-lung machine were eliminated if the baby was surface cooled,[14] and if bypass was briefly used for cooling, removed for the intracardiac work. (Though relatively unobtrusive in larger children and adults, in small hearts these cannulae get in the operator's way.) And the open heart is dry. (On bypass, small vessels send blood from the aorta to the lungs, which returns to the heart via the pulmonary veins. While surgeons use "suckers" to remove it, both the blood and suckers obscure a workspace where millimeters count.) Finally, the heart is completely relaxed, rendering its interior maximally accessible. John Lewis (and others) mostly used modest cooling,[15] which provides too little time for complex operations. Deep hypothermia—down to about 20 °C—gives surgeons a longer leash, enabling more than mere hole-patching. Improved equipment—such as fine sutures originally used for adult coronary bypass, better light sources, magnifying loupes, and other aspects of bypass—have greatly lowered its risk for newborns and reduced deep hypother-

[8] Kirklin and DuShane (1961).

[9] Pulmonary artery banding involves narrowing the pulmonary artery using a cloth or silicone band, which reduces the (abnormally high) pulmonary blood flow and pressure.

[10] Müller Jr and Dammann Jr. (1952).

[11] A perusal of the pulmonary artery pressures of their patients suggests that many of them would not have been operated so soon today, or perhaps at all (Horiuchi et al. 1963).

[12] Hikasa et al. (1967, 1968).

[13] The Seattle surgeons were K. Alvin Merendino, David Dillard, and Hitoshi Mohri. The Seattle group *began using* deep hypothermia in August 1965. Barratt-Boyes did so in July 1969, and Castañeda in January 1973 (Mohri et al. 1969; Rittenhouse et al. 1974; Hikasa et al. 1967; Dillard et al. 1967; Barratt-Boyes et al. 1972; Castañeda et al. 1974).

[14] With surface cooling, the patient is placed in an ice bath to lower the body temperature.

[15] John Lewis used "moderate" hypothermia (cooling to about 29 °C [84.5 °F]), with an average circulatory arrest time of four-to-five minutes. Swan also mostly used the same, good for six to eight minutes of circulatory arrest, although he, and other surgeons, occasionally used deep hypothermia (Lewis et al. 1957; Swan et al. 1955; Swan and Paton 1961; Shumacker Jr. 1992, p. 291).

mia's utilization today, but in neonatal surgery's neonatal period, this strategy was a game-changer.

Though not driving neonatal hypothermia's lead Conestoga wagon, two pioneers get a major share of credit for its promotion. Brian Barratt-Boyes—Sir Brian as of 1971—was the first. Shumacker states that Barratt-Boyes was the most important exponent of deep hypothermia. But note that the Seattle group did extensive experimental and clinical work defining the physiology of deep hypothermia, and Subramanian in Buffalo (New York) was another prominent early cooler.[16]

If one could somehow quantify a hospital's fame and multiply it by its mileage from leading American or European centers, easily the highest number would go to New Zealand's Green Lane Hospital, thanks to Barratt-Boyes. *The Independent* described him as "aggressive, autocratic, patriarchal, and tough"; he was also technically superb and attracted a galaxy of trainees from far and wide. Hitoshi Mohrio,[17] one of Horiuchi's collaborators in Sendai, visited Barratt-Boyes and together they laid the groundwork for the New Zealander to introduce deep hypothermia into his practice, starting in July 1969.[18] Babies as small as 2.9 kilograms (a little over six pounds) were repaired.[19] Ironically, Barratt-Boyes long suffered from cardiac disease and had had four heart operations, succumbing after having two valves replaced by Toby Cosgrove, a cardiac surgeon's cardiac surgeon at the Cleveland Clinic.[20]

Aldo Ricardo Castañeda was the other (Fig. 11.2). The 1974 paper that drew me to Boston was his first regarding hypothermia, and it was his later neonatal arterial switch work that had major impact. Babies whose aorta is connected to the right ventricle, and pulmonary artery to the left ventricle, have "transposition of the great arteries." By the 1980s, surgeons has gotten good at rearranging the circulation to accommodate this defect, with an operative risk of less than 10%. But the procedure (the *atrial* switch operation, two types were developed, one by Ake Senning in Sweden and the other by William Mustard in Toronto)) didn't actually return the patient to the wild type, and serious complications may occur years later. The *arterial* switch operation does connect the arteries with the correct ventricles and is theoretically superior, but it is technically challenging. Its initial mortality risk was presumably higher than the atrial switch's, at least early on a surgeon's learning curve. Furthermore, *only possibly*—no guarantee—would the newer operation improve long-term results; it was plausible that outcomes would eventually prove *worse* with the new procedure. Other surgeons had performed the arterial switch in

[16] Mee (1991); Sano (2007); Vida et al. (2006); Shumacker Jr. (1992), p. 291; Rittenhouse et al. (1974); Subramanian and Wagner (1973).

[17] Mohri worked on deep hypothermia in Seattle from 1964–1976 (Prabook (2024), https://prabook.com/web/hitoshi.mohri/201542)

[18] Paton (1992).

[19] Barratt-Boyes et al. (1972).

[20] Richmond (2006); Paton (1992). See also the interview with Richard Jonas, a Barratt-Byes trainee and surgeon of considerable accomplishment himself, conducted by the World Society of Pediatric and Congenital Cardiac Surgery (2010).

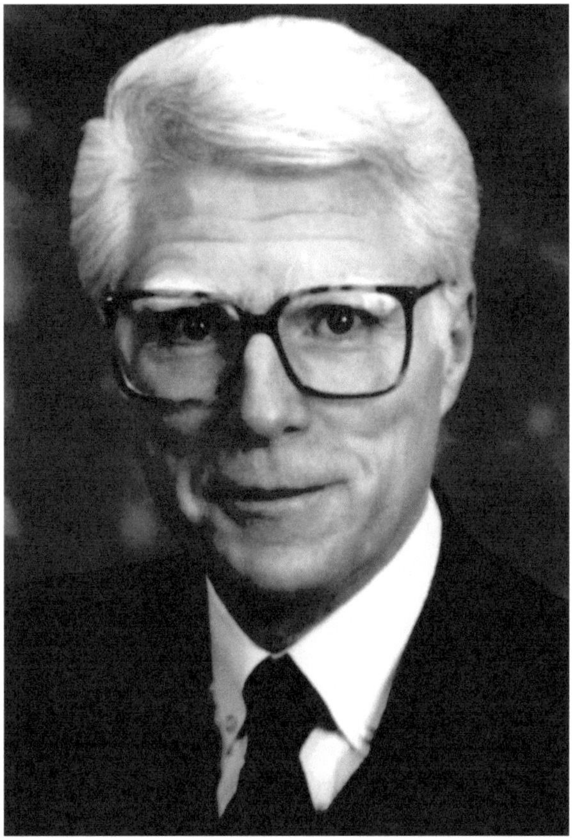

**Fig. 11.2** Aldo R. Castañeda MD PhD with permission of the Boston Children's Hospital Archives

older patients, but such candidates were few and often at high risk.[21] If the "switch" was as big an advance as intuition promised, offering it to newborns seemed imperative. But Castañeda and his colleagues had a tough choice, different from that confronting Blalock and Lillehei: We've got an excellent, if imperfect operation; dare we subject our patients to a higher immediate risk of dying in the *hope* of eventual benefit?[22] This conundrum is endemic in congenital cardiology. Unlike the effects of a new antibiotic or pain reliever, which can be quickly assessed, novel procedures or drugs intended to improve function over decades may take that long to evaluate. Decisions must be made on what are, in the final analysis, theoretical rather than empirical considerations.

Even if the *only way* that therapy can ever be improved requires a leap of faith, that refusing to risk being wrong neuters the very idea of innovation; Castañeda was, nevertheless, acutely aware of the underlying ethical considerations. He brought the family intimately into the decision-making process, explaining the

[21] Jatene et al. (1982).

[22] Bull et al. (2000); de Laval (2001).

options and giving them final say. Armed with a cogent rationale, more than adequate self-confidence, and a trust-inspiring bedside manner, he approached the father of his first candidate who, as luck would have it, was an engineering professor. He easily grasped the theoretical arguments and decided to swap the hope of a better long-term outcome for a higher operative risk. Like Gross and Blalock and Fontan, Castañeda was both lucky and good—his initial patient survived, as did thirteen of his first fourteen; goodness knows what would have become of his switch program were it sullied by even a few early deaths.[23]

More than lucky, better than good—Castañeda was an unusual master of his craft, and more. During my half-summer in Boston, I was dazzled by his supple, fluid movements as he guided eyelash-sized needles through obliging tissue and, with fingers a blur, stroked hair-thin sutures into anchoring knots. Always in control and seldom hesitating, if Castañeda were a painter, he would be Jackson Pollock, continuously, sinuously, drizzling paint onto a canvas, rather than Leonardo, tediously brushing well-contemplated strokes. He was as graceful in the real world as in the singular realm of the operating theater, though not salesman smooth. In fact, he was often blunt and assertive. And brutally and publicly self-critical, without varnish or euphemism. He occasionally used "lousy" to describe a surgical result of his, and related—to me on one occasion and with a wry smile—that he had once written a referring doctor expressing his dismay at not having done a better job for his patient, only to have the letter presented in court as evidence for the plaintiff![24]

But he was also sincerely and flatteringly engaging. Nobodies—like me—he looked in the eye and connected with, at least for a few moments, showing more consideration than might actually be merited. His artistry in the operating room was taken as a given: What comes up time and again in people's recollections of Aldo is his inclusiveness. That Castañeda was a highly effective surgeon gave him standing, but it was his respect and generosity for those in his orbit that rendered him a superlative leader.[25] The origins of this proclivity are unclear to me—cardiac team building during his training in Minnesota, as we saw in Chap. 7, was nothing to write home about—and presumably goes back to his childhood in war-ravaged Europe.

Castañeda was born in Nervi, Italy in 1930, to a Guatemalan father and Nicaraguan mother in Europe while the former attended medical school. They moved to Munich in 1935, and the family, being enemy aliens, was not allowed to leave Germany during the war. Castañeda saw his home destroyed in an air raid, and suffered a Nazi regime suffused with anything but respect for the individual. One suspects that this experience drove this emerging young man, endowed with a strong moral compass,[26] in precisely the opposite direction. Fulfilling college requirements in Switzerland after the war, he moved to Guatemala for medical school (1951). His

[23] World Society of Pediatric and Congenital Heart Surgery, Aldo Castañeda interview (2010); Castañeda et al. (1984); Open Pediatrics (2016).

[24] Van Praagh (2010); Lock (2017).

[25] Lock (2017).

[26] Castañeda's strong moral sense is well reflected in his presidential address to the American Association for Thoracic Surgery in 1994 (Castañeda 1994).

surgical residency was at the University of Minnesota, and then Castañeda was recruited to Boston Children's Hospital in 1972 as the chief of cardiovascular surgery in succession to Robert Gross.[27]

Whatever its source, Castañeda's quiver had all the arrows: technical excellence and a relentless commitment to continuously improve; self-assurance without self-absorption; a deeply collegial spirit; and *art*. Dean Acheson had observed that it was Winston Churchill's art that enabled him to accomplish great things,[28] and—on a rather more modest scale—so did Castañeda's. Good looks complemented by a discerning wardrobe; finely sculpted and expressive hands that *looked* like they could only be connected to a surgeon nonpareil; his capacity to communicate with colleagues in five languages; and *savoir faire*: it is no surprise that this rare concoction powerfully attracted people to his sprawling camp.

Castañeda's last, and greatest, project started late in life and a world away from Boston. Retiring from Children's in 1994, he worked three years at a clinic in Grenolier, Switzerland before returning to Guatemala in 1997. Then 67, Castañeda had posted himself in that difficult country not to retire but to build, from scratch, a pediatric heart surgery program. Few Guatemalan children had access to cardiac surgery; the rare family with means would travel to the US or Europe for such care. The only provider of pediatric heart surgery in Central America, Castañeda's Unidad de Cirugia Cardiovascular Pediatrica de Guatemala, is financed on a frayed shoestring, partly from donations from admiring colleagues. But the dividends on the modest investment were astronomical: In its first eight years, more than 1200 patients had operations, with nearly 90% surviving.[29]

One of Castañeda's former trainees, a distinguished cardiac surgeon himself, told me that he would walk through a wall of fire for Castañeda. He would have to join a crowd.[30]

All of the dogs died, usually within an hour postop, except for one which survived for two, but: "Because of the desperate nature of hypoplastic left heart syndrome and the lack of a useful palliative or corrective operation, clinical trial of this procedure seems warranted."—Hurley Knott and Donald Doty.[31]

Fascination with the hypoplastic left heart goes back quite a ways. Maude Abbott's classic atlas[32] includes illustrations of a tiny left heart and a diagram of the blood's purported movement therein. But with arrows indicating flow across "atretic" (unformed) aortic and mitral valves, her drawing is confusing, and one wonders whether Dr. Abbott's mind wasn't elsewhere when she scratched it out.

[27] Vida et al. (2006).

[28] Acheson (1969), pp. 595–596.

[29] Vida et al. (2006); Larrazabal et al. (2007); Van Praagh (2010); Lock (2017).

[30] Discussions with Dr. John Lamberti (August 2020).

[31] Knott and Doty (1977).

[32] Abbott (1936/2006).

This malformation had been described long before her,[33] but the modern landmark exposition of hypoplastic left heart syndrome (HLHS) was produced in 1958 by Jackie Noonan and Alexander Nadas, two distinguished pediatric cardiologists.[34] Nadas, in his 1957 textbook, couldn't imagine a remedy, and even 20 years later, most practitioners regarded HLHS as inoperable.[35]

But not everybody. In 1959, Frank Redo and Robert Gross operated upon a two and one-half month old with HLHS and a patent duct, enlarging the opening in the atrial septum.[36] They knew only that the baby had mitral atresia before operating—the full diagnosis was made at autopsy—and did not appreciate that, with opening the septum, too much blood would flood the lungs; the infant died soon after the operation. While hardly providing a road map to the Norwood, these surgeons had at least learned the crucial importance of limiting pulmonary blood flow. Sachchida Sinha and colleagues in Chicago inched HLHS surgery forward, proposing banding the branch pulmonary arteries to reduce flow.[37] Assuming that the duct would remain open, they never engaged the most difficult part of what was required for a successful procedure. But by 1970, Glen Cayler and colleagues, at a hospital in Sacramento, had mapped out all the essential elements of neonatal palliation:

1. A large atrial septal defect
2. A large communication between the aorta and the ventricle
3. An adequately sized ascending aorta and arch
4. Restricting pulmonary flow by pulmonary artery bands
5. Ensuring adequate coronary flow (which is actually a restatement of number three).

Reporting a single seven-month survivor, they knew that their palliation would be too short-lived to be truly satisfactory but speculated that a "curative" procedure was on the horizon.[38]

The Californians were prescient. The Fontan was in the air,[39] causing people to think differently: Now one could envision something like a "repair," thus upping the ante for an effective operation. At the University of Iowa, Donald Doty and Hurley

[33] Gehrmann and colleagues (2002) claim that the first complete description of HLHS was by K. Bardeleben, in 1851. But his description was hardly typical of this malformation, or even physiologically tenable, as the ascending aorta and arch were a "thin solid cord"; perhaps his dissection was not careful enough to reveal the tiny lumen of the vessel.

[34] Keith et al. (1978), p. 547; Noonan and Nadas (1958).

[35] Nadas (1957).

[36] The date of operation is not given, but their two other cases (neither HLHS) were done in 1959 (Redo et al. 1961).

[37] Sinha et al. (1968).

[38] Cayler et al. (1970); Van Praagh et al. (1971); Saied and Folger Jr. (1972); Moody et al. (1972).

[39] Shortly thereafter, Van Praagh and associates described an operation—albeit for a different malformation—that met Cayler's requirements and noted that it could be applied to HLHS. Other workers, such as Abraham Saied and Gordon Folger at the Medical College of Georgia were also acutely aware of the pernicious effects of excessive pulmonary flow although not everyone was so enlightened.

Knott sewed closed the mitral valve of dogs, excised the atrial septum, inserted a conduit from the pulmonary artery to the aortic arch, and directed all venous blood into the pulmonary arteries. Eight dogs were operated upon, and all were dead within two hours. Even without the advantage of hindsight, this is not terribly surprising. It was known at the time that the Glenn shunt is poorly tolerated in very young patients; how could Doty expect that directing *all* venous blood through the lungs would work any better?[40] But Doty, undeterred, tore a page from Francis Fontan: Satisfied that he had worked out the technique, Doty proceeded to perform his operation in five infants.[41]

What was he thinking?

I can only speculate, but I return yet again to the perfidy of animal models. Their unreliability grants considerable skeptical license, sometimes even enough to ignore them (as did Fontan). And there is also another, adjacent, issue: interpretation of any sort of experimental observation is often colored by underlying assumptions and beliefs. A fuzzy penumbra often encircles empirical data, especially those emanating from complex systems and investigations, affording considerable latitude in their interpretation.[42] Robert Skidelsky, in *Money and Government*, quoted the influential economist Milton Friedman: "I was interested in science qua science, and I have tried—successfully I hope—not to let my ideological viewpoints contaminate my scientific work.... (But) I felt deeply concerned with the course of events and I wanted to influence them so as to enhance human freedom. *Luckily, these two aspects of my interests appeared to me as perfectly compatible.*"[43] One doesn't need to be half as smart as Friedman to know better than that—preexisting bias *does* contaminate data interpretation and conclusions drawn. What proclivity licensed Dr. Doty to shrug off pretty compelling clinical and experimental evidence? I suspect that it was a surgeon's optimism—their tribe surely being the most optimistic of medicine's many—that led him to intuit, deep in his bones, that he could, somehow, make this procedure work.

But physiology had its way. All five babies quickly died,[44] which Doty attributed to high resistance to flow in the lungs.[45] The idea of a *staged* approach—a neonatal operation where the right ventricle propelled blood through the lungs, followed later by a Fontan—apparently had not occurred to him. But by 1979 it had, and he managed a hospital survivor by providing pulmonary flow via a (restricted) communication between the systemic circuit and the lungs.[46]

---

[40] Glenn et al. (1965); Willman et al. (1974); Williams et al. (1975, 1976).

[41] Knott and Doty (1977); Doty and Knott (1977).

[42] Strevens (2020), pp. 24–74.

[43] Skidelsky (2018), p. 177; emphasis mine.

[44] Doty's manuscript was submitted in March 1977, so it seems likely that at least the first patient was operated upon in 1976.

[45] Doty and Knott (1977).

[46] Doty et al. (1980).

Such was the state of the art when Bill Norwood, then a junior colleague of Castañeda, engaged the problem. That phrase, though, may imply too wide an appreciation of what had been done and learned. We've seen that Glenn didn't know of Carlon's or the Russians' cavopulmonary shunts; nor almost anybody of Azzolina's; nor Kreutzer of Fontan's procedure (Chap. 9). Word didn't always get around, or maybe get taken seriously. It is hard to know exactly what the Boston team had derived from previous workers, and how much was reinvented there.

In any case, the tougher challenge is translating ideas into substance. How *does* one arrange for the correct amount of pulmonary flow? Doty's solution turned out to be evanescent—the connection into the lungs narrowed quickly, causing the baby's death after a scant twelve weeks. And the aorta: A good way to enlarge the ascending aorta and the arch, and connect it to the right ventricle, had yet to be invented. Doty's was incomplete and didn't optimally open the aorta, and the conduit eventually needed replacement. And how to configure the renovation so as to not compromise a subsequent Fontan-like procedure? Turning theoretical requirements into an actual structure was Norwood's charge. For this, he had three advantages relative to most of the rest of the field.[47]

Norwood was a surgeon of rare technical gifts. He was ambidextrous and therefore had—this is admittedly an exaggeration—roughly twice as many deft fingers at his disposal than almost anybody else. He had his way inside a neonate's chest in a way that few surgeons could. And successful surgery demands more than driving a stich, or incising an artery, with sub-millimeter precision. The operator manipulates a still heart, empty of blood and collapsed; when it starts up again, it swells and contracts, and its geometry changes. What was moments ago an exquisite connection is now too narrow, blood flow critically restricted, and the procedure at immediate risk of failure. Or a "repaired' valve leaks like a sieve. Like all great neonatal surgeons, Norwood had an uncanny three-dimensional sense and could envision how an essentially two-dimensional structure would add a third at operation's end. Imagining how tissue should be sculpted and doing it are very different propositions; Norwood was brilliant at both.

His second advantage was the team. Postoperative care prior to the 1970s was typically primarily the responsibility of the surgeon, and at night and during off hours, his trainees. But the surgeon is often unavailable, and residents cycle through the system, moving on as soon as they get reasonably good at complex care. Castañeda, talent magnet that he was, attracted the first pediatric cardiac intensive care team anywhere, as near as I can tell. Roberta Williams, a young cardiologist at Children's, was its primogenitor cardiac intensivist, and Dolly Hansen, an anesthesiologist, another key contributor.[48] Other cardiologists soon joined, most notably Peter Lang. This modest band would grow over time, developing and accreting the

[47] This section is largely based upon discussions with: Drs. Edward L. Bove, John Lamberti, Peter Lang, Stephen Sanders, and Roberta Williams, as well as the papers cited. See also World Society of Pediatric and Congenital Heart Surgery (2010).

[48] Odegard and Rockoff (2020).

very specialized expertise that could spell the difference between a patient on the knife edge surviving, or not. And they added ideas, enthusiasm, and encouragement.

Finally, $E_1$ prostaglandin had arrived just as Norwood took the bit. We looked at this development in Chap. 10 and placed it central in the story of single ventricle rescue, especially babies with HLHS. $E_1$ prostaglandin became the initial treatment—and life saver—for babies with HLHS, as well as babies with cyanotic congenital heart disease.

Prior to this medication, there were two types of HLHS patients. Newborns with closing ducts were the majority; they were very sick, often desperately so, and their metabolic status was so compromised that they seldom survived with or without the stress of surgery. A handful of others were older, with an open duct but too much or too little pulmonary blood flow, also increasing operative risk. Because medically opening the duct with prostaglandin improved the condition of the first group, Norwood had access to more babies, in better shape, than previously available.

But these advantages would have amounted to little without imagination and persistence. If fifty chicks pecking once at fifty shells didn't crack the problem of cardiopulmonary bypass or Fontan palliation (Chaps. 7 and 9), neither did they solve the puzzle of HLHS. (Don Doty appears to have been the only other early HLHS aficionado who kept pecking away.) Sticking with this problem took backbone. Critics at Boston Children's—and indeed throughout congenital cardiology—feared that attempts at palliation offered far greater prospects for patient (and family) suffering than a good life. Even in 1980, when an operation for HLHS was still a chimera, Don Doty wrote that the ethical and moral implications of pursing this therapy deserved serious contemplation, and doubts about the wisdom of performing Norwood palliation persisted long after its technical feasibility was a fact.[49] In two physician surveys (1999 and 2007), for example, fewer than half of those responding would have certainly chosen an operation, rather than end-of-life care, were they to have a baby with HLHS.[50] Marathon runners are cheered on every step along the course; Norwood's route ran through as many protests as cheers.

Persistence-driven iteration was the essence of the Norwood's invention. As if anticipating future curiosity about their procedure's creation, Norwood and colleagues provided something unusual.[51] Their very first (reported, at any rate) case—a non-survivor—had the superior vena caval flow directed into the right pulmonary artery, similar to Doty's failed attempts to conduct all venous return straight into the lungs.[52] As just noted, it's hard to see the rationale for this arrangement—perhaps

[49] Doty et al. (1980).

[50] Kon et al. (2013); Paul et al. (2016). Neonatologists, intensivists, cardiologists, and surgeons were surveyed. In 1999, 39% said that they would choose surgery, 28% palliative care, and 33% were uncertain; in 2007, 45% would choose surgery and 35% were uncertain. There is a considerable literature dealing with caregivers' thoughts and attitudes regarding offering surgery for babies with HLHS—larger, I believe, than for any other similar issue in congenital cardiology.

[51] Norwood et al. (1980, 1981); Lang and Norwood (1983). This summary comes with a grain of salt. The relevant papers do not jibe perfectly with respect to the number of variants performed.

[52] Norwood et al. (1980).

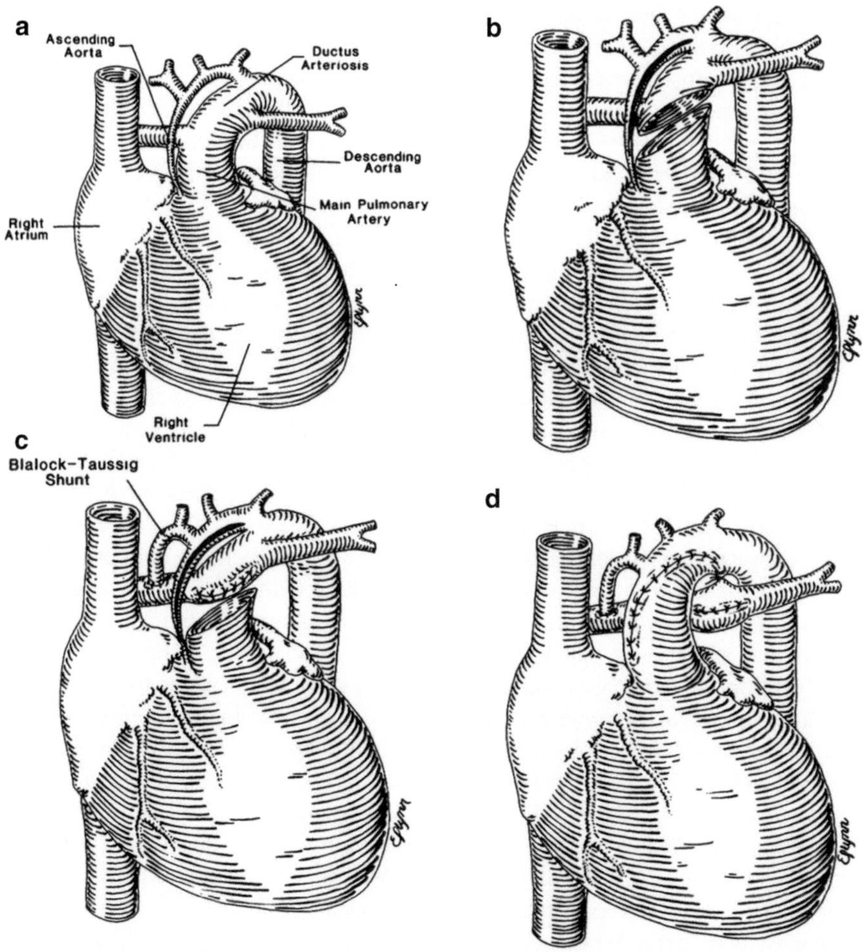


**Fig. 11.3** After at least 6 iterations of the operation by Dr. Norwood and colleagues, this is the final "standard" model. Note the still useful Blalock-Taussig-Thomas shunt (B-T-T) 41/2 decades after its invention. Lang (1983). (Reprinted with permission of the American Heart Association)

that is why it merited no diagram in Norwood's first report and went unmentioned in his 1981 paper. Figure 11.3 illustrates the final standard model after a number of iterations.[53]

Their papers discussed the reasons for some of the modifications. For example, sewing a conduit from the pulmonary artery to the aorta distorted the latter, so the conduit was moved to the right ventricle. The ventricle-to-aorta connection was ultimately crafted using the pulmonary artery and aorta, thus avoiding non-growing materials, and improving flow to the coronary arteries. These and other

[53] Norwood et al. (1980, 1981).

improvements were made as Norwood and colleagues saw what worked, what didn't, and what might be improved. Some were *ad hoc*: The decision to make one modification was literally made in the operating room. What was not mentioned are the intensive care techniques that the team had to discover and apply to nurse patients through the difficult postoperative hours and days. Physiology and pharmacology were welded and wielded to adjust blood flow to the body and the lungs; they learned how to manage mechanical ventilation in such patients; they discerned indications of an inadequate operation requiring investigation and rectification. HLHS rescue was a process continuing well after the surgery itself. Even after the Norwood worked well enough to seem like therapy—rather than yet another failed attempt at same—it was still low-yield. Of Norwood's first sixteen reported patients, only three were still alive six to nineteen months after the operation.[54] (Hospital survival at the best centers today is over 90%.)

Norwood provided the blueprint, but crafting the Norwood defied protocolization; other surgeons made this operation work only through failure and iteration, much as had the Boston surgeon. Ed Bove at the University of Michigan, a widely acknowledged master of the Norwood as well as the arterial switch, had such miserable early results that on at least one occasion the intensive care unit nurses didn't even bother to prepare a post-operative bed for the HLHS baby in the operating room. Physiology had to be learned, technique refined, and innumerable problems solved. In some real sense, every surgeon who developed facility with this procedure had to invent it for himself.[55]

What are the major lessons of this chapter? For one, we've seen the craft of surgery outrun the laboratory. Cardiac surgery's earliest, highest, and most *general* hurdles could be largely addressed in the dog lab (e.g., how to sew one blood vessel to another; inventing a machine to pump and oxygenate blood; technical maneuvers to bypass the right ventricle). These sorts of fundamental problems usually submitted to substantial solution using animal models, even if much remained to be learned. But as surgeons mastered simple stuff, they tackled more complicated malformations, which brought *special* challenges, like those bedeviling Doty and Norwood. Operations for HLHS and the arterial switch (and those for other defects) required moving the lab into the clinical arena because no good animal models existed or could be created. While some craft can be exported from the lab into the clinic—Thomas and Blalock, for example, learned from Carrel's anastomotic techniques—other varieties can only be developed by treating and learning from the actual anatomic deformities. As we've pointed out, medical innovation is, like gold, where you find it; workers have advanced the field from venues as disparate as autopsy tables, dog and basic science labs, the clinic, and even the social milieu.

As the craft matured, so too did the ethical environment. In Lewis and Lillehei's day, the ethics of medical innovation were "ambiguous," as the former put it, or perhaps even less well-formed than that. That has changed, and surgeons and their

[54] Norwood et al. (1981).

[55] Telephone discussion with Edward L. Bove, May 2020.

medical colleagues feel the need, and are obligated, to be transparent with families about therapeutic options (including novel treatments), risks, and possible benefits. Some currently fear that increasingly stringent ethical and regulatory standards are hamstringing progress, but as Castañeda and many others have showed, partnerships with patients and families enable new—and risky—treatments to be offered.[56] Congenital cardiology continues to innovate, even if with a little less celerity than in Lillehei's day.

Most importantly, we engaged a point made by Mary Beard in *Confronting the Classics*: The Classics live on in our cultural landscape, even if their influence is subtle and its provenance obscure. What were widely appreciated poems, plays, and sculpture in their day have mostly faded into the background, yet remain vital parts of the contemporary warp and woof. It's the same for congenital cardiology. Our discipline operates, and advances, not only via seminal breakthroughs, but also thanks to developments whose sources are difficult or impossible to ascertain. Helen Taussig, for example, invented some of the clinical skills required for the Blalock-Taussig-Thomas shunt to become therapy, but also inherited others long since flattened into the landscape. As an apprentice surgeon, Lillehei was taught ancient ways of manipulating tissue, whose origins are obscure. It is impossible to precisely pinpoint the origins of the Boston team's collection of the surgical manipulations, physiology, and pharmacology needed for HLHS rescue, yet this expertise is deeply embedded in the way we treat these patients today. People with durable new ideas, like Van Praagh and Anderson (Chap. 8), may influence via refinement rather than revolution, contributing incremental advances which eventually merge into the background. In fact, Coceani, Olley, and the Auckland team's invention of a duct-opening agent had a monumental impact but secured little acclaim for its inventors and soon became yet another drug that practitioners use reflexively, as though it had always been there. *Reimagining a Child's Heart* is preoccupied with seminal advances and their authors—partly for the obvious reasons, partly because the archeology of much of current practice is tough or impossible digging. But the distinction between disruptive creations and the current landscape is merely a temporal one. Ductal ligation, the Blalock-Taussig-Thomas shunt, open heart surgery—at first, they *did* stand out. People in the institutions where they were performed followed the developments and generated a buzz; a sense of something new and special permeated their space. News filtered through professional networks and the lay media, and prestigious prizes were awarded. But these breakthroughs stand out no longer. As special as they still are, they have become routine, even mundane, and vanished into the terrain, at least for people working in the field. Historians—and people, like me, interested in history—re-hoist these solo trees, these Lone Pines, above ground level to examine the fabric of therapy creation, even while knowing that their ultimate purpose is to form the anchoring landscape for the many Lone Pines to come.

[56] It seems to me that innovation—even radical—still proceeds, even if sometimes more slowly and at greater expense.

# References

Abbott ME (1936/2006) Atlas of congenital cardiac disease. McGill-Queen's University Press, Montreal

Acheson D (1969) Present at the creation: my years in the State Department. W.W. Norton & Co., New York

Barratt-Boyes BG, Neutze JM, Seelye ER, Simpson M (1972) Complete correction of cardiovascular malformations in the first year of life. Prog Cardiovasc Dis 15:229–253

Beard M (2013) Confronting the classics. Profile Books, London, UK

Bull C, Yates R, Sarkar D, Deanfield J, de Laval M (2000) Scientific, ethical, and logistical considerations in introducing a new operation: a retrospective cohort study from pediatric cardiac surgery. BMJ 320:1168–1173

Castañeda AR (1994) The making of a cardiothoracic surgeon: an Appolonian quest. J Thorac Cardiovasc Surg 108:806–812

Castañeda AR, Lamberti J, Sade RM, Williams RG, Nadas AS (1974) Open heart surgery during the first three months of life. J Thorac Cardiovasc Surg 68:719–731

Castañeda AR, Norwood WI, Jonas RA, Colon SD, Sanders SP, Lang P (1984) Transposition of the great arteries and intact ventricular septum: anatomical repair in the neonate. Ann Thorac Surg 38:438–443

Cayler GG, Smeloff EA, Miller GE (1970) Surgical palliation of hypoplastic left side of the heart. N Engl J Med 282:780–783

de Laval M (2001) Lessons from the arterial switch operation. Lancet 357:1814

Dillard DH, Mohri H, Hessel EA II, Anderson HN, Nelson RJ, Crawford EW et al (1967) Correction of total anomalous pulmonary venous drainage in infancy utilizing deep hypothermia with circulatory arrest. Circulation 35–36(suppl):I-105–I-110

Doty DB, Knott HW (1977) Hypoplastic left heart syndrome: experience with an operation to establish functionally normal circulation. J Thorac Cardiovasc Surg 74:624–630

Doty DB, Marvin WJ Jr, Shieken RM, Lauer RM (1980) Hypoplastic left heart syndrome: successful palliation with a new operation. J Thoracic Cardiovasc Surg. 80:148–152

Gehrmann J, Krasemann T, Kehl HG, Vogt J (2002) Hypoplastic left syndrome: the first description of the pathophysiology in 1851; translation of a publication by Dr. Bardeleben from Geissen, Germany. Chest 120:1368–1371

Glenn WWL, Ordway NK, Talner NS, Call EP Jr (1965) Circulatory bypass of the right side of the heart. VI. Shunt between superior vena cava and distal right pulmonary artery; report of clinical application in thirty-eight cases. Circulation 31:172–189

Hikasa Y, Shirotani H, Saromura K et al (1967) Open heart surgery in infants with an aid of hypothermic anesthesia. Arch Jap Chir. 36:495–508

Hikasa Y, Shirotani H, Saromura K et al (1968) Open heart surgery in infants with an aid of hypothermic anesthesia (II). Arch Jap Chir 37:399–412

Horiuchi T, Koyamada K, Matano I, Mohri H, Komatsu T, Honda T et al (1963) Radical operation for ventricular septal defect in infancy. J Thorac Cardiovasc Surg 46:180–190

Jatene AD, Fontes VF, Souza LC, Paulista PP, Neto CA, Sousa JE (1982) Anatomic correction of transposition of the great arteries. J Thorac Cardiovasc Surg 83(1):20–26

Keith JD, Rowe RD, Vlad P (1978) Heart disease in infancy and childhood, 3rd edn. Macmillan Publishing Co., Inc., New York

Kirklin JW, DuShane JW (1961) Repair of ventricular septal defect in infancy. Pediatrics 27:961–966

Kirklin JW, Donald DE, Harshbarger HG, Hetzel PS, Patrick RT, Swan HJC, Wood EH (1956) Studies in extracorporeal circulation. I. Applicability of Gibbon-type pump-oxygenator to human intracardiac surgery: 40 cases. Ann Surg 144:2–8

Knott HW, Doty DB (1977) Experimental bypass of the left ventricle. J Thorac Cardiovasc Surg 74:436–439

Kon AA, Prsa M, Rohlicek CV (2013) Choices doctors would make if their infant had hypoplastic left heart syndrome: comparison of surgery data from 1999 and 2007. Pediatr Cardiol 34:348–353

Lang P, Norwood WI (1983) Hemodynamic assessment after palliative surgery for hypoplastic left heart syndrome. Circulation 68:104–108

Larrazabal LA, Jenkins KJ, Gauvreau K, Vida VL, Benavidez OJ, Gaitán GF, Castañeda AR (2007) Improvement in congenital heart surgery in a developing country. Circulation 116:1882–1887

Lewis FJ, Winchell P, Bashour FA (1957) Open repair of atrial septal defects: results in sixty-three patients. JAMA 165:922–927

Lillehei CW, Cohen M, Warden HE, Read RC, Aust JB, DeWall RA, Varco RL (1955) Direct vision intracardiac correction of the tetralogy of Fallot, pentalogy of Fallot, and pulmonary atresia defects: report of first ten cases. Ann Surg 112:418–442

Lock JE (2017) Are the spin doctors winning? Cong Heart Dis 12:697–698

Mee RB (1991) Current status of cardiac surgery in childhood. Prog Pediatr Surg 27:148–169

Mohri H, Dillard DH, Crawford EW, Martin WE, Merendino KA (1969) Method of surface-induced deep hypothermia for open-heart surgery in infants. J Thorac Cardiovasc Surg 58:262–270

Moody DS, Gallen WJ, Friedberg DZ (1972) Congenital aortic atresia: report of long survival and some speculations about surgical approaches. J Thoracic Cardiovasc Surg 63:726–731

Müller WH Jr, Dammann JF Jr (1952) The treatment of certain congenital malformations of the heart by the creation of pulmonic stenosis to reduce pulmonary hypertension and excessive blood flow. Surg Gyne Obst 95:213–219

Nadas AS (1957) Pediatric cardiology. W.B. Saunders Co., Philadelphia

Noonan JA, Nadas AS (1958) The hypoplastic left heart syndrome: an analysis of 101 cases. Pediatr Clin N Am 5:1029–1056

Norwood WI, Kirklin JK, Sanders SP (1980) Hypoplastic left heart syndrome: experience with palliative surgery. Am J Card 45:87–91

Norwood WI, Lang P, Castañeda AR, Campbell DN (1981) Experience with operations for hypoplastic left heart syndrome. J Thorac Cardiovasc Surg 82(4):511–519

Norwood WI, Lang P, Hansen DD (1983) Physiologic repair of aortic atresia-hypoplastic left heart syndrome. N Engl J Med 308:23–26

Odegard KC, Rockoff MA (2020) "The mother of pediatric cardiac anesthesia": an interview with Dr. Dolly D. Hansen, a pioneering woman in medicine. Paediatr Anaesth 30(9):964–969

Open Pediatrics. Interview with Dr. Aldo Castañeda 2016. Accessed October 21, 2024. https://www.youtube.com/watch?v=voTxtx72niU

Paton BC (1992) Sir Brian Barratt-Boyes. Clin Cardiol 15:694–695

Paul EA, Orfali K, Stare TJ (2016) Hypoplastic left heart syndrome: exploring a paradigm shift in favor of surgery. Pediatr Cardiol 37:1446–1452

Prabook. Hitoshi Mohri. Accessed October 21, 2024. https://prabook.com/web/hitoshi.mohri/201542

Redo SF, Farber S, Gross RE (1961) Atresia of the mitral valve. Arch Surg 82:678–694

Richmond C. Sir Brian Barratt-Boyes. The Independent, March 16, 2006. Accessed October 21, 2024. https://www.the-independent.com/news/obituaries/sir-brian-barrattboyes-6106628.html

Rittenhouse EA, Mohri H, Dillard DH, Merendino KA (1974) Deep hypothermia in cardiovascular surgery. Ann Thoracic Surg 17:63–98

Saied A, Folger GM Jr (1972) Hypoplastic left heart syndrome: clinicopathologic and hemodynamic correlation. Am J Cardiol 29:190–198

Sano S (2007) Recent development of congenital heart surgery in neonates and small infants. Nihon Geka Gakkai Zasshi 108:339–343

Shumacker HB Jr (1992) The evolution of cardiac surgery. Indiana University Press, Bloomington

Sinha SN, Rusnak SL, Sommers HM, Cole RB, Muster AJ, Paul MH (1968) Hypoplastic left ventricle syndrome: analysis of thirty autopsy cases in infants with surgical considerations. Am J Cardiol 21:166–173

Skidelsky R (2018) Money and government: the past and future of economics. Yale University Press, New Haven

Strevens M (2020) The knowledge machine. Liveright, New York

Subramanian S, Wagner H (1973) Correction of transposition of the great arteries in infants under surface-induced deep hypothermia. Ann Thorac Surg 16:391–401

Swan H, Paton BC (1961) The current status of hypothermia in cardiovascular surgery. Prog Cardiovasc Dis 4:228–258

Swan H, Virtue RW, Blount SG Jr, Kircher LT Jr (1955) Hypothermia in surgery: analysis of 100 cases. Ann Surg 142:382–400

Van Praagh R (2010) Aldo Ricardo Castañeda, MD, PhD: what is he really like? Thorac Cardiov Surg 58:318–319

Van Praagh R, Bernhardt WF, Rosenthal SA, Parisi LF, Fyler DC (1971) Interrupted aortic arch: surgical treatment. Am J Cardiol 27:200–211

Vida L, Sade RM, Stellin G (2006) Aldo R. Castañeda. Cardiol Young 16:221–228

Williams WG, Rubis L, Trusler GA, Mustard WT (1975) Palliation of tricuspid atresia. Potts-Smith, Glenn, and Blalock-Taussig shunts. Arch Surg 110:1383–1386

Williams WG, Rubis L, Fowler RS, Rao MK, Trusler GA, Mustard WT (1976) Tricuspid atresia: results of treatment in 160 children. Am J Cardiol 38:235–240

Willman VL, Barner HB, Mudd G, Fagan LF, Kaiser GC (1974) Superior vena cava-pulmonary artery anastomosis. J Thorac Cardiovasc Surg 67:380–386

World Society for Pediatric and Congenital Heart Surgery. Interviews with Leading Figures in Congenital Cardiac Care. 2010. Accessed October 21, 2024. https://wupchs.education/interviews-leading-surgeons

# Afterword

Thomas Jonathan Kulik MD, age 69, passed away suddenly and unexpectedly on January 6, 2021.

As many of you know, Tom was working on a book regarding congenital heart disease, stimulated in part by his interest in history and his fascination with therapy for the final gordian knot of congenital cardiology – the hypoplastic left heart syndrome. Publishing this book was a professional goal that Tom was unable to complete before his untimely death. Tom was very excited and proud of his book, and we learned later that he was making edits on the day that he passed. I am forever indebted to Dr. Macdonald Dick (Mac), our friend and a colleague of Tom, for his dedication, editorial skills, and know how to move Tom's book towards publication. I hope you enjoyed reading *Reimagining a Child's Heart. The Lone Pines of Congenital Cardiology.*

Tom had a unique personality. He was a loving husband and a wonderful father to his beloved daughter Elise. He was a creative, generous, kind, and philanthropic person. On the other hand, Tom held himself (and often others) to high expectations. Tom was driven, hardworking, and conscientious. He was an avid reader on a variety of subjects. He had a thirst for knowledge and was ready to talk about any topic from medicine, sports cars or politics, sometimes with a dry sense of humor or a hint of sarcasm.

Tom was very intentional with his time with Elise, rarely passing upon an opportunity to nurture her mind. They played "tricky games" on long walks, solved riddles on ski lifts, and listed state capitals on paper napkins while waiting for dinner. As Elise grew older, the conversations expanded and deepened. Among Elise's favorite memories of Tom are their conversations through which he encouraged her to think critically and creatively and to engage with whatever idea lay before her. Even though Tom had a very busy professional life, he took time to enjoy life as well. Tom was a dedicated cyclist and car enthusiast. He loved to travel, especially to Italy (as long as I was making all the arrangements), and home to Colorado to reconnect with family and friends, and to hike and ski his favorite spots around


T. J. Kulik, M. Dick, *Reimagining a Child's Heart*,
https://doi.org/10.1007/978-3-031-88608-9

Ouray and Telluride. Tom was especially proud to have hiked Mt. Sneffels of the San Juan Mountains, Colorado successfully.

During his funeral eulogy, given by one of his close colleagues Dr. Ravi Thiagarajan, Tom was described as a "devoted physician providing excellent and compassionate care to critically ill children and their families. His research, discoveries, and scientific writings have helped understand, treat, improve lives, and bring hope to children with heart and lung disease. Tom was a gifted teacher whose thoughtful and methodical approach made complex concepts of heart disease understandable and interesting. He successfully mentored a large number of aspiring pediatric cardiologists across this nation who have now gone on to become important contributors themselves".

Tom's life was cut short and he is sorely missed by his family, friends, colleagues, patients and families.

Newton, MA, USA Linda Kulik

# Introduction to the Appendices

Tom, as was known by many, was a car guy. He appreciated high performance engines such as his Ferrari – and the human heart. As noted in the Foreword, Tom initially intended to have these appendices as chapters intermingled in the body of the text. Tom spent many hours reading about and thinking about medical innovation, and engineering innovation, constantly mulling them over contrasting, comparing, evaluating the strengths and weaknesses of each. This section is for those readers who are interested in how Tom thought about engineering and medical innovation and how he related it to the development of surgical therapy for a congenital heart disease.



T. J. Kulik, M. Dick, *Reimagining a Child's Heart*,
https://doi.org/10.1007/978-3-031-88608-9

# Appendices

## Appendix 1

> I die by the help of too many physicians.
> –Alexander the Great, 323 BC[1]

> God heales, and the Physitian hath the thankes.
> –Proverb popularized by George Herbert, 1640[2]

> The medical treatment of malformation of the heart must consist, first, in the hygienic management of the patient … secondly, in the avoidance of the various causes which may aggravate the existing defects in the conformation of the heart … and, thirdly, in the relief of the urgent symptoms when they arise.
> –Thomas B. Peacock 1858[3]

> Of the over-all benefit that ensued (from using penicillin to treat battle injuries in several thousand men) there can be no doubt. Apart from the general diminution in the infection rate, and the probable effect of that on subsequent mortality, we can recall many instances where the man's life was beyond question saved solely because this drug was available.
> –J.S. Jeffrey and Scott Thompson 1944[4]

The *number* of available therapies and how *well they work* has changed remarkably over the millennia, the last hundred years having provided many more effective interventions than all the previous years. But *what* therapies do in the broad, general sense has changed little. In fact, the general motifs referred to in the quotes

[1] Porter (1997, p. 66).

[2] This quotation appears to have been first published in *Outlandish Proverbs*, a volume of sayings whose collection was attributed to Herbert and published in 1640, some 7 years after his death in 1633.

[3] Peacock (1858, p. 141).

[4] Jeffrey and Thompson (1944).



T. J. Kulik, M. Dick, *Reimagining a Child's Heart*,
https://doi.org/10.1007/978-3-031-88608-9

above—therapy as harmful, as supportive, as management and palliation, or as powerful and effective—are as descriptive today as throughout history. What has changed is the *shift in the prevalence of these* classes of treatments.

Therapeutic interventions are many and immensely varied. One way to lay eyes on this vast landscape is to scan the 999 pages of the American Medical Association's Current Procedural Terminology (CPT) codebook, a listing of descriptive terms and identifying codes for the diagnostic and therapeutic services that physicians provide.[5] While it is near impossible to determine the number of distinctly different types of surgical procedures (there are many minor variations on standard operations), the fact that the surgery section alone sprawls over 352 pages gives some indication of the immense variety of procedures developed over the years. And therapy via medications hardly lags behind. As of 2013, 1453 drugs had been approved by the Food and Drug Administration, with the total number of available medications (including non-approved and experimental) now running to over 17,000.[6]

Whether therapy be aspirin to quench a headache, a cast to oblige a fractured arm to lie low, or a surgical intrusion deep inside the brain or heart, there is a solitary common denominator: Therapy ideally aims to restore—to use the words of the biologist—the wild type phenotype. *Phenotype* is the way an organism looks and functions; *wild type* refers to the typical form and function of an organism in nature. The most satisfactory therapy fixes a problem(s) in the body and returns function to normal.[7] But early therapies, and most applied even today, are far from true fixes.

## Parental Therapy

Hippocratics' "therapeutic stance was 'expectant': they waited and watched their patients, talking, winning trust, and giving a helping hand to the 'healing power of nature' (*vis medicatrix naturae*) emphasized in the text *On Ancient Medicine*. (They believed) that 'our natures are the physicians of our diseases.'"[8]

Intentionally applied at least as far back as Hippocrates (c. 460–377 BCE) and likely for much longer, many therapies work by *supporting the body while it heals itself*. Though the metaphor is imperfect, I shorthand this to *parental* therapy. Parents sustain their children as they grow into adults, but their development largely evolves independent of the support (putting aside the powerful role of parental influence on shaping the adult). There is no analogy outside of medicine for this

[5] Ahlman et al. (2015).

[6] Gaffney (2014), Law et al. (2014), and Drugbank Online (2024).

[7] Not all medical interventions cure illness. Prevention constitutes perhaps the most important medical technology. This book is focused on interventions which return the body to normal function, although preventative and curative interventions share many of the same fundamental characteristics.

[8] Porter (1997, p. 59).

type of therapy, for the obvious reason that machines do not fix themselves, though self-repairing materials are already approaching practical application.[9]

A shell of plaster or plastic which aligns and immobilizes a broken arm while the body mends the bone is *parental* therapy. The cast is invaluable for keeping the bone appropriately lined up, speeding healing and reducing pain, but the bone, not the doctor, does the mending. At a considerably more technically demanding level lies mechanical support of the circulation, which temporarily substitutes for the heart and lungs. Venous blood is removed from the body, oxygen added and carbon dioxide removed, and the blood pumped back into the body. This is a project, involving multiple devices, medications, and procedures. Its success is predicated upon the idea that whatever led to the need for this support will end, with the body itself being the prime contractor for much or all of the repair work.

Justin was 14 years old when he was rushed by his mother, early one August morning, to the local emergency room. He had chest pain and shortness of breath, a rapid heart rate, and hands of ice. His was a previous history of good health, although 10 days prior he had a runny nose, fever, and cough, and 2 days before the emergency room, he had chest pain and shortness of breath when walking to class. His blood pressure was low and he was struggling to breathe, so intravenous medications were started and a mechanical ventilator was used to take over his breathing. He was transferred with lights and siren to a large pediatric hospital.

At the receiving hospital, an echocardiogram (an ultrasound of the heart) showed that the structure of Justin's heart was normal, but its pumping action was severely diminished. Viral myocarditis was the diagnosis. Although many people with myocarditis ultimately enjoy a complete recovery, in a few cases the heart is so critically weak at the height of the illness that, without special therapy, death intervenes before recuperation. Indeed, Justin's blood pressure was inadequate despite the intravenous medications, and he developed an abnormal heart rhythm which further reduced his heart's output. Cannulae (tubes about a half an inch in diameter) were urgently placed in a large vein and artery so that venous blood flowed from Justin's heart to a pump, which drove the blood though a device to pick up oxygen and remove carbon dioxide, and then back into the body. This extracorporeal membrane oxygenation (ECMO a variant of cardiopulmonary bypass – heart-lung machine) bought Justin time: It augmented the volume of blood pumped blood by his heart to a quantity sufficient to meet the needs of the body while the heart recuperated.

Seven days after initiation of ECMO, Justin's heart had recovered enough that this therapy could be discontinued. He required oral medications for his heart for a few more days, but by the eighteenth day of his hospitalization, his heart function was normal, his heart medications discontinued, and he was discharged to home.[10]

Mechanical ventilation is a much more common and generally more recognized form of parental therapy. Mechanical ventilators are sophisticated pumps which are used to move air into and out of the lungs for people unable to do this for

[9] Bolimowski et al. (2016).

[10] This narrative reflects the clinical course of a patient I encountered a few years ago.

themselves. This be may in conjunction with surgery, after serious injury, or with severe pneumonia or other lung malfunction. The ventilator does not heal the lungs; it keeps the patient alive while the body does. Mechanical ventilation is often used to support a patient during and after cardiac surgery, especially for operative palliation for a single ventricle patient.

In the end, all supportive treatments do the same: Taking advantage of the body's talent for self-repair, they facilitate healing (e.g., by keeping a fractured bone from moving) or even preserve life itself (ECMO being the most extreme example), while the body works on the ultimate fix.

## Managers

This brings us to a second analogy: the medical practitioner as a *manager*. Management means making interventions to favorably alter the course of a disease that cannot be eliminated. One such strategy is to adjust in the way the body operates to improve its function or reduce symptoms. Consider treatment of congestive heart failure (CHF). Most patients with CHF have weakness of their heart (muscle, as opposed to heart valves) which is seldom amenable to repair and tends to worsen with time. Despite this, medications and other therapies afford more capacity for work and play and prolong lives.[11] These artifacts don't fix the "root cause" of CHF, *they work by telling one or more tissues or organs to do more, or less, of what they are already doing*. For example, diuretics (water pills) direct the kidneys to produce more urine, which reduces fluid accumulation in the lungs and elsewhere. Angiotensin converting enzyme (ACE) inhibitors reduce the activity of the enzyme that catalyzes the production of angiotensin II, a naturally produced hormone which can be counterproductive in a patient with CHF. Similarly, "beta blockers" are drugs which support the function of the failing heart by binding to beta receptors in the heart and thereby reducing a negative effect of another class of hormones (catecholamines) on the heart.

But it's important to appreciate that management's effect is often pretty modest, even for the best available therapies. Consider the effect of enalapril, a commonly prescribed ACE inhibitor. In 1991, an important clinical trial (SOLVD study)[12] found that adults with CHF were more likely to live longer, or not to be hospitalized for heart failure, than those taking placebo (inactive substitute), which caused a certain amount of excitement in the cardiology community at the time. But that the rate of these events was still far higher than one would hope. Two years after starting the SOLVD trial, 44% of the placebo group in the study had died or required hospitalization, compared with a still substantial 34% of the enalapril group. Two decades later, a clinical trial of a newer medication for CHF (a combination drug of

[11] One medical historian surveyed the 1824 *Pharmacopoeia* of the Royal College of Physicians of London and found that, of the hundreds of drugs listed, only opium, foxglove (digitalis), and purgatives were actually effective (Porter 2006, pp. 116–177).

[12] SOLVD Investigators (1991).

sacubitril and valsartan) was compared with enalapril. While the newer agent reduced the rate of death due to cardiovascular cause and first hospitalizations for heart failure compared with enalapril (21.8% vs. 26.5% over about three and a half years), there was still a considerable risk of these events even with the more effective medication.[13]

"The wisdom of the body" is a phrase well-worn and well-deserved—but if the body is so smart, why does it need to be told what to do? Why doesn't it self-adjust its production of urine (or angiotensin II or catecholamines) to optimize its function? Very clever at self-regulation under something like normal circumstances, the body's response to illness can be poorly calibrated and perverse. For example, the kidneys are ordinarily very efficient at adjusting their output, taking into account fluid taken in and lost. But when a weak heart pumps less blood than normal, the kidneys are fooled into thinking there is too little fluid on board, and they decrease their output. The body benefits from accumulating water insofar as this augments its blood volume, increasing its heart's output. But fluid retention is useful only up to a point, and then becomes a big part of the problem. The story is similar for angiotensin II and catecholamines. These hormones help adjust blood pressure and force of contraction of the heart in the healthy person, but with heart failure can actually reduce the amount of blood pumped and damage the heart over the long run.[14]

And the body is capable of greater self-directed havoc than clinging onto fluid, inflammation being perhaps the most egregious example.[15] Various cells and proteins defend organisms by killing invading microorganisms and cancer cells, but this can be a nasty two-edged sword. Cell damage and death inflicted by inflammation is a major or even sole part of many life-threatening illness. The irony is that, for some diseases whose proximal cause is an infectious agent (for example, an infection of the heart called viral myocarditis, or rheumatic fever), the sickness is actually caused partly (myocarditis) or wholly (rheumatic fever) by the inflammatory response to the invading organism, not by the bug itself. With rheumatic fever, it's as though the streptococcus bacteria incites a riot—without flinging a single rock or bottle—then quietly slips out of town while the inflammation crowd roils on.[16] Even more frustrating, with many diseases the provocation for the inflammation is unknown. An ever-increasing array of drugs, ranging from venerable aspirin to steroids, to sophisticated new "biologics," direct this system to back off, and can be exceedingly helpful in reducing the destructive effects of too much or wrongly directed inflammation. But they don't eliminate its underlying cause.

Medications that are used to manage generally act as *messengers*, transmitting information from the practitioner to cells and organs, directing them to do more or

[13] McMurray et al. (2014).

[14] Colucci and Braunwald (2005, pp. 509–534).

[15] Because inflammation causes dysfunction in nearly every tissue in the body, it may be medicine's most widely issue tackled today; calendar year 2017 saw 42,949 references in PubMed linked to "inflammation."

[16] Rose (2016) and Carapetis et al. (2016).

less of what they are already doing. They seldom bring anything truly new to the game, but they are useful for ameliorating even if not eliminating sickness.

Other management tools work differently. In Chap. 6, you met the Blalock-Taussig-Thomas shunt, an exceedingly valuable surgical procedure used to treat—not repair—various forms of congenital heart disease. This operation increases the amount of oxygen in the blood to a level required for ordinary activities and even life itself, but the shunt causes problems of its own, and it restores neither the oxygen level nor capacity for activity to normal. Chronic renal dialysis is another example; a machine does life-prolonging filtering and fluid management, while the dysfunctional kidneys persist.

Replacement drugs fall in this category. Some achieve something very close to normal function; for example, thyroid hormone replacement can be considered a type of repair, making allowance for the inconvenience of having to take the drug and monitor its effect. Others are lifesaving but so difficult to use and imperfect in their effect (for example, insulin replacement does not eliminate long term complications of diabetes) that a useful way to think about them is as managers.

Management isn't always about physical stuff. *Information* can be used to make a patient better: Simply advising a patient what foods to avoid effectively alleviates various conditions. Exercise prescriptions help patients avoid ill-effects of dangerous activities while encouraging healthy activities.

To summarize, many of the implements in the hands of practitioners reduce symptoms and lengthen life without eliminating the abnormality. Some alter natural processes, some physically alter the body to improve function, others replace deficient production of normal endogenous substances. Even sound advice belongs in this catalogue. While for many diseases this is all we've got, the aim of medical innovators is to eventually replace all the managers with mechanics.

Finally, we circle back to the idea of therapy as a fix. By way of analogy, practitioners aspirationally aim to do the same as mechanics and other people who repair broken objects.

## Mechanics

What might be called the *mechanics analogy* for therapy comes readily to mind. Mechanics remove, repair, and replace to restore the wild type of objects. While the physical actions of a mechanic are usually nothing like those of a physician, both aim to make their system of interest perform normally. Consider a crude example: A mechanic scours rust and sludge from a motor, and it runs better; a physician gives an antibiotic to eradicate an infection, and the patient runs better. Sandpaper and elbow grease have little in common with penicillin, but both accomplish fundamentally the same thing (eliminate harmful stuff from the system of interest). And in some cases—for example, when a surgeon repairs or replaces a faulty heart valve, as a plumber might in a house—the analogy is even more obvious.

The problem is, the mechanics model of therapy trades on a *good understanding*[17] of the object to be repaired, as well as the ability to mend or create, and install identical replacement parts.[18] But the medical practitioner is challenged by a nature-made structure whose architecture is exceedingly complex and tenuously understood. Despite centuries of anatomic and physiological investigations, elucidating thousands of convoluted biochemical pathways and mapping the genome, our understanding of the human machine remains frustratingly incomplete.

While we have discovered—even down to their three-dimensional shapes—thousands of the molecular components of cells, we often only dimly perceive how they associate with each other, and how these interactions add up to a functioning cell. Just as tentative is our understanding of how cells and organs associate and coordinate their activities. Consider cardiac embryogenesis—a number of investigators have sharply delineated the macro and microscopic architecture of the evolving organ, and fingered scores of genes and molecules crucial to its formation, but we still have only a very preliminary notion of exactly how these parts come to associate to culminate in a beating organ.[19]

It is these *interactions between the component parts*—not the shear diversity of parts—that makes the human inconceivably complex. Genes and the proteins they code for do not function in isolation, or even in restricted domains; it is the web-like intersection of *many* molecules, biochemical pathways, and systems of pathways that ultimately determines the organism's phenotype. When biologist and biochemist Hans Westerhoff calculated the number of theoretically possible interactions between the ~30,000 human proteins, his computer spat out $10^{121202}$, a number which vastly exceeds the number of atoms in the known universe (~$10^{80}$). If one makes certain simplifying assumptions, the number of "real" interactions (those essential to understanding the system) may be as few as ~100,000—still an imposing figure.[20] More recently, network analysis was used to formulate a map of interactions between 13,460 biologically relevant proteins. This human "interactome" showed 141,296 interactions, a gross underestimate, as the true number is likely at least five-fold higher.[21]

The reductionist approach to biological investigation—studying one or a limited number of components of the system at a time—has been invaluable in setting the stage for many modern therapies. But this information will have to be supplemented by new ways of thinking about, analyzing, and synthesizing complex data to develop a sufficiently rich comprehension of human biology. What these strategies will be is

[17] I've overstated how well we understand some of the engineering artifacts that we create, which is especially true early in our experience operating them. Books have been written about engineering failures which boil down to incomplete understanding of the object designed. Still, well-functioning manmade objects operate in a way consistent with their intended function, and with experience we come to deeply understand their characteristics.

[18] Petroski (1992, 1994).

[19] Moorman and Christoffels (2003) and Clowes et al. (2014).

[20] Westerhoff et al. (2010).

[21] Loscalzo et al. (2017, pp. 19, 31) and Menche et al. (2015).

still unclear, but the rapidly evolving novel approaches to analyzing complex systems will surely play an important role.[22]

Furthermore, there are many yarns in the biological tapestry which haven't yet caught our eye, if recent history is any indication. For example, nucleic acids have been scrutinized for half a century, with research activity exploding in the early 1970s with the discovery of restriction enzymes and the development of gene cloning. Yet even though ribonucleic acid (RNA) had been extensively studied regarding its role in protein synthesis since the early 1950s,[23] it wasn't until 1998 that a fundamental and important function of RNA—*RNA interference*, which helps regulate protein production in the cell—was unearthed. This finding was so unexpected and exciting that one expert later related that "quite a few (researchers) in the field can tell you where they were the first time they heard of RNAi,"[24] and the 2006 Nobel Prize in Physiology or Medicine was awarded to its discoverers.

Ditto for nitric oxide. This discovery was of such wholesale importance that the American Association for the Advancement of Science named nitric oxide Molecule of the Year in 1992, and its elucidation as a signaling molecule led to a Nobel Prize in Physiology or Medicine in 1998. This simple molecule, composed of one atom each of nitrogen and oxygen, eluded detection despite over a century of intensive investigation of the physiological phenomena with which it is intimately associated. And it isn't as though it lurks about in obscure nooks and crannies—nitric oxide emanates from cells in every corner of the body. Scientists first clearly sensed its presence only in about 1980, and another 7 years passed before it was unequivocally identified as a key player in a variety of physiological processes.[25]

And if recent discoveries of new molecules, as vital as they are but previously unnoticed, don't surprise you, consider this: In 2018, researchers first uncovered a new type of *cell* (pulmonary ionocyte), new sub-classes of previously known cells, and novel transitional cells in the lining of the trachea. Curious people have been using microscopes—using light, then electrons, and finally manipulating light in special ways to yield ever-better definition of the thin slip of tissue under inspection—for hundreds of years, intent on identifying each and every type of cell in the body. And still the pulmonary ionocyte escaped detection until newer, highly sophisticated techniques led to its discovery.[26] One imagines that similar discoveries, to be made in other precincts of the body, patiently await their turn.

Since every year brings new and increasingly powerful means of probing tissues and organs and illuminating their components and function, maybe eventually there will be no more surprises. But for now, and certainly decades to come, doctors face

---

[22] Kitano (2002), Kaltenbach et al. (2009), Westerhoff et al. (2010), and Loscalzo et al. (2017). Tom did not have the time to consider the recent rise of artificial intelligence; he would have greatly enjoyed the opportunity to ponder AI. Similarly, mRNA as a therapeutic tool emerged after Tom's time.

[23] Watson et al. (2004, pp. 30–31).

[24] Zamore (2006).

[25] Furchgott and Zawadzki (1980).

[26] Montoro et al. (2018).

the challenge of fixing a machine lacking a complete set of blueprints, a fragment of an owner's manual, few spare parts, and many of whose components are tough or impossible to safely access. Though useful, the mechanics model is an incomplete way of thinking about this problem because it does not explain effective therapy in the face of very limited knowledge of the machine.

The mechanics concept also breaks down when confronted with medical problems which are exceedingly well-understood but poorly treated. Sickle cell disease is a classic example. In this inherited blood disease, red blood cells tend to transform their shape—from deformable discs to stiff sickles or bananas—and thus become fragile and prone to clogging up tiny blood vessels. A beautiful series of basic and translational investigations, scrutinizing this disease at the cellular, molecular, and genetic levels, culminated in a deep understanding of its fundamental nature: Abnormal hemoglobin (the major protein in these cells) causes the sickling, and by the late 1950s the precise defect in the protein (substitution of one type of amino acid for another in the chain which makes up hemoglobin) was clearly established. Alas, despite understanding the "root cause" perfectly, nearly 60 years elapsed before definitive treatment—via genetic manipulations—began to emerge.[27] It is possible to treat sickle cell disease using bone marrow transplantation, but this is available for only a small minority of patients and entails significant risk and burden. Modifying the activity and structure of genes to correct sickle cell disease has recently gathered steam and holds great promise for correcting it in all patients (see Appendix 4). There are multiple reasons why even extensive knowledge of an illness may not lead to cure, one of which relates to the human machine's myriad microscopic component parts, which are often inaccessible and hence difficult or impossible to repair or replace.

It's hard to find a good mechanic, and we are especially grateful for the relatively few that may be the most important. These medicines kill bacteria, or at least inhibit their replication. Aided by the immune system, in the vast majority of instances they restore the wild type phenotype (state of good health). They are usually one and done—a single course of therapy for a limited time, then discontinued—although prolonged treatment is sometimes needed.

A different kind of mechanic is levothyroxine, which is given to someone with an insufficient amount of thyroid hormone in their blood: T4 needs to be given chronically, as this medication does not remedy the underlying failure of the thyroid gland to produce enough thyroid hormone. Replacing a faulty heart valve with a mechanical substitute is a variation on this theme.

But while the mechanics model applies well for some therapies, it only goes so far. It implies that all useful therapies fix the problem—retrieve the wild type—but many only ameliorate, not eliminate, disease. No single ventricle-*specific* treatment lies in this category, although a few often used to treat these patients qualify (e.g., antibiotics and a few types of surgical procedures that can be curative, such as removal of an infected appendix).

[27] Frenette and Atweh (2007), Ribeil et al. (2017), and Demirci et al. (2018).

This is the aspirational category—next to prevention, what could be better than to eliminate or completely repair an ailment? Medical progress is reckoned, in part, by the number of treatments that fall in the mechanics category or the other categories. The boundaries are porous and overlapping on purpose. For one thing, there is sometimes ambiguity in where a treatment best fits. Take eyeglasses—even if they turn a nearsighted person's vision into Ted Williams', considering the inconvenience involved with wearing them, they might as well be regarded as management as mechanics. Some mechanics-type therapies (e.g., repair or replacement of a heart valve) may function well for a while, but also require long-term blood thinning agents and close monitoring, and often do not last as long as the wild type item. So, if more replacements will be needed down the road, this is in a sense management as well as repair.

Other treatments span all three categories. For example, ibuprofen is used to treat pericarditis, an inflammation of the sack surrounding the heart which can lead to a deadly accumulation of fluid. This disease usually eventually disappears on its own, but this medication reduces pain and may speed its resolution. Ibuprofen therefore works like a mechanic (hastening the resolution), a manager (reducing the pain), and a parent (supporting the body by reducing the chance of dangerous fluid build-up while awaiting resolution). For yet other treatments, the category depends upon the ailment and circumstances. Analgesics are among the very oldest actually effective medications[28]; where do they fit? If a single dose of aspirin or ibuprofen vanquishes a headache, that's a mechanic. On the other hand, if chronic use is required to suppress arthritic pain, ibuprofen acts more as a manager. And if analgesia is required to get a patient through a limited period of post-operative pain, facilitating deep breathing and other healing activities, it's functioning in the parental mode.

But considering category overlap and occasional ambiguity in where a treatment best fits, it's hard to find a therapy which doesn't find a comfortable place in this scheme. In the Introduction, I suggested that one can think of therapy invention as multiple kinds of knowledge, ideas, and technique woven into a tapestry. The vast body of *all* medical therapies also constitutes a tapestry of sorts, a broad fabric that displays three fuzzily edged patterns, rather like the Monet haystacks, or fit a Zen diagram.

There are at least two reasons why this three-category notion of therapy deserves a few more minutes of reflection. For one, the features of the medical landscape are easier to discern knowing that only a few basic themes underlie virtually all therapies. It's a way to help non-practitioners wrap their arms around this massive subject. More importantly, this construct also makes "all too concise and too clear"[29] the overweening fact that medical therapy is about *working with, not imposing stuff on,* the body. Drugs, procedures, and medical regimens must acceptably *interface* with the body and rely upon its collaboration to work. This concept doesn't often

[28] Porter (2006, pp. 116–177).

[29] Thanks to Bob Dylan for this turn of phrase.

bubble to the top of accounts of the latest medical breakthroughs; on the contrary, the excitement is with the artifact that is the medicine or procedure. But it is essential to appreciate that the junction between treatment and its object is where successful therapy rotates, as will be discussed in Appendix 4.

Having discussed what therapies do, let's consider *how* they do it. Engineering and therapeutic artifacts share several fundamental characteristics:

1. *Both have to conform to the same natural physical constraints* (the properties of materials and how they behave, physical constants, etc.). Obvious and unsurprising.
2. *Many of the fundamental physical processes that medical artifacts execute are similar or identical to those performed by engineering artifacts.* For example, therapeutic artifacts serve as *conduits* or *pathways* for fluid transport (artificial blood vessels, surgical procedures which alter blood flow inside or outside the heart), *valves* (artificial heart valves), *filters* (dialysis machines), and *pumps* (artificial hearts).

The same is also true for the largest and most diverse class of therapeutic artifacts—medications. As we've seen, drugs generally do not enable the body to do something that it otherwise couldn't. They function as messengers, as a means of telling the body to do more, or less, of what it is already doing, depending upon what the prescriber thinks will improve the patient's condition. We've already met diuretics, ACE inhibitors, and beta blockers, and other examples are too many to cite. But perhaps one more medication, commonly used in the management of single ventricle patients, might be mentioned: Epinephrine, a naturally occurring hormone which is used as a medicine, binds to beta adrenergic receptors to ask the heart to beat stronger and faster, and to alpha-adrenergic receptors to cause contraction of small blood vessels; this drug is often very helpful in supporting the circulation after surgery or with other types of stress.

Of the ten most often prescribed medications, all but two inhibit molecular substances or structures in the body—endogenous enzymes, transporters, channels and pumps—or stimulate endogenous receptors; replacements for thyroid hormone and insulin are the two exceptions.[30] Though not all drugs act in this way, the majority of drugs[31] are, in a sense, molecular one-way fiber optic cables which transmit signals from the practitioner to the patient's tissues.

But there is a big difference between therapeutic and engineering artifacts, which is key to understanding the nature of therapy and why it is so difficult to create: *interface*.

Let's start with engineering. To a greater or lesser extent, all engineering artifacts have to interface with an external environment of natural features, man-made artifacts, and people. The challenge of designing a device that not only performs a

[30] Antibiotics are an important exception, as they do not work by altering the body's physiology; most kill by binding to specific proteins in the bacteria (as distinct from the body's cells) and altering the biology of the bug.

[31] Hardman et al. (2001, pp. 1203–1205).

given task but does so in its operating environment can be formidable. A cell phone, for example, has a physical existence independent of its environment, but lots of interaction with external factors. The human user interface is critical to its function, as is its connection with the cellular network, and its power ultimately comes from an outside source. In a similar way, an automobile, although capable of careening forward with a brick on the gas pedal, is only useful by virtue of a driver being able to control it. Moreover, it must also successfully interface with the surface it rolls over, resist adverse weather, and get its power externally.

Closer to the other end of the scale of independence, a bridge has to fit into its natural environment and resist winds and weather, but its interface with the pedestrian crossing it is very straightforward. Tunnels which transport water from areas of more water to less have a less complex relationship with their environment. Although they must reach accommodation with the rock and soil through which they are driven, and the water coursing through them, they have little or no direct interface with more complex entities.[32]

Therapeutic artifacts are different. *They have no functional existence outside the body.* Medicines are inscrutable liquids and pills sitting on the shelf. If one wanted to ascertain what possible therapeutic effect(s) a substance might have without actually giving it to a human, sophisticated laboratory studies may yield a clue, but only giving it to people would provide a complete and reliable answer. Medicines have therapeutic function *only* in the context of interacting with the body. Surgical procedures obviously cannot exist at all outside the context of the patient. Even therapies consisting of mechanical objects—say, an artificial heart valve or tube to replace a blood vessel—are useful, and their effectiveness definitively measured, only after having been placed inside the body. It isn't just that therapeutic artifacts need to interact with their environment as part of their "job"—interface *is* their job.

I pointed out that engineering artifacts, too, need to interact with their environment, but the level of intimacy is much less. Even for the cell phone, whose human interface is quite crucial to its success, the user intersection is, in the physical sense, only superficial. The phone does not find its way inside the body, and absent catastrophic malfunction (say, the battery igniting), does not physically perturb the human.[33] Medicines, on the other hand, usually find their way into virtually every space in the body, potentially affecting many cells and tissues, including those not intended. Surgical procedures often have effects which ramify far beyond the tissues manipulated. Stress related to the procedure itself affects the function of the

[32] I do not want to trivialize the problem of interface for engineering objects, since this can be crucial to their function. For example, the catastrophic 1928 failure of the St. Francis dam appears to have resulted from the interface between the dam and the canyon into which it was constructed (Petroski 2004, pp. 200–205). And designing objects to survive in highly stressful environments—for example, deep undersea or in outer space—requires great expertise. But at least the engineer usually has some idea of what she is up against; the medical innovator will not know how her artifact will grate against the patient until the therapy is actually tried.

[33] I leave out poorly defined effects of electromagnetic radiation on the brain, the effects of using computer screens on sleeping, and the like.

body as a whole, but even after that has subsided, the surgical re-arrangement itself may negatively impact remote tissues (see Fontan discussion below and in Chap. 9).

Interface not only explains how medical interventions work, but also helps illuminate the yang of therapy's yin: Therapies can also cause *harm*, up to and including life-depriving injury. Every artifact is linked with a risk of adverse effect(s), making a consideration of the risk-to-benefit ratio of any therapy fundamental to all medical decision making.

The idea here is that even if no adverse event is ever experienced, the risk of such is not normally present; hence therapy itself causes a reduction—even if only small—of the wild type. For example, mechanical heart valves can incite blood clots and infection (among other adverse events), and the blood thinners used to reduce the risk of the former increase the risk of bleeding.

The reasons for these adverse effects are many, but failure of interface is often the culprit. Consider the situation where severe malfunction of the heart necessitates its replacement. In principle, this should be eminently doable, either using a biological substitute (heart transplantation) or an artificial heart. Transplantation is indeed a commonly used form of therapy, but since the donor heart is not an exact replacement for the ailing one (subtle differences in its proteins cause it to be recognized as being "foreign" by the recipient), the interface of the donor heart with the recipient is tenuous. Chronic anti-rejection medications, which cause adverse events themselves, are required, and acute and chronic rejection of the "replacement" organ can occur. (A paucity of donor hearts also severely limits the usefulness of transplantation.)

One might think that an artificial heart—which would not be subject to rejection or supply limitations—would be easy to invent, since the heart is mostly a pump and people have been building pumps for thousands of years. It would be, were it not for the difficulty of creating a device which can perform the basic function required *and* not rub up against the body's other complex systems, some of which include: (a) The coagulation system stops bleeding resulting from injury, but it also makes the blood prone to form life-threatening clots upon contact with artificial surfaces. (b) "Biofilms" form on mechanical devices placed within the stream of blood, and with the film comes a tendency for bacteria to set up shop on the artifact. (c) People are ordinarily highly mobile, and artificial organs which restrict this can hardly be regarded as gracefully interfacing with the body, or as fully satisfactory forms of therapy.

While there are several types of artificial pumps which can fit inside the human chest, it has been a daunting task to design one which does not damage the red blood cells, provoke the formation of blood clots, or run an appreciable risk of becoming infected. Providing power for an artificial heart also means a cumbersome connection with a power supply outside the body, since so far we lack the technology to utilize the body's source of energy (chemicals in the blood). The bottom line is that, because of the need for compatible interface, a really good artificial heart has yet to be developed.[34]

Failure of interface also underlies many medication-associated adverse effects.[35] Consider penicillin, an antibiotic whose primary action is to inactivate a key bacterial enzyme and thereby destroy a bacteria's cell wall. Ideally, bacteria would be penicillin's only target, but the body senses and reacts to this drug by forming antibodies which, in a small but significant percentage of individuals, may set up allergic reactions, ranging from inconsequential rash to lethal anaphylaxis (systemic collapse, largely a breathing difficulty).[36] Many other drugs can provoke immune responses, inflaming otherwise healthy tissues.[37] Other medications induce toxic effects by generating "reactive oxygen species," molecules which damage cellular components and cause cell death. The antibiotic vancomycin, for example, can cause kidney damage at least in part in this way.[38] Some medications damage the liver by causing chemical reactions that cause liver cells to die or increase the activity of enzymes whose products damage this organ.[39]

Artifacts can interface in other harmful ways. For example, mechanical ventilators damage lungs when the pressure needed to move air into the lungs is high, as occurs with certain diseases. Surgical procedures can fail, or deliver disappointing results, because of what amounts to a failure of interface. Procedures which inadvertently introduce bacteria into the body have interfaced badly, possibly even lethally.[40] Leaving aside the problem of infection, surgery for single ventricle hearts still sometimes fails for lack of interface. Though the Fontan operation (Chap. 9), in principle, should benefit all patients who meet certain criteria, an occasional person benefits much less, or even would have been better off with an alternative form of palliation. The reason(s) for this is often unclear, but in some cases seems to be related to the patient being unusually sensitive to one of the predicted consequences of the operation (higher than normal venous pressure; see Chap. 9).

Not all adverse effects are due to failure of interface, at least not in such a straightforward way. It's hard to boil these other mechanisms down to only a handful of themes, but one common denominator explains many: The sheer complexity of the human body makes it difficult to alter the function of only the target(s) of choice. Often other functions are affected deleteriously. In some cases, the body's proclivity to contrive multiple uses for a single molecule or class of molecules is responsible.

Take aspirin, which has been an invaluable therapeutic artifact for nearly 150 years. Prostaglandins mediate pain, fever, and inflammation, and aspirin relieves

---

[34] Stawiarski et al. (2021).

[35] Xie et al. (2011).

[36] Hardman et al. (2001, pp. 1203–1205).

[37] Dougan (2017).

[38] Bamgbola (2016).

[39] Vinken (2015).

[40] Shryock (1947/1979, pp. 280–281) and Zimmerman and Veith (1993, p. 479).

these signs and symptoms by inhibiting the prostaglandin-generating enzyme cyclooxygenase. But platelet aggregation—important for stanching bleeding—is inhibited as well, since aspirin also blocks synthesis of thromboxane $A_2$ (which stimulates platelets to stick together), thereby increasing the risk of bleeding. And it can cause stomach irritation and ulcers by inhibiting prostaglandins $I_2$ and $E_2$.[41] ACE inhibitors, which decrease angiotensin II by inhibiting an enzyme called angiotensin converting enzyme, have analogous knock-on side-effects. In addition to forming angiotensin II, ACE breaks down bradykinin. Adverse effects of ACE inhibitors, one common (cough), the other rare (angioedema, giant hives), are due at least in part to ACE inhibitors increasing bradykinin.[42]

Corticosteroids present a final example. These important, naturally occurring anti-inflammatories are useful but notorious for their side effects, especially with long-term use.[43] This is not surprising, since they alter the expression of over 2700 genes in one type of human cell, and when added to TNF$\alpha$ (an endogenous inflammatory substance), over 5600 genes are affected.[44] Considerable time and effort have gone into trying to eliminate corticosteroids' undesired effects, but their patient interface remains fraught.[45] Not all unfavorable drug interactions stem from messing with hundreds or thousands of genes; as we've seen, inhibiting or stimulating a single type of enzyme can trigger unwanted side effects. But I offer these important drugs as an example of how medical interventions can ramble down countless thoroughfares and side streets, and not only to those leading to the intended address, constantly challenging those who aspire to create new—*and safe*—therapy.

To summarize, three leitmotivs broadly describe the ways that therapies are helpful: eliminating the sickness, making an incurable illness more tolerable, and supporting the body while it heals itself. We also discussed how many therapeutic artifacts work—for example, by replacing malfunctioning components, adjusting the speed of various bodily processes, and temporarily substituting for critical organ function. We confronted the fact that therapies, even when effective, can also cause harm, sometimes so much as to obviate any positive results. Most importantly, the interface between the artifact and the body is at the core of all therapy and explains both its successes and its failures.

In Appendix 2, we will see that that the histories of engineering and medicine suggest that the former has been a considerably more powerful generator of useful artifacts than the latter. There are identifiable reasons for this potency gap, and—less obviously—reasons *why the gap is not even greater*. It turns out that while medical innovators confront serious design hurdles that engineers do not, they also enjoy certain advantages, elements which make possible most of the therapies we use today.

---

[41] Hardman et al. (2001, pp. 687–696).

[42] Israili and Hall (1992) and Straka et al. (2017).

[43] Schäcke et al. (2002).

[44] Lannan et al. (2012).

[45] Chow and Simons (2018).

## References for Appendix 1

Ahlman JT, Boudreau AJ, Connelly J et al (2015) CPT 2016: current procedural terminology. American Medical Association, Chicago

Bamgbola O (2016) Review of vancomycin-induced renal toxicity: an update. Ther Adv Endocrinol Metab 7(3):136–147

Bolimowski PA, Bond IP, Wass DF (2016) Robust synthesis of epoxy resin-filled microcapsules for application to self-healing materials. Phil Trans R Soc A 374:20150083

Carapetis JR, Beaton A, Cunningham MW et al (2016) Acute rheumatic fever and rheumatic heart disease. Nat Rev Dis Primers 2:1–24

Chow CC, Simons SS (2018) An approach to greater specificity for glucocorticoids. Front Endocrinol 9:76

Clowes C, Boylan MGS, Ridge LA et al (2014) The functional diversity of genes required for mammalian cardiac development. Genesis 52:713–737

Colucci WS, Braunwald E (2005) Pathophysiology of heart failure. In: Zipes DP, Libby P, Bonow RO, Braunwald E (eds) Braunwald's heart disease: a textbook of cardiovascular medicine, 7th edn. Elsevier, Philadelphia

Demirci S, Uchida N, Tisdale JF (2018) Gene therapy for sickle cell disease: an update. Cytotherapy 20(7):899–910

Dougan M (2017) Checkpoint blockade toxicity and immune homeostasis in the gastrointestinal tract. Front Immunol 8:1–8

Drugbank Online. Accessed 14 Nov 2024. https://go.drugbank.com/stats

Frenette PS, Atweh GF (2007) Sickle cell disease: old concepts, new discoveries, and future promise. J Clin Invest 117:850–858

Furchgott RF, Zawadzki JV (1980) The obligatory role of endothelial cells in the relaxation of arterial smooth muscle by acetylcholine. Nature 288:373–376

Gaffney A (2014) How many drugs has FDA approved in its entire history? Regulatory Focus. Accessed 14 Nov 2024. https://www.raps.org/News-and-Articles/News-Articles/2014/10/How-Many-Drugs-has-FDA-Approved-in-its-Entire-Hist

Hardman JG, Limbird LE, Gilman AG (2001) Goodman & Gilman's the pharmacological basis of therapeutics, 10th edn. McGraw-Hill, New York

Israili ZH, Hall WD (1992) Cough and angioneurotic edema associated with angiotensin-converting enzyme inhibitor therapy. Ann Int Med 117:234–242

Jeffrey JS, Thompson S (1944) Penicillin in battle casualties. Br Med J 2(4356):1–4

Kaltenbach H, Dimopoulos, Stelling J (2009) Systems analysis of cellular networks under uncertainty. FEBS Lett 583:3923–3930

Kitano H (2002) Systems biology: a brief overview. Science 295:1662–1664

Lannan E, Galliher-Beckley AJ, Scoltock AB, Cidlowski JA (2012) Proinflammatory actions of glucocorticoids: glucocorticoids and TNFα coregulate gene expression in vitro and in vivo. Endocrinology 153(8):3701–3712

Law V, Knox C, Djoumbou Y, Jewison T, Guo AC, Liu Y et al (2014) DrugBank 4.0: shedding new light on drug metabolism. Nucleic Acids Res 42(1):D1091–D1097

Loscalzo J, Barbasi A-L, Silverman EK (eds) (2017) Network medicine: complex systems in human disease and therapeutics. Harvard University Press, Cambridge

McMurray JJV, Packer M, Desai AS et al (2014) Angiotensin-neprilysin inhibition versus enalapril in heart failure. N Engl J Med 371:993–1004

Menche J, Sharma A et al (2015) Disease networks: uncovering disease-disease relationships through the incomplete interactome. Science 347(6224):1257601

Montoro DT, Haber AL, Biton M et al (2018) A revised airway epithelial hierarchy includes CFTR-expressing ionocytes. Nature 560(7718):319–324

Moorman AFM, Christoffels VM (2003) Cardiac chamber formation: development, genes, and evolution. Physiol Rev 83:1223–1267

Peacock TB (1858) On malformations, &c., of the human heart. John Churchill, London. Reprinted in The Classics of Medicine Library. Birmingham, AL: Gryphon Editions, Ltd.; 1981
Petroski H (1992) To engineer is human: the role of failure in successful design. Vintage, New York
Petroski H (1994) Design paradigms: case histories of error and judgment in engineering. Cambridge University Press, Cambridge
Petroski H (2004) Pushing the limits: new adventures in engineering. Vintage, New York
Porter R (1997) The greatest benefit to mankind: a medical history of humanity. W.W. Norton & Co., New York
Porter R (ed) (2006) The Cambridge history of medicine. Cambridge University Press, Cambridge
Ribeil J-A, Hacein-Bey-Abina S, Payen E et al (2017) Gene therapy in a patient with sickle cell disease. N Engl J Med 376:848–855
Rose NR (2016) Viral myocarditis. Curr Opin Rheumatol 28:383–389
Schäcke H, Docke W-D, Asadullah K (2002) Mechanisms involved in the side effects of glucocorticoids. Pharmacol Ther 96:23–43
Shryock RH (1947/1979) The development of modern medicine. University of Wisconsin Press, Madison
SOLVD Investigators (1991) Effect of enalapril on survival in patients with reduced left ventricular ejection fractions and congestive heart failure. N Engl J Med 325:293–302
Stawiarski K, Stulak JM, Ramakrishna H (2021) HeartMate 3: analysis of recent trial data. J Cardiothorac Vasc Anesth 35:3105–3107
Straka BT et al (2017) Effect of bradykinin receptor antagonism on ACE inhibitor-associated angioedema. J Allergy Clin Immunol 140:242–248
Vinken M (2015) Adverse outcome pathways and drug-induced liver injury testing. Chem Res Toxicol 28(7):1391–1397
Watson JD, Baker TA, Bell SP, Gann A, Levine M, Losick R (2004) Molecular biology of the gene. CSHL Press, Woodbury
Westerhoff HV, Verma M, Nardelli M, Adamczyk M, van Eunen K, Simeonidis E, Bakker BM (2010) Systems biochemistry in practice: experimenting with modeling and understanding, with regulation and control. Biochem Soc Trans 38:1189–1196
Xie J, Talaska AE, Schacht J (2011) New developments in aminoglycoside therapy and ototoxicity. Hearing Res 281:28–37
Zamore PD (2006) RNA interference: big applause for silencing in Stockholm. Cell 127:1083–1086
Zimmerman LM, Veith I (1993) Great ideas in the history of surgery. Norman Publishing, San Francisco

## Appendix 2 – Through Engineering's Lens – Why Compare Therapy Invention With Engineering Invention

When pondering medical therapeutic achievements, I find it hard not to compare—and enviously contrast—them with engineering trophies. The power of engineers to manipulate the environment, from pico to mega, is astonishing, and no less so for its being on constant display. The smart phone may be its most ubiquitous demonstration, but there are many equally mind-boggling examples of man's command of molecules and materials: brute force intelligently applied to rock, igneous and metamorphic, grinding a tunnel 35 miles long under the Swiss Alps (Gotthard rail tunnel)[46]; devices that translate a fraction of a microsecond into the position of your

[46] Fabbri (2004, p. 4).

shadow on the sidewalk (Global Positioning System); satellite pictures of your (and pretty much everyone's) rooftop, free of charge (Google Earth); safe, rapid, nonstop air travel for almost 10,000 miles (commercial airliners).

There may be no better example of technology's capacity to delight and amaze than the Hubble Space Telescope.[47] The Hubble has produced a trove of unprecedented images, including of a galaxy born over 13 billion years ago, near the temporal edge of the universe. Almost 95 inches in diameter, this observatory's primary mirror is crafted of special glass ground to a precision of 1/800,000 of an inch—roughly the diameter of 200 silicon atoms. Its path enforced by Earth's gravity, the Hubble rushes through space at 5 miles a second, yet it needs to stay precisely aimed at the tiny sliver of the firmament being studied. This is managed by gyroscopes, sensors and reaction wheels so good that what they do is equivalent to fixing a laser beam, for 24 hours straight, on a dime 400 miles distant. Postage stamp-sized charge-coupled devices, each stuffed with 640,000 pixels, serve as its retinas, retinas a billion times more sensitive than those of humans. If you were the Hubble, your eyes could separate a shining pair of auto headlights 5000 miles away.[48] This hardly scratches the surface of the body of engineering that underlies this most sobering of light collectors, although a litany of its magnificent engineering is really beside the point. What is most profound about this orbiting observatory is not its gee whiz technology but the naked fact that it reveals so inconceivably much of this inconceivable universe.

While one can imagine engineering feats that will never be realized, our imaginative failure is more likely to be in quite the opposite direction—failure to anticipate what will, next week, next month, or next year spring from the mind of man.

Situated in dubious contrast is medical invention. As much progress as has been made in the last century in extending human life and alleviating suffering, room for improvement seems to overwhelm past achievements. Uncured aliments are too many to count. For example, mortally benign but seriously debilitating chronic back pain is only unreliably cured despite miserably afflicting millions. Many even more enervating conditions, not to mention life-threatening ones, remain dug in, despite monumental efforts to dislodge them. Indeed, single ventricle palliation offers a good example: Although it is an invaluable advance, it is still far from ideal therapy.

Confronting this capacity chasm between engineering and medical invention, one therefore wonders: How do *engineers* create their stuff, and how is this similar, and not, to how medical innovators create theirs? Are medical therapies analogous to the objects that engineers create? Most importantly, can we learn something about medical invention in general—not only single ventricle palliation—by peering at it through the window of engineering invention?

The fine ends of the roots of conflating biological organisms and mechanical objects extend back at least as far as the ancient Egyptians and Romans; thinking about life as a mechanical process is reflected in their creation of automata—objects

[47] The Webb telescope came after Tom; no doubt he would have opined in wonder on that as well.

[48] See hubblesite.org for this and further information on the telescope's capabilities.

that look like and imitate certain functions of living organisms.[49] The tendrils thickened by the 17th and 18th centuries, when work from many foundational thinkers and experimenters (e.g., Rene Descartes, William Harvey, Giovanni Borelli, Marcello Malpighi, Stephen Hales, Herman Boerhaave, Julien Offray de la Mettrie) converged; life forms were viewed as functioning like machines, or even as a machine. "I do not recognize any difference between machines made by craftsman and the various bodies that nature alone composes" declared Descartes,[50] venturing perhaps further than some of his contemporaries, but nevertheless reflecting the general tenor of the times.[51] To be sure, there were competing theories about life in the eighteenth and nineteenth centuries.[52] *Vitalism*—the now jettisoned idea that the living differ fundamentally from the inanimate, with some sort of ill-defined vital force infiltrating the living—competed strongly for many years with the mechanical view.

Centuries before, Leonardo da Vinci applied hydrodynamic principles to study blood flow across the heart's aortic valve, and mechanical principles to the movement of muscles and bones.[53] As years, decades, then centuries of biological investigations accrued, ever more penetrating observations led to many more comparisons between the operations of the body and machines. For example, Wilfreid F.H.M. Mommaerts, in a sweeping historical review of how people laid the foundations of cardiac mechanics, observed that the "[h]eart and other muscles may be said to be engines. They transform the energy of chemical reactions, 'metabolism,' into mechanical energy, often into work." He also pointed out that certain mechanical characteristics of heart muscle can be modeled as if it were a spring.[54] Indeed, as illustrated in Fig. 1, pressure-volume loops—of surprisingly similar shape—are used by engineers to characterize the performance of piston engines, and by cardiologists and physiologists, the performance of the heart. And it isn't just organs of obvious mechanical function like the heart that bear uncanny resemblance to engineering devices. When, in the 1940s and early 1950s, investigators first extracted an understanding of how nerves work, equations describing the propagation of signals in *undersea cables* proved very useful in describing signal transmission in nerves.[55]

As biologists and chemists elucidated the structures and functions of molecules, and aggregations of them, describing them as machines was perhaps inevitable. The cell has been described as a "collection of protein machines" by one prominent biologist, and other workers concur: "A look under the hood of the eukaryotic protein synthesis machine reveals the use of fuel to power molecular motors, clocks,

---

[49] Channel (1991, pp. 30–46).

[50] Pasipoularides (2013) and Porter (1997, p. 218).

[51] Channel (1991, pp. 30–46), Pasipoularides (2013), Hurst et al. (2003, p. 29), Porter (2006, pp. 140–141), and Del Negro (2001, pp. 181–183).

[52] Porter (1997, pp. 247–251).

[53] Keele (1961), Porter (2006, p. 137), Jastifer and Toldeo-Pereyra (2012), and Isaacson (2017, pp. 401–424).

[54] Fishman and Richards (1964, pp. 128, 138–142).

[55] Katz (1966, p. 73) and George et al. (2015).

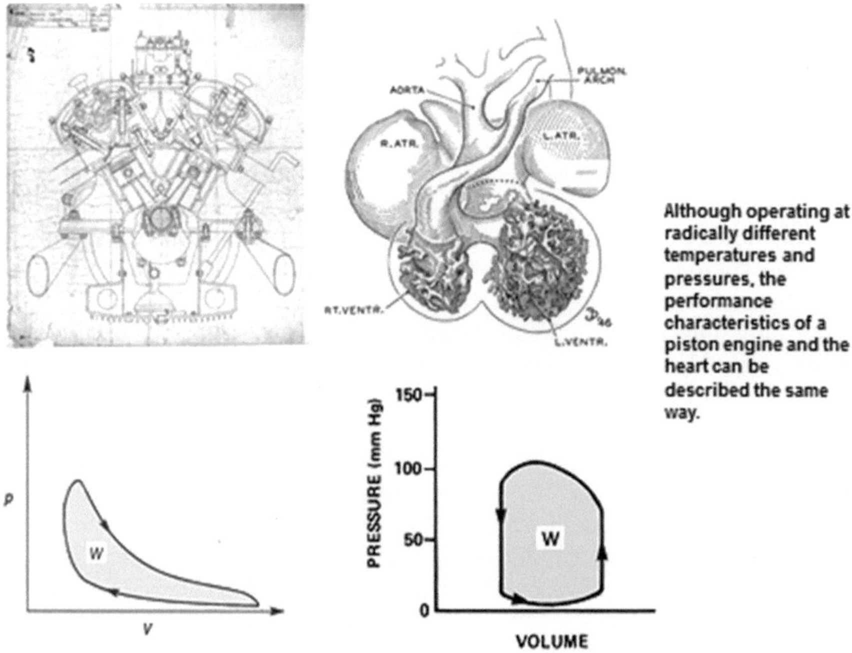


**Fig. 1** Suite of four diagrams (cross-section Colombo Ferrari engine, Carnegie heart, P-V loop for engine, P-V loop for heart)On the upper left is a blueprint of the embryonic form (it was subsequently much refined) of one of the most successful automobile engines ever, the Ferrari type 125; on the right, the embryonic form of perhaps the most successful biological engine ever, the human heart. When engineers want to characterize how their piston engines work, they simultaneously measure the pressure and volume inside a cylinder and generate the pressure-volume loop in the lower left. Physiologists characterize the performance of the heart in much the same way, measuring pressure and volume inside the ventricle, and likewise generate a pressure-volume loop (bottom right). Although the these loops are not identical—pressure is generated in very different ways in the two engines—they are uncannily similar, despite the profound differences in structure and composition which distinguish an engine from a heart. Could it be that thinking about how engineers create their machines can help us understand how medical innovators invent ways to fix biological machines? W = work performed

and springs for achieving speed and accuracy."[56] To be sure, machines at the molecular scale aren't just miniscule versions of ordinary devices. Globular proteins, for example, spin about their various axes millions of times per second, and enzymes contact their substrate molecules hundreds of thousands of times in the same interval.[57] Not many engineering artifacts (excepting electronic devices' manipulation of electron flow) have that sort of operating profile! Differences in relative speeds, the types of energy utilized, the impact of thermodynamic influences, and other factors

[56] Alberts (1998) and Staley and Guthrie (1998).

[57] Alberts (1998).

weaken the analogy between cellular and most artificial machines, but the close kinship between the biological and mechanical still compels.

One can go overboard on the people-as-machines conceit. Indeed, thought has more recently veered away from the classical mechanical construction, becoming preoccupied with the difficult puzzles of how molecules, cells, and whole organisms self-organize and self-regulate. At the cellular and sub-cellular levels, these processes can differ radically from those utilized by man-made devices.[58] My argument is not that living things are simply machines, but that taking an engineering view of the challenge of beneficially interfacing with living organisms (i.e., providing medical therapy) fits comfortably into the slipstream of many centuries of thinking about the human body. In fact, an analogous, if mirror image, argument has already been made: Technological invention in many ways mimics biological evolution. Andreas Wagner and William Rosen[59] point out that many process motifs observed in evolution—for example, trial and error within populations, descent with modification (cultural inheritance of technology), and exaptation (parts of a system) used for new purposes—are also common engineering innovation strategies. If engineering, in effect, looks to evolution for avenues of invention, so might the obverse occur: Innovators working with evolved biological systems appeal to engineers for the same.

Much more than philosophical ruminations and analogies confirms that engineering and medical invention have much in common:

1. Medical inventors and engineers develop stuff—"artifacts", more formally—to solve problems, and these artifacts are often quite similar. A synthetic tube used to replace a blood vessel or an artificial replacement for a malfunctioning heart valve are obvious examples, but engineering and medical artifacts can mimic each other in more subtle ways. For example, we have seen that most medications function as signaling devices, allowing doctors to adjust the body's physiology in beneficial ways, just as engineering devices send information and control machines.
2. Medical and engineering innovators solve problems of several distinct types, and these *problems are surprisingly similar*. The most common engineering problems are the lack of a device to fill a current need (e.g., why Edison invented the light bulb) and inventions that extend the utility of currently existing devices (e.g., developing more fuel-efficient gas engines). As a lengthy discussion of engineering problems is not important for us here, I won't dwell on it, although more details are provided in Appendices 3 and 4. But I'd like to offer two examples of how even relatively arcane types of engineering problems also challenge medical innovators. When *imbalances between related technologies* occur, improvements in one kind of technology can stimulate advances in other, interacting technologies.[60] For example, small computers grew more powerful and

[58] Channel (1991, p. 9), Kirschner (2000), Nicholson and Gawne (2015), and Loscalzo et al. (2017).

[59] Wagner and Rosen (2014).

[60] Laudan (1984).

personal in the 1980s, but they were clunky to use. Development of the graphical user interface—why you can execute many functions on your computer by point-and-click, rather than typing—provided a much more efficient and user-friendly interface, greatly expanding the utility and adoption of the personal computer. In *Steve Jobs*, Walter Isaacson recounts Jobs's reaction as he drove home from Xerox's PARC, where he had experienced a demonstration of this innovative technology—*the mouse*: "'This is it!' he shouted, emphasizing each word. 'We've got to do it!' It was the breakthrough that he had been looking for: bringing computers to the people."[61]

Perhaps the most profound imbalance in the history of medicine was early nineteenth century surgery's rapidly increasing technical sufficiency, which was severely constrained by the lack of anesthesia to make operations tolerable and by the need for asepsis, to prevent deadly postoperative infections. Only when these two problems were solved in the mid-to-late 1800s did surgery leap into the modern era.[62] More closely related to the story at hand, Flavio Coceani, the biologist we encountered in Chap. 10, took the first step toward solving exactly this type of problem when he discovered that prostaglandin $E_1$ keeps the ductus from closing in a newborn. In the 1970s, surgeons were beginning to develop the techniques and knowledge needed to treat neonates with complex cardiac malformations, but with closure of the ductus in the first day or so, many of these babies died or become so sick that operation had little chance of success. By preventing ductal closure, prostaglandin $E_1$ keeps the neonate alive and stable, giving the newly advancing surgical technology a chance to be successfully applied. This therapeutic artifact thus served to ameliorate an imbalance between the capacity to provide effective surgical therapy and the ability to keep the patient alive and in good shape until an accurate diagnosis is made and surgery performed.

Potential rather than actual failures of technology (*presumptive anomaly*) is another type of problem solved by engineers. Historian Edward Constant proposed that a presumptive anomaly "occurs in technology not when a conventional system fails in any absolute or objective sense, but when assumptions derived from science indicate that under some future conditions the system will fail (or function badly) or that a radically different system will do a better job." Invention of the turbojet engine was in large part impelled by the realization that, as advances in airframe and aerodynamic design enabled higher aircraft speeds, a piston engine driving a propeller would no longer be sufficient.[63] The history of congenital heart surgery provides a striking example of the power of presumptive anomaly to drive therapy invention and dissemination, despite serious theoretical and practical concerns.

---

[61] Isaacson (2011, pp. 94–97); Jobs quote p. 97.

[62] Shryock (1947/1979, pp. 280–281), Zimmerman and Veith (1993, p. 479), and Gawande (2012).

[63] Constant II (1980, p.15).

Babies whose aorta and pulmonary artery arise from the opposite ventricles as normal (*transposition of the great arteries*) soon die of severe hypoxemia without treatment. Transposition was treated for many years with great success (operative survival was about 95%) with the *atrial* switch operation. Worry about late complications (which usually occur only many years after the surgery)[64] induced pioneering surgeons in the early-to-mid 1980s to consider using a newer, much less familiar procedure (the *arterial* switch operation) which—*in theory*—would be associated with fewer late complications. But the novelty of the new operation meant that, for the first babies operated upon, the likelihood of surviving the operation was *less* than for the traditional procedure.[65] That is, the hope of securing a healthier patient 30 or 40 years after operation (again, based on cogent but largely theoretical supposition, not actual experience) was the justification for ditching a therapy with a roughly 5% operative mortality for one with a surely (if impossible to quantify) higher risk of death until the bugs could be worked out. (Most surgeons did quickly ascend the learning curve of the arterial switch; operative mortality is now less than it was for the atrial variety of surgery, and, as hoped, long-term outcomes are much better.) The power of the idea of presumptive anomaly drove surgeons to "switch the switches" despite the technical, philosophical, and even ethical concerns involved.[66]

3. Medical innovators and engineers utilize a *variety of types* of knowledge and technical expertise, only some of which have scientific provenance. Academic engineers have many times emphasized this,[67] though seldom with the élan of British journalist John Lanchester: "Science and technology: we tend to think of them as siblings, perhaps even as twins…When it comes to the shiniest wonders of the modern world—as the supercomputers in our pockets communicate with satellites—science and technology are indeed hand in glove. For much of human history, though, technology had nothing to do with science. Many of our most significant inventions are pure tools, with no scientific method behind them. Wheels and wells, cranks and mills and gears and ships' masts, clocks and rudders and crop rotation…none had any connection with what we think of today as science."[68]

It isn't just that some inventions lie outside the realm of science. Creation of even heavily basic science-informed objects also requires multiple other types of knowledge. There are those who think that, boiled-down, engineering *is* applied basic science[69]; but others believe that the crucial role which engineering-specific knowl-

[64] Myocardial dysfunction (weakness of the heart muscle), arrhythmia, and leakage of the tricuspid valve are of greatest concern.

[65] Bull et al. (2000).

[66] Stark (1984), Bull et al. (2000), and de Laval (2001).

[67] Vincenti (1990), Lewis (2004), Petroski (1996), and McClellan III and Dorn (2015, pp. 7–8).

[68] Lanchester (2017, p. 22).

[69] Layton Jr. (1974) and Auyang (2004, p. 17).

edge plays in artifact design powerfully argues that engineering is a distinct activity.[70] Engineers have even been known to get a little cranky when assaulted by the notion of engineering as applied science: "Aeroplanes are not designed by science, but by art in spite of some pretense and humbug to the contrary. I do not mean to suggest for one moment that engineering can do without science, on the contrary, it stands on scientific foundations, but there is a big gap between scientific research and the engineering product which has to be bridged by the art of the engineer."[71]

A key idea in this book is that, while basic science increasingly informs new therapies, many other types of knowledge are required for medical invention. Engineering is much the same: Artifact design is derived in part from scientific knowledge, but also from knowledge and intellectual approaches very distinct from those of science. Aeronautical engineer and historian Walter Vincenti[72] discerned multiple distinct (though at times overlapping) forms of knowledge used in engineering.[73]

Both activities—science and technology—operate within social and regulatory structures, and grapple not only with physical limitations, but also with constraints imposed outside of physics and biology. The nature of society's impact on medical innovation has changed over time. For thousands of years, cultural and religious inclinations against dissecting human cadavers inhibited this crucial first step in discovering how the body functions. Only in the mid-fourteenth century did the Papacy, desperate to find a way to staunch the Black Death, first sanction post-mortem examinations, and not until 1537 did Pope Clement VII approve teaching of anatomy by human dissection.[74] We are long past societal proscriptions which strike at the very foundation of medical innovation (understanding the system of interest), but headwinds persist. Modern clinical research is heavily encumbered by regulatory requirements[75] which impose substantial administrative, financial, and temporal costs.[76]

While ultimately serving a vital purpose, these prohibitions and proscriptions are sufficiently burdensome that some have even called for massive overhaul of the

---

[70] Layton Jr. (1974), Laudan (1984), Gutting in Laudan (1984), Staudenmaier (1985, p. 114), Lewis (2004), and Vincenti (1990).

[71] J.D. North (1922), quoted in Vincenti (1990, p. 4).

[72] Walter Vincenti is an emeritus professor of aeronautical engineering at Stanford University and past chairman of Stanford's Program in Values, Technology, Science, and Society. The Society for History of Technology awarded his 1990 book a prize for best book, and Vincenti an award for lifetime achievement in the understanding of technology's past. I've saved details of Vincenti's observations for Appendix 4 but suffice it to say here that we will encounter many examples of knowledge, some of it pretty homely, that were vital to the creation of single ventricle palliation.

[73] Vincenti (1990).

[74] Porter (2006, pp. 136–143).

[75] Strict regulation of studies involving human subjects is relatively new; the Declaration of Helsinki on medical research was formulated only in 1964, with regulatory structures following several years later. The Food and Drug Administration specifies what is acceptable conduct of many aspects of clinical trials aimed at culminating in FDA approval.

[76] Porter (1997, pp. 649–651) and Grady (2015).

existing system.[77] The Food and Drug Administration (FDA) also greatly impacts medical innovation by specifying the characteristics that drugs need for FDA approval, and how drug safety and efficacy is demonstrated.[78]

Nor are engineers immune from the impress of non-technical factors, and how social factors impact engineering can be pretty surprising. In *Twenty-First Century Jet: The Making and Marketing of the Boeing* 777, Karl Sabbagh illustrated how the work of engineers is shaped by the non-engineering world, including decisions that one might have thought would be made purely on the basis of technical considerations. Boeing engineers initially planned to use a special aluminum-lithium alloy to save weight in the 777, gross poundage being a big issue in aircraft design. Unfortunately, when the alloy is machined small cracks form around the cut edges of the part. The engineers were confident that these "cracks were not a problem—at least not in any physical sense. …[But the senior engineer on the project] had another worry, one that was psychological rather than physical. He did not want a plane where, in the future in some far-off airfield, a maintenance engineer could be inspecting the interior of a wing or the fuselage and come across cracks in the metal, however benign they turned out to be." After considerable deliberation, the aluminum-lithium was thus scrapped, despite its technical superiority to conventional metals.[79] (Tom, of course, missed the recent spate of airline structural issues occurring in 2023 and 2024; he surely would have opined on them.)

Many other sorts of non-technical factors bedevil engineers, none more than regulations. While they grapple with fewer federal regulations limiting and complicating their testing procedures than medical innovators, the things engineers invent must conform to myriad safety, environmental, and other constraints.

One could endlessly cite examples of this, but I will limit myself to one. In 1971, the automobile manufacturer Porsche set out to design an entirely new car, the first "clean sheet" effort in the firm's history. They had had huge experience and success with air-cooled, rear-engine cars—in fact, they built their formidable reputation on just such vehicles—but for their new car, they chose a design with a water-cooled engine situated in the front. There were multiple reasons for this radical break from prior practice, but the need to meet upcoming environmental and safety regulations was among the most compelling. Ernst Fuhrmann, Porsche's Managing and Technical Director, explained: "The only nightmare for our engineers," referring to the design effort for the 928 Porsche, "was the new (environmental and safety) legislation in the United States. …The worst thing was that no one knew exactly what these laws would be like or when they would take effect. … We therefore chose a concept that would be more similar than before to the majority of cars built, for it would be to this majority—and not just to the air-cooled rear engine—that the new laws would be most applicable."[80] Even for a company like Porsche, populated by

[77] Grady (2015) and Schneider (2015).

[78] Hwang et al. (2017) and US Food and Drug Administration (2013). There is a vast literature on this subject.

[79] Sabbagh (1996, pp. 98–105).

[80] Ludvigsen (1977, pp. 834–836).

enthusiast-engineers building automobiles for enthusiast-drivers, and having a penchant for developing interesting and unusual technology, strategic engineering decisions are often shaped as much by legislators as engineering principles.

If it's true that engineering and medical innovation share much, they are not the same. In fact, what is most compelling about thinking about one in the context of the other is that, despite their many similarities, they part company in two crucial domains: the nature of the artifacts themselves, and the role that models and testing play in their creation. Examining both of these aspects shows how holding these elements up against each other reveals the nature of the hard edges which separate the stunning power of engineering invention from the slower pace of medical developments. It also demonstrates that medical inventors enjoy certain *advantages*, relative to engineers, which are crucial to successful therapies. Before we get there, let's take a close look at the sufficiency gulf which has long separated engineering and medical artifacts. In the Appendix 3, I hope to make the case that, while engineers have long been pulling rabbits out of the hat, medical innovators have had to suffice with something more like smoke and mirrors.

## References for Appendix 2

Alberts B (1998) The cell as a collection of protein machines: preparing the next generation of molecular biologists. Cell 92:291–294

Auyang SY (2004) Engineering: an endless frontier. Harvard University Press, Cambridge

Bull C, Yates R, Sarkar D, Deanfield J, de Laval M (2000) Scientific, ethical, and logistical considerations in introducing a new operation: a retrospective cohort study from pediatric cardiac surgery. BMJ 320:1168–1173

Channel DF (1991) The vital machine: a study of technology and organic life. Oxford University Press, New York

Constant EW II. (1980) The origins of the turbojet revolution. Johns Hopkins University Press, Baltimore

de Laval M (2001) Lessons from the arterial switch operation. Lancet 357:1814

Del Negro G (ed) (2001–2003) The university of Padua: eight centuries of history. Signum Padova Editrice s.a.s, Padua

Fabbri D (2004) The Gotthard Base Tunnel: project overview. Lombardi Engineering Group. Accessed 17 Nov 2024. https://www.coursehero.com/file/41100536/Pubb-0394-L-The-Gotthard-Base-Tunnel-Project-overviewpdf/

Fishman AP, Richards DW (1964) Circulation of the blood. Men and ideas. Oxford University Press, New York

Gawande A (2012) Two hundred years of surgery. N Engl J Med 366:1716–1723

George S, Foster J, Richardson G (2015) Modelling in vivo action potential propagation along a giant axon. J Math Biol 70:237–263

Grady C (2015) Institutional review boards. Chest 148(5):1148–1115

Hurst JW, Conti CR, Fye WB (2003) Profiles in cardiology. Foundation for Advances in Medicine and Science, Mahwah

Hwang TJ, Franklin JM, Kesselheim AS (2017) Effect of US Food and Drug Administration's cardiovascular safety guidance on diabetes drug development. Clin Pharmacol Ther 102:290–296

Isaacson W (2011) Steve jobs. Simon and Schuster, New York

Isaacson W (2017) Leonardo da Vinci. Simon and Schuster, New York

Jastifer JR, Toldeo-Pereyra LH (2012) Leonardo da Vinci's foot: historical evidence of concept. J Investig Surg 25:281–285
Katz B (1966) Nerve, muscle, and synapse. McGraw-Hill, New York
Keele KD (1961) Three early masters of experimental medicine: Erasistratus, Galen, and Leonardo da Vinci. Proc R Soc Med 54:577–588
Kirschner M (2000) Molecular "vitalism". Cell 100:79–88
Lanchester J (2017) How civilization started. The New Yorker, 18 Sept 2017
Laudan R (ed) (1984) The nature of technological knowledge: are models of scientific change relevant? D. Reidel Publishing Co., Dordrecht
Layton ET Jr (1974) Technology as knowledge. Technol Cult 15:31–41
Lewis EE (2004) Masterworks of technology: the story of creative engineering, architecture, and design. Prometheus Books, Amherst
Loscalzo J, Barbasi A-L, Silverman EK (eds) (2017) Network medicine: complex systems in human disease and therapeutics. Harvard University Press, Cambridge
Ludvigsen K (1977) Porsche: excellence was expected—the complete history of the sports and racing cars. Princeton Publication, Princeton
McClellan JE III, Dorn H (2015) Science and technology in world history: an introduction, 3rd edn. Johns Hopkins University Press, Baltimore
Nicholson DJ, Gawne R (2015) Neither logical empiricism nor vitalism, but organicism: what the philosophy of biology was. Hist Philos Life Sci 37(4):345–381
Pasipoularides A (2013) Historical perspective: Harvey's epoch-making discovery of the circulation, its historical antecedents, and some consequences on medical practice. J Appl Physiol 114:1493–1503
Petroski H (1996) Invention by design: how engineers get from thought to thing. Harvard University Press, Cambridge
Porter R (1997) The greatest benefit to mankind: a medical history of humanity. W.W. Norton & Co., New York
Porter R (ed) (2006) The Cambridge history of medicine. Cambridge University Press, Cambridge
Sabbagh K (1996) Twenty-first-century jet: the making and marketing of the Boeing 777. Scribner, New York
Schneider CE (2015) The censor's hand: the misregulation of human subjects research. MIT Press, Cambridge
Shryock RH (1947/1979) The development of modern medicine. University of Wisconsin Press, Madison
Staley JP, Guthrie C (1998) Mechanical devices of the sliceosome: motors, clocks, springs, and things. Cell 92:315–326
Stark J (1984) Transposition of the great arteries: which operation? Ann Thorac Surg 38:429–430
Staudenmaier JM (1985) Technology's storytellers: reweaving the human fabric. The Society for the History of Technology and The MIT Press, Cambridge
US Food and Drug Administration (2013) Guidance for IRBs, clinical investigators, and sponsors. Accessed 17 Nov 2024. https://www.fda.gov/files/about%20fda/published/IRB-Responsibilities-for-Reviewing-the-Qualifications-of-Investigators%2D%2DAdequacy-of-Research-Sites%2D%2Dand-the-Determination-of-Whether-an-IND-IDE-is-Needed-%28Printer-Friendly%29.pdf
Vincenti WG (1990) What engineers know and how they know it: analytical studies from aeronautical history. The Johns Hopkins University Press, Baltimore
Wagner A, Rosen W (2014) Spaces of the possible: universal Darwinism and the wall between technological and biological function. J R Soc Interface 11:20131190
Zimmerman LM, Veith I (1993) Great ideas in the history of surgery. Norman Publishing, San Francisco

## Appendix 3 – In the Rearview Mirror – Comparing Success of Engineering and Therapeutic Artifacts

Roman-built in the first century BCE, the Pont du Gard is a segment of an aqueduct that (in its prime) stretched 31 miles and carried over ten million gallons a day, snaking its way from a spring near Uzès, France to Nîmes

> Benjamin Rush … formulated the body of theory that most fully represented the essence of medical orthodoxy in America during the first third of the nineteenth century… [I]t assumed that there was really only one disease … (and) that only a single type of treatment was necessary: a generously applied combination of bloodletting and purging.
> –James Cassedy[81]

There are two main ideas in Appendix 3, the first being that engineers are better at artifact creation than medical innovators, and the second that medical innovators are dependent upon powerful *therapy facilitators*—properties inherent in the human body, or in other organisms—that innovators exploit when creating other impossible therapies. We will address them in that order.

We have already seen how challenges of interface bedevil medical therapies, but there are other important factors, as I hope will be apparent in the next few pages. But let's start with a disclaimer: Comparing the creative power of engineering apples with therapeutic oranges isn't actually possible, at least not in any rigorous or quantitative way. What is the greater achievement, manipulating steam to pump water from a mine, or using cinchona bark to cure malaria? Long-distance telephony, or opening, repairing, and then closing a human heart? But if precision in comparison is impossible, the notion of differential potency is not new. Roy Porter noted how much more advanced were the physical sciences, compared with the biological, in the Enlightenment.[82] Richard Shryock emphasized the unsettling gap between engineering and medical achievement in the early Victoria era: "There was the increasing contrast between practical success in physical science, and the continued failure of medicine to contribute to human welfare on anything like the same scale. Everyone appreciated, by 1850, the significance of the steam engine and of the electric telegraph… Except for Jenner's immortal discovery (of smallpox vaccination), what did medicine have to offer which was comparable to these?"[83]

For me, this notion is partly visceral. I am taken (too much?) with the contrast between the furious pace of technological advancement and the patience-demanding tempo of medical progress. Perhaps my perceived differential between engineering and medical sufficiencies is actually a difference in *satisfaction*: Our bar for the healing arts is stratospheric (we won't be gratified until we can all live, very healthily, for a very long time), but we derive great utility, pleasure—and even satisfaction—from the technology we've evolved over the millennia, even if we can imagine

[81] Cassedy (1984, p. 53).

[82] Porter (1997, p. 248).

[83] Shryock (1947/1979, pp. 248–249).

even better. But history also supplies a persuasive argument: It is all too easy to display examples of relentless technological achievement, dating back millennia, contemporaneous with a compendium of medical "therapies" that, on balance, surely did more harm than good. Even if it cannot be shown that the engineer's portfolio is exactly greatly more effective than the doctor's, I believe that this idea can serve as a useful premise for exploring factors which both hamper and facilitate therapy invention.

I start with very brief sketches of four engineering artifacts culled from the Western catalogue of technological achievement, all created before the nineteenth century. A host of alternatives, including many from other geographies and cultures, could substitute, but these selections strike me as especially attractive examples of technology's immense power, extending back even thousands of years. A highly condensed and hardly flattering sketch of the concurrent medical landscape follows. I did not advance past the eighteenth century, hoping, I confess, to make my argument sharper, given that the gulf between engineering and medical sufficiencies was at its widest prior to the late 1800s, when medicine first picked up real steam. And since ever more penetrating ways of defining human anatomy, physiology, and genetics are drawing the edges of this gap together, this argument may be of mostly historical interest a few decades down the road. But even if so, there is still much to learn about the loom on which medical therapy is fashioned by comparing and contrasting these two artifact-creating endeavors.

A few years before BCE sidled, unaware, into CE, Roman architect and engineer Marcus Vitruvius Pollio wrote *De Architectura*, today known as *Ten Books on Architecture*. Among other things, Vitruvius described ancient Greek and Roman technological artifacts: multiple varieties of hoisting machines, employing blocks and sheaves; devices for moving large loads across the land, such as marble from quarry to building site; machines of various types for raising water, including a "pump of Ctesibius", utilizing a piston in a cylinder; water wheels, mills, and screws; steelyards (balances); a "hodometer," for measuring distance traveled by land and by water; water organs; sundials; and water clocks. The ordnance detailed is as ingenious as anything currently flung between adversaries: catapults, ballistae, many varieties of siege machines; scaling machines; movable towers; a boring machine; "tortoises" to fill ditches; a battering ram; a device to defend against helepolis (movable siege towers); and fire darts.[84]

What Vitruvius did not describe were massive Egyptian pyramids constructed over 2000 years prior, nor the aqueduct in Jerwan, Iraq, constructed 700 BCE, which included a bridge spanning over a thousand feet,[85] nor the early segments of the Great Wall of China. More complex is the system of Roman aqueducts, begun 312 BCE. Though mostly running underground, they also employed massive aboveground bridges, many of which still stand. But more astonishing than the sheer size of the supra-terranean segments is the precise engineering that went into this com-

[84]Vitruvius (1914).

[85]Kirby et al. (1990, pp. 15–16, 25–32).

plex system: the slope of the canals was carefully calibrated (and executed) to be steep enough for water to move freely but not so rapidly as to erode the stone walls directing it. The system was designed to limit hydraulic pressure so that its channels and pipes would not burst; settling chambers were incorporated to contain silt[86]; and distribution tanks were constructed at their termini. At one point, the aqueducts directed 300 million gallons of water each day into Rome alone,[87] and even today the Eternal City's magnetic Trevi Fountain is supplied from the Acqua Vergine Antica, built by Agrippa in 19 BCE.[88] Only 2000 more years will reveal whether our modern water distribution systems will last as long as some segments of the Roman construction already have.

One could recall any number of effective and useful engineering artifacts created during the millennium after Rome hit its peak, but from a purely aesthetic standpoint, Gothic cathedrals are hard to beat. "Maximum height and maximum light"[89] were the desiderata for the designers of these twelfth and thirteenth century churches, admitting that "church" is a pitifully incomplete descriptor. *Universe of Stone*, Philip Ball's biography of Chartres Cathedral surely comes much closer to conveying the substance of these magnificent structures. "[S]piritual … rational … social … and technological [elements] came together in twelfth-century Europe to produce a series of buildings that are unparalleled in the West, and to which frankly we are now quite unable to offer any rivals."[90] Even if not everyone subscribes to the last half of Ball's declaration, Gothic cathedrals' persisting impact, on countless believers and non-believers alike, certify them as some of our most deeply affecting technological achievements. And technological artifacts they most certainly are—medieval engineers had to integrate distinctive design elements in a way unprecedented to achieve their beautiful effect. Their aesthetics cannot be peeled off of their engineering.

The charge for height and light, given the lack of advanced building materials (such as steel), was ingenious design. Wanting to avoid the risk of fire attached to wood, medieval master masons—the architects and engineers of their day—were pretty much limited to stone as the major structural material for their cathedrals. Stone mightily resists compression (that is, it's great at bearing weight), but is weak in tension (when stretched). But the loads in structures like these are more than compressive: the weight of the roof tends to bulge out the supporting walls, putting the stone under tension, and this force also tends to separate one block from the other. One can thicken the walls to solve this problem, but bulk gets in the way of light. To build a stable structure while maximizing room for windows, engineers employed three design strategies. Peaked arches—rather than the earlier (Romanesque) semi-circular variety—direct a larger fraction of their load straight

[86] Kirby et al. (1990, pp. 63–68).

[87] Rodà (2016).

[88] Flood (2004).

[89] Lewis (2004, p. 47).

[90] Ball (2008, p. 6).

down, rather than laterally. Ceilings were constructed using ribbed vaults, which direct their loads into slender piers, leaving plenty of room for great swatches of glass and the light it welcomes. And the piers could be thin yet sufficiently strong, since flying buttresses, erected outside the walls of the cathedral, subtracted some of the horizontal load without getting in the way of rays filtering into the building.[91]

Gothic cathedrals are more than places of shelter or congregation; they are gathering places with an agenda, beautifully demonstrating the power of engineering to provide far more than physical benefit. These churches' poignant message to medieval Catholics—and modern nonbelievers and believers alike—derives from more than management of loads and tensions, but without competent and imaginative engineering, that message could never have been delivered.

Engineering genius predating the American revolution was not limited to artifacts of monumental size or static demeanor. As people scratched ever deeper into the earth, extracting coal and metal-bearing ore, water settled its way into their mines,[92] defying the power of men and horses to pump the shafts dry.[93] Thomas Savery invented the first successful (if barely so) steam engine, patented in 1698, which was used to evacuate water from mines. Far more efficient than Savery's device, if still not very (less than 0.5%), was Thomas Newcomen's steam-powered pump, invented in 1712. Revolutionizing mining, this machine soon found enthusiastic use in England and the continent. Draining mines at Dannemora in 1734, the Newcomen pump was doing as much work as 528 horses in 24 hours; at a French coal mine, 48 hours each week of steam-driven pumping replaced 50 men and 20 horses, working 24/7 in shifts; and in 1775, a Newcomen engine pumped out the dry docks at Kronstadt, doing a year's worth of work of two huge windmills in only 2 weeks.[94]

Newcomen's pump was soon exceeded by Scottish inventor James Watt's more efficient (though still only 2–3%) steam engine (1775). When ways were found to convert its reciprocating motion to rotary, it was pressed into service in a variety of different kinds of mills, blast furnaces, and factories. Mobile steam did not lag far behind, and Robert Fulton and Robert Livingston introduced a commercially successful steamboat in 1807.[95]

Steam was not the first non-human, non-animal motive force; water and wind power antedated it by many years and still remained the major sources of power in the eighteenth century.[96] But steam could be used where and when they were unavailable, and sometimes provided greater power. Steam engines evolved greatly after the low-pressure Newcomen and Watt inventions—high pressure units were far more efficient and powerful—but even the early machines were tremendous

[91] Salvadori (2002, pp. 206–224) and Lewis (2004, pp. 47–67).

[92] Leinhard (2006, pp. 58–59).

[93] Kirby et al. (1990, pp. 152–153, 162).

[94] Kirby et al. (1990, pp. 157–158, 162–166, 180).

[95] Kirby et al. (1990, pp. 164–167, 172, 180, 251–252).

[96] Lienhard (2000, p. 93).

multipliers—of coal and ore mined; of cotton woven into cloth; of iron, copper, and lead produced; and of the output of a wide variety of other industrial goods. Engineering power powered the Industrial Revolution, with huge and persisting impact.

I'd like to round out this very narrow-angle view of pre-eighteenth century technology with an artifact much closer to human scale. Dava Sobel's *Longitude* describes the invention of an eighteenth-century masterpiece you could easily heft in one hand.[97] British Parliament passed the Longitude Act of 1714, offering large monetary rewards to spur development of a practical tool to determine longitude at sea. One way for a ship's captain, confronted by unbounded liquid sapphire, to determine his longitude is to compare the local time (knowing that noon is when the sun is at its highest) with the time at a known longitude. But you need a clock that tells you the reference time, the more accurately the better.[98] Although clocks far antedate the eighteenth century, none could cope with the "Shocks and Motions,"[99] fluctuations in temperature, humidity, and barometric pressure that run with any long ocean voyage.

Englishman John Harrison, a "very sober … industrious, and … modest"[100] clockmaker pondered what might work for the works of such an artifact for 4 years, then took another five to create his first iteration of a marine clock (1736). "H-1" erred by only a few seconds over 24 hours at sea, but Harrison was a perfectionist. He turned back to work, and 23 years later, he produced the "H-4": Five inches in diameter and weighing only three pounds, this handsome piece was crafted with a silver case, flawless black on white enamel dial, and a movement decorated with hand-carved scrollwork sprinkled with the heads of blued screws. Fit to be a bespoke ornament for a czar or emperor, its most beautiful feature was its unerring rhythm—H-4 lost only 5 seconds on an 81-day voyage from Portsmouth, England to Port Royal, Jamaica. This artifact, anticipating the modern global positioning system which transforms time into location, was the leading edge of a technology which facilitated transoceanic transportation and saved innumerable cargoes and lives at sea.

Early creators of medical artifacts were no less ingenious or industrious than their engineer counterparts.[101] In fact, the scope of medical and surgical interventions stretching back to ancient Egypt and other geographic areas is astonishing. Even before recorded history, as archeological evidence demonstrates, prehistoric peoples bored holes in the skull (trephination), set broken bones, and reduced dislocations. It seems certain that they availed themselves of medicines, plant-based and

[97] Sobel (1995).

[98] Sobel (1995, p. 58). To be accurate within a half degree of longitude, the mariner needs a clock which gains or loses no more than 3 seconds in 24 hours (about 2 minutes in a 6-week voyage).

[99] Sobel (1995, p. 80).

[100] Sobel (1995, p. 80).

[101] The practice of medicine has displayed and continues to have substantial geographical variation. The discussion below, and throughout this book, is largely focused on Western medicine, and is not necessarily reflective of medicine in other regions.

others, although the lack of a written record leaves the details to our imagination.[102]

Practicing among the rising pyramids, ancient Egyptian physicians reduced and immobilized bone fractures,[103] dabbed on salves, wound on bandages, and passed out medications (tree resins, extracts of plants, parts of animals, and minerals). More than 700 drugs and 800 formulae were listed in the Ebers papyrus (1550 BCE),[104] and many were added to practitioners' catalogues as the centuries wore on. Serious people took these medications very seriously long before they actually understood them; in London, the Royal College of Physicians produced a pharmacopeia as far back as 1618.[105]

More impressive is the thick catalogue of surgical procedures, some remarkably precocious.[106] Ancient Egyptians performed surgery, mostly simple (e.g., for wounds, abscesses, and circumcision) and manipulated dislocations.[107] (Up until the late nineteenth century, wound care, amputations, and "therapeutic" bloodletting were the most important contributors to the surgical book of business.) Sophisticated plastic surgery, including moving skin on a pedicle from the forehead to repair a deformed nose (rhinoplasty) was executed as early as 700 to 600 BCE, as was cataract removal.[108] Nasal polyps and tonsils were extirpated, hemorrhoids cauterized, amputations performed, hernias fixed, tracheotomies performed (incising the windpipe in the neck for patients with obstruction to their airway higher up), and bladder stones ejected well before the Common Era. By the 1700s, certain tumors, such as breast malignancies, were extirpated. One surgeon, in an unsuccessful attempt to save a dying man, even dared to ligate a bleeding aneurysm of the distal aorta in the early nineteenth century.

But if medical innovators were as clever and daring as engineers, were they as effective? How well did their artifacts actually work? Innovative and bold does not necessary certify useful or even appropriate by today's lights. Trephination, for example, may have been lifesaving for the occasional patient with bleeding between the brain and the skull, but for pretty much everyone else, it could only have decreased their misery by shortening their life. In 1667, surgeon Richard Lower innovated: He and colleagues transfused 9 or 10 ounces of … *sheep's blood* into Arthur Coga, a mentally unstable ex-clergyman. Human-to-human transfusion was thought too dangerous for the donor, and Lower and collaborators rationalized this experiment as being possibly helpful to Coga, should it cure his mental illness (it didn't). However important such experiments were for advancing the field, they

[102] Nutton in Porter (2006, p. 46).

[103] Hirschfeld (1938, p. 1).

[104] Porter (1997, p. 48).

[105] Weatherall in Porter (2006, p. 215).

[106] Wangensteen and Wangensteen (1978), Porter (1997, 2006), and Zimmerman and Veith (1993).

[107] Porter (1997, pp. 46–50).

[108] Saraf (2006), Banerjee et al. (2011), and Grzybowski and Ascaso (2014).

certainly didn't advance the cause of Mr. Coga (except for the 20 shillings he got for participating).[109]

But surgical technical virtuosity, if impressive even by today's standards, was scattered and uneven; the fact that one surgeon described advanced treatments (e.g., rhinoplasty) well before Hippocrates does not mean that this procedure was widely available at the time, or even very effective. Indeed, the very high rate of devastating post-operative infections before the application of asepsis greatly limited the ultimate utility and application of surgical artifacts.[110] James Young Simpson, a nineteenth century Scottish obstetrician, estimated that "The man laid on an operating table in one of our surgical hospitals' was 'exposed to more chances of death than the English soldier on the field of Waterloo."[111] Historian James Cassedy pointed out that when observers in the early to mid-1800s finally got around to careful analysis of surgical results in the United States, the results were unexpectedly sour. Amputation was attended by a substantial mortality rate, deformity often attended healed bone fractures, lithotomy (removal of bladder stones) killed 20%, and ovariotomy was too often unsuccessful.[112]

The agony of surgery without anesthesia often mooted the surgeon's proficiency at manipulating tissue—it must have taken powerful motivation for most to submit when faced with the ordeal of the procedure.[113] Surgery—its practitioners, beneficiaries, and victims—desperately needed anesthesia and measures to reduce the risk of infection, both of which barely arrived in the mid-1800s.[114]

The state of ingestible artifacts was hardly more advanced. *Positive Therapeutics* was published in 1913 by two medical doctors, William F. Waugh and W.C. Abbott. The authors launch this 700+ page tome with expressions of dismay from various observers regarding the state of medicine and Galenic (plant-based) medicines, a few of which include: "[Medicines] have destroyed more lives than war, pestilence, and famine combined" (John Mason Good); "Let us no longer wonder at the lamentable want of success which marks our practice, when there is scarcely a sound physiological principle among us" (Marshall Hall); "Physicians have slain more than war. The public would be better off without professed physicians" (Dr. Eliphalet Kimball); "How rarely do our medicines do good! How often do our medicines make our patients really worse! … in most cases the sufferer would be safer without a physician than with one" (Dr. Ramadge); and "[T]he prevailing mode of practice is productive of vastly more evil than good" (Dr. Coggswell). Oliver Wendell Holmes opined that drugs are healthy for neither man nor beast: "Mankind has been drugged to death, and the world would be better off if the contents of every

109 Yale (2015).

110 Porter (2006, pp. 198–200).

111 Schwarcz (2017).

112 Cassedy (1984, pp. 83–89).

113 Gawande (2012).

114 Shryock (1947/1979, pp. 174, 281) and Zimmerman and Veith (1993, p. 465).

apothecary shop were emptied into the sea, though the consequences to the fishes would be lamentable."[115]

To be sure, Waugh and Abbott's disdain for the current state of medical therapy was not universal. One of medicine's master clinicians and teachers, William Osler, had a distinctly contrary view in 1905: "Though used less frequently, medicines are now given with infinitely greater skill; we know better their indications and contra-indications; and we may safely say (reversing the proportion of 50 years ago) that for one damaged by dosing, one hundred are saved."[116] And it turns out that the authors of *Positive Therapeutics* had an axe to grind—their book shills the salutary effects of the purified active ingredients of plant-based medications (mostly a class of chemicals called alkaloids) and assorted other substances, the very types of drugs manufactured by Abbott's Abbott Alkaloidal Co. in Chicago.[117]

A handful of sharp and true arrows did lay at the ready in doctors' quivers before the mid-nineteenth century[118]: Quinine (good for treating malaria) was wrested from the bark of the cinchona tree in 1822; morphine from opium (1804); and earlier still, willow bark (containing an aspirin-like substance) was used to remedy rheumatic fever. Ingestion of the *Colchicum autumnale* plant (a source of colchicine, a medication still used today) as a remedy for gout goes back much further to the sixth century CE.[119] Of special interest are the leaves of the foxglove plant (*digitalis purpurea*), used to treat patients with fluid accumulation in their tissues, abdomen, and chest. William Withering, a Birmingham (England) physician, accumulated extensive experience prescribing digitalis, in the form of powdered leaves of the plant (or an infusion extracted from the same), and shared 10 years of observations in *An Account of the Foxglove, and Some of its Medical Uses, &c.* (1785).[120]

Withering's book is evergreen not because "dig" is a wonder drug, but because he made the then-unusual effort to rigorously determine the effective use and utility of his artifact. At the time, prescribing drugs "depended upon a mixture of authority, tradition, and philosophy,"[121] but Withering brought real evidence and analysis to bear. Numerical, rigorous studies of treatments at Withering's time were unusual, and there was a tendency to report only good results and ignore adverse events. More accurate and informative reports of efficacy and safety slowly gathered in the 1800s.[122] Withering prescribed an empirically derived optimal preparation and dosing of the leaves and, focusing on its diuretic properties, offered a detailed (if non-quantified) account of the results, both good and bad. The conditions where the drug delivered benefit, and those for which it was useless, were described, and complica-

[115] Waugh and Abbott (1913).

[116] Osler (1905).

[117] Made in Chicago Museum (n.d.).

[118] Halberstein (2005), Tong et al. (2016), Weatherall in Porter (2006, pp. 211–237).

[119] Shryock (1947/1979, pp. 161–162), Porter (1997, p. 270), Hartung (1954), and Tong et al. (2016).

[120] Withering (1785/1979).

[121] Weatherall in Porter (2006, p. 214).

[122] Cassedy (1984, pp. 68–91).

tions related to the medicine were discussed. Withering included all 163 cases of his own ("I have mentioned every case in which I have prescribed Foxglove, proper or improper, successful or otherwise", p. vi), *all* being key: Selecting individual patients for reporting could bias the account (usually suggesting better efficacy than real). He even declined to describe his most recent experience prior to publication, for lack of sufficient follow-up.[123] (Contemporary authors having only a limited amount of clinical material often include pretty much every available patient up to the time of manuscript preparation—the adjective "short term" in front of "results" being the fig leaf over the private parts of incomplete and thus barely useful information.) Withering made as convincing a case for therapeutic profile of this artifact, still in use, as could be found at the time.

But, as Roy Porter put it, "The [late 19th century's] pharmacopeia was a bag of blanks," with a limited number of exceptions. One medical historian surveyed the 1824 *Pharmacopoeia* of the Royal College of Physicians of London and found that, of the hundreds of drugs listed, only opium, foxglove (digitalis), and purgatives were actually effective.[124] Or worse, live rounds aimed at the patient: Many of the prescribed agents were toxic. For example, in the mid-1800s, calomel (mercurous chloride) was widely used as a purgative,[125] even while more perceptive physicians apprehended its net effect: "Hundreds of physicians have treated (congestive miasmatic fevers) with calomel, relying on it as a specific … but experience has shown that it is rather a specific in destroying, rather than in saving life."[126] While many of the agents advertised in *Positive Therapeutics*[127] have retained a place in modern therapeutics, the mere fact that compounds of arsenic merited 26 pages, and strychnine 78, suggests the wide gulf which separated early twentieth century medicine from that 50 years hence. (It also speaks volumes that, after trashing alternative medicines, the rationale proffered in *Positive* for using more potent agents was mostly only based on authority and physiologic and anecdotal observations.)

Perhaps nothing better reveals the unfavorable risk-benefit balance of pre-twentieth century medicine than bloodletting. Hippocrates approved of bloodletting to remedy an excess of blood, one of the four humors (along with yellow bile, black bile, and phlegm) whose balance was thought key to good health,[128] but its use goes back to at least to the Egyptians.[129] Lances and other special instruments were invented to incise veins, and anything from a few to many ounces of blood were allowed to vacate the ailing premises, depending upon the patient's condition and the physician's intuition.[130] (Leeches were alternative blood-removal agents.)

---

[123] Withering (1785/1979, p. 199).

[124] Porter (1997, p. 674); Shorter in Porter (2006, pp. 116–177).

[125] Cassedy (1984, pp. 76, 97–99).

[126] Hort (1847/1848).

[127] Waugh and Abbott (1913).

[128] Porter (1997, pp. 57–58).

[129] Wangensteen and Wangensteen (1978, p. 246).

[130] Thomas (2014).

Bloodletting was used pretty much whenever and for whatever the problem might be, including insanity. (Actually, I exaggerate: Galileo taught Pisan medical students astrology so they would know when *not* to bleed a patient,[131] Galen approved its use even to treat hemorrhage,[132] and bleeding was indulged as a seasonal tonic for those without specific complaint.[133] Its indiscriminate use was perhaps inevitable, since well into the nineteenth century practitioners had little comprehension of the nature of most diseases and lumped many together.[134]

Doctors were sincere and their patients all-in. Benjamin Rush, introduced in this Appendix's prologue, was his generation's preeminent U.S. physician (a sort of American Swiss army knife, he was also a founding father, politician, reformer, civil servant, and educator). Desperately ill and on what turned out to be his death bed, doctors removed ten ounces of his blood, after which Rush fainted and slept for several hours. Upon his groggy awakening, he demanded yet more blood to be let, to which his reluctant doctors finally relented, helping Rush to soon depart this mortal coil.[135] George Washington, also in his final hours, insisted that an overseer open his vein and allow copious flow even before his physicians arrived.[136]

Today, we only rarely intentionally remove blood (while replacing the volume lost with blood cell-free fluid), for certain unusual blood diseases, and for people with very specific congenital heart conditions. Leeches are still occasionally used to relieve blood-congested tissues with poor venous drainage. But from a twenty-first century perspective, it is hard to imagine that the vast majority of historical bloodletting was physiologically helpful, and easy to conclude that it was more often injurious.

Why this practice persisted for well over two millennia (even, albeit at a much-reduced rate, into the twentieth century) is perplexing. Very intelligent, acutely observant practitioners such as Osler found merit in this intervention, suggesting that in certain circumstances it was of actual value, especially in an era lacking the alternative therapies we use today, such as powerful diuretics. Possibly, in some patients, the loss of blood volume subtracted fluid from the lungs, with positive

[131] Heilbron (2010, p. 46).

[132] Porter (1997, p. 76).

[133] Wangensteen and Wangensteen (1978, pp. 246–254), Cassedy (1984, p. 75), and Petroski (1992, pp. 9–10).

[134] Cassedy (1984, pp. 53, 70) and Weatherall in Porter (2006, p. 214).

[135] Rutkow (2010, pp. 30–40).

[136] Chernow (2010, p. 807). To be sure, not all physicians blood let much. Erasistratus, one of the most famous of ancient physicians (roughly first half of the third century BCE) eschewed its use (Dobson 1927), and Austin Flint, Henry Heberden, and Henry Bowditch were three of several influential clinicians in the eighteenth and nineteenth centuries who soft-pedaled this therapy (Fye 1993; Cassedy 1984, pp. 68–70). And the lay public could be skeptical. Giorgio Vasari, the Tuscan Renaissance artist who authored *Lives of the Most Excellent Painters, Sculptors, and Architects* in the mid-1500s, complained that doctors "unwisely bled [Raphael], so that he began to faint from weakness just when he needed a restorative" in his final hours (Rowland and Charney 2017, p. 203).

results.[137] And there must have been a few souls, perched on the very edge of physiology, who benefited from what would be flagrant malpractice today: An 1825 case report of a foot soldier with an unrepairable carotid arterial injury suggested that intentional bloodletting, causing hypotension (low blood pressure) may have been instrumental in slowing bleeding from the wound and saving the soldier's life.[138] The fact that most ailments resolve on their own surely led to many false conclusions with respect to the efficacy of bleeding. The placebo effect is yet another explanation, but bloodletting's tenacity may have derived as much from sociology as physiology: "It is wrong (said Aristotle, rightly) to remove the foundations of a science unless you can replace them with others more convincing"[139]; something beats nothing, every time.

Medicine always had *something* to offer, but engineering was far more likely to actually deliver the goods: Manipulation of massive volumes of water; capacious and stunningly beautiful public buildings; vast quantities of material clawed from the surface and innards of the earth and then transformed into objects of practical value; the concepts, knowledge, and machines needed to reckon one's position thousands of miles from any terrestrial guidepost. And this is only one paragraph of the first page of technology's vast inventory; not mentioned are the paper, glass, dams, windmills, water mills, bridges, ships, tunnels, printing presses, and many other practical artifacts developed well before the nineteenth century. Simultaneously, medical practitioners had many medicines, but few were efficacious (and many pernicious), along with operations that made a posting at Waterloo seem comfortable and safe in comparison. Staying out of the way of the natural healing process (as Hippocrates well knew) was usually the best that the practitioner could do.

As I noted above, bringing the comparison between medicine and engineering into the twenty-first century complicates it a little because medicine now has many therapeutic artifacts that actually work. Medicines to kill most bacteria and even a few viruses; many replacement drugs, devices, organs, and even genes; definitive therapies for some malignancies; surgical procedures for complex congenital and acquired malformations that (often) work amazingly well—these constitute only a partial listing of modern medical artifacts. One might conclude that therapy creation has, with a great upward heave, finally caught up over the last 75 years. But lining up the intimidating technological masterpieces mentioned in previous chapters against the many serious afflictions which remain dug in, it still seems that medical artifact invention remains in the rearview mirror of our engineering colleagues. To know why is to understand the essence of therapy invention and is the subject of our next Appendix.

[137] Bertin in Fye (1993, p. 74), McMichael (1948), and Taussig (1947, pp. 548, 565).

[138] Delpech (1825).

[139] Heilbron (2010, p. 269).

## References for Appendix 3

Ball P (2008) Universe of stone: a biography of Chartres Cathedral. Harper, New York

Banerjee AD, Ezer H, Nanda A (2011) Susruta and ancient Indian neurosurgery. World Neurosurg 75(2):320–323

Cassedy JH (1984) American medicine and statistical thinking, 1800–1860. Harvard University Press, Cambridge

Chernow R (2010) Washington: a life. Penguin Books, New York

Delpech (1825) Case of a wound of the right carotid artery, cured by frequent bleeding, the application of ice, and the internal use of digitalis. Lancet:210–213

Dobson JF (1927) Erasistratus. Proc R Soc Med 20:825–832

Flood S (2004) Aquaducts and the Trevi Fountain. Accessed 19 Nov 2024. https://depts.washington.edu/hrome/Authors/floods/TheTreviFountain/pub_zbarticle_view_printable.html

Fye WB (1993) Red-Joseph-Hyacinthe Berth*. Clin Cardiol 16:273–274

Gawande A (2012) Two hundred years of surgery. N Engl J Med 366:1716–1723

Grzybowski A, Ascaso FJ (2014) Sushruta in 600 B.C. introduced extraocular expulsion of lens material. Acta Ophthalmol 92:192–197

Halberstein RA (2005) Medicinal plants: historical and cross-cultural usage patterns. Ann Epidemiol 15:686–699

Hartung EF (1954) History of the use of colchicum and related medicaments in gout: with suggestions for further research. Ann Rheum Dis 13:190–200

Heilbron JL (2010) Galileo. Oxford University Press, Oxford

Hirschfeld B (1938) The history of the treatment by extension of fractures of long bones. MD thesis, University of Nebraska Medical Center. Accessed 20 Nov 2024. https://digitalcommons.unmc.edu/cgi/viewcontent.cgi?referer=&httpsredir=1&article=1662&context=mdtheses

Hort WP (1847/1848) An inquiry whether there is in the Southern States, a specific disease that can properly be called congestive fever; with cases and remarks. New Orleans Med Surg J, Devoted to Medicine and the Collateral Sciences 4:58

Kirby RS, Withington S, Darling AB, Kilgour FG (1990) Engineering in history. Dover Publications, New York

Leinhard JH (2006) How invention begins: echoes of new voices in the rise of new machines. Oxford University Press, Oxford

Lewis EE (2004) Masterworks of technology: the story of creative engineering, architecture, and design. Prometheus Books, Amherst

Lienhard JH (2000) The engines of our ingenuity: an engineer looks at technology and culture. Oxford University Press, Oxford

Made in Chicago Museum (n.d.) Abbot Laboratories, est 1888. Accessed 20 Nov 2024. https://www.madeinchicagomuseum.com/single-post/abbott-alkaloidal-co/

McMichael J (1948) Heart. Annu Rev. Physiol 10:201–223

Osler W (1905) Counsels and ideals: from the writings of William Osler. Oxford University Press, London

Petroski H (1992) To engineer is human: the role of failure in successful design. Vintage, New York

Porter R (1997) The greatest benefit to mankind: a medical history of humanity. W.W. Norton & Co., New York

Porter R (ed) (2006) The Cambridge history of medicine. Cambridge University Press, Cambridge

Rodà I (2016) Aqueducts: quenching Rome's thirst. National Geographic History Magazine. Accessed 20 Nov 2024. https://www.nationalgeographic.com/history/history-magazine/article/roman-aqueducts-engineering-innovation

Rowland I, Charney N (2017) The collector of lives: Giorgio Vasari and the invention of art. W.W. Norton, New York

Rutkow I (2010) Seeking the cure: a history of medicine in America. Scribner, New York

Salvadori M (2002) Why buildings stand up: the strength of architecture. W.W. Norton & Co., New York

Saraf S (2006) Sushruta: rhinoplasty in 600 B.C. Internet J Plast Surg 3:1–4
Schwarcz J (2017) James Simpson, chloroform pioneer, took the pain away. McGill University Office for Science and Society. Accessed 19 Nov 2024. https://www.mcgill.ca/oss/article/health-history-science-science-everywhere/joe-schwarcz-james-simpson-chloroform-pioneer-took-pain-away
Shryock RH (1947/1979) The development of modern medicine. University of Wisconsin Press, Madison
Sobel D (1995) Longitude: the true story of a Lone Genius who solved the greatest scientific problem of his time. Bloomsbury USA, New York
Taussig HB (1947) Congenital malformations of the heart. The Commonwealth Fund, New York
Thomas DP (2014) The demise of bloodletting. J R Coll Physicians Edinb 44:72–77
Tong DC, Wilson AW, Layland J (2016) Colchicine in cardiovascular disease: an ancient drug with modern tricks. Heart 102:995–1002
Vitruvius (1914) The ten books on architecture (trans: Morgan MH). Harvard University Press, Cambridge
Wangensteen OH, Wangensteen SD (1978) The rise of surgery: from empiric craft to scientific discipline. University of Minnesota Press, Minneapolis
Waugh WF, Abbott WC (1913) Positive therapeutics, 3rd edn. The Abbott Press, Chicago
Withering W (1785) An account of the foxglove and some of its medical uses: with practical remarks on dropsy and other diseases. M Swinney, for G.G.J. and J. Robinson, Paternoster-Row, Birmingham/London. Reprinted in The Classics of Medicine Library. Birmingham, AL: Gryphon Editions, Ltd.; 1979
Yale E (2015) First blood transfusion: a history. Daily.jstor.org. Accessed 20 Nov 2024. https://daily.jstor.org/first-blood-transfusion/
Zimmerman LM, Veith I (1993) Great ideas in the history of surgery. Norman Publishing, San Francisco

## Appendix 4 – Inventing Therapy – Challenges of Therapy Creation

*Interface*, *access*, *ignorance*, and *testing limitations*—these are the facts of life with which medical innovators must grapple. We have already touched upon them in previous Appendices, but I will say a little more about them before we arrive at the last and the most important sand in therapy inventions' gears.

### Interface

As you recall from Appendix 1, *all* artifacts must interact appropriately with their environment, but the engineer's territory is usually more straightforward and forgiving than the biological domain. Medical artifacts aim to influence a complex, highly-evolved, and—this is most important—finely-calibrated system, leaving ample room for medicines and procedures to upset this fine-tuning as they interact with the human machine. As we've noted, engineering artifacts do not perform in a space with nearly so many different moving and meshing molecular parts—when they interface with biological systems, it is only superficially, so there are fewer ways for engineering artifacts to wreak havoc.

We've seen how medicines—a class of therapeutic artifacts with ancient provenance—provoke adverse effects, but even the most modern, technologically advanced agents, designed to interact very close to or directly on a specific dysfunctional component, are prone to do likewise. For example, innovators seeking a cure for sickle cell disease have identified therapeutic opportunities which operate very close to the genetic defect—inserting the wild-type hemoglobin gene or a modified, sickling-resistant hemoglobin gene, modifying the abnormal hemoglobin gene or reducing its expression or increasing expression of co-existing normal genes. But early efforts at gene therapy for certain other disorders caused leukemia because of inadvertently causing activation of cancer-causing genes, or provoked vicious immunological responses, with catastrophic effects.[140] Even twenty-first century medicine, with opportunities for modifying even the very blueprints of our molecular bits and pieces, operates in a space with lots of room for unintended consequences.

## Access

Although some engineering artifacts need to find their way to remote or demanding locations, getting to their site of action is usually straightforward. For a medical artifact, whose functional existence, as you recall, requires intimate interaction with the body, access can be problematic. This was all too often the case for surgical ailments before anesthesia, ways of managing the cardio-respiratory system, and other advances enabled surgeons to safely penetrate deep into the body. More recently, avenues for access have been expanded by catheters and guided using X-ray imaging (and even computer navigation systems), which all permit interventions within organs while minimizing injury to adjacent tissues. An example: Catheters threaded from an artery in the leg up into blood vessels in the brain can treat aneurysms and blood clots. Another example is the deployment of tubular laparoscopic instruments that are placed within the abdominal cavity through small incisions to access diseased tissues such as the appendix, prostate, or kidney. Through these tubular devices, using fiberoptics embedded within them, images of internal structures are displayed on a monitor, and specially designed surgical instruments can be inserted through the device to remove diseased tissue. But even today, geographic constraints can foil otherwise easy interventions. Bleeding into small airways deep in the lungs, for example, can be exceedingly difficult to treat, simply because one cannot manipulate tissue at the site of hemorrhage without seriously injuring the lung.

Thornier access issues revolve around replacing, or suppressing, faulty parts at the molecular level. I previously discussed the daunting number of components, and their vastly greater number of interactions, which make up cells and organisms, but said nothing about their *spatial* arrangement; they are not a soup of innumerable atoms and molecules meandering about. While some components are widely and

---

[140] Demirci et al. (2018) and Wilson (2009).

more or less randomly distributed (say, sodium ions),[141] many others are arranged in precise structures. For example, the heart's contractile cells (cardiomyocytes) are stuffed with arrangements of proteins of striking order and beauty, called sarcomeres. And many proteins are specifically incorporated into intricate "organelles" that are far smaller than the cells they occupy.

Deficient molecules which circulate in the blood can often be readily replaced (for example, thyroid hormone), but we often cannot incorporate normal proteins in a functional way into tissues. In theory, sickle cell disease could be cured simply by replacing the defective protein. But one cannot infuse hemoglobin into the blood, since it needs to find its way into very restricted and special spaces—the innumerable tiny red blood cells—and stay out of all others.[142] Other examples are proteins arranged in tight order in cells or organelles. Defective proteins in these structures can be the cause of disease, but it is usually impossible to insert replacements.[143] And even for ailments where it is not necessary to direct an artifact to a microscopic location, access can be a problem. For example, some medications cannot cross the "blood brain barrier," making them hard or impossible to use in treating conditions in the brain; some drugs are broken down in the stomach, or very rapidly metabolized in the blood, complicating their administration.

While a number of potential solutions utilizing genetic artifacts are being explored, getting the artifact into enough of (only) the correct type of cells has proven difficult. Viruses are the most commonly used vectors for introducing therapeutic genetic materials into cells, but often only small quantities are delivered, or their expression is only short-lived. Much work remains before we will know to what extent genetic therapies offer a solution for access limitations.

## Ignorance

Incomplete understanding of the system of interest (our bodies) is a third factor. Up through much of the nineteenth century, this ignorance was, for many reasons, profound. I have given some inkling in the previous appendices of the body's myriad parts (at the cellular and molecular levels) and, more crucially, the virtually innumerable interactions between these components. What I didn't mention are the many external influences, such as the food we eat, the microorganisms we host, the

[141] Actually, not even water is evenly and randomly distributed, nor ions such as sodium and potassium. Indeed, precisely controlled differences in the concentration of sodium and potassium ions inside and outside neurons and muscle cells are key to controlling their activation. Doctors can easily adjust the amounts of these ions in the blood, and the body takes care of the local concentration differences.

[142] In 2023, the FDA approved a molecular technique (CRISPR) to correct the defective gene causing the human disease and thus provide a cure for it. Tom knew of CRISPR and its potential.

[143] There are some exceptions. For example, for some lysosomal storage disorders—where there is a dysfunctional enzyme in organelles called lysosomes—intravenously infused replacement enzyme will naturally find its way into the lysosome (Parenti et al. 2013).

things we do, and so on, but these also add to the mix. And that the system is opaque to the naked eye, since most organs are situated within the body, with much of the action taking place in tiny structures whose ways and means defy easy observation. Even as smart and discerning an observer as William Harvey, who first clearly mapped the blood's circulation, found elucidation of what is today's Physiology 101 nearly impossible: "When I first [set out to discover the motions and uses of the heart,] I found the task so truly arduous, so full of difficulties, that I was tempted to think, with Fracastorius, that the motion of the heart was only to be comprehended by God."[144]

The tools for probing the system of interest—conceptual, cultural, and physical—were slow to develop. Ancient Egyptians looked to religion to explain the world. Because they attributed sickness to gods and supernatural forces,[145] a low ceiling was thrown over investigations needed to advance the healing arts. Hippocrates and his school of practitioners advanced thinking immeasurably by looking to natural causes, not disapproving and angry deities, as the cause of sickness.[146] The significance of this conceptual leap cannot be overestimated: Perceiving that man is subject to the same natural forces as everything else is the necessary prelude to rational discovery. But their overarching theory of disease—an imbalance of yellow and black bile, phlegm, and blood—was wildly incorrect and even fanciful by modern standards; meanwhile, the normal body function was little understood.

Because defining an object's structure is often key for understanding its function, cultural prohibitions against human dissection until the sixteenth century were a terrible drag on medicine's evolution. Nearly 2000 years passed between Hippocrates and *De humani corporis fabrica* (1543), the atlas which ushered in the modern era of human anatomical description. Andreas Vesalius (1514–1564), a professor of anatomy at the University of Padua,[147] authored this landmark contribution, which arguably first crossed the threshold of modern medical research. *Clinico-pathological correlation*—a way of learning about the causes of diseases by relating a patient's clinical characteristics in life to findings at autopsy—emerged as a seminal advance two centuries later. Giovanni Battista Morgagni, also a professor of anatomy at Padua, condensed 50 years of toil into *De Sedibus et causis morborum per anatomem indagatis* (Of the seats and causes of diseases investigated through anatomy) in 1761.[148] (If you were searching for a hat trick of medical history's most deeply foundational books, *De Sedibus*, *De humani*, and Harvey's *De Motu* would do very nicely.) This physically and intellectually hefty work demonstrated the power of

144 Harvey (1628).

145 McClellan III and Dorn (2015, pp. 69–70) and Porter (2006, p. 48).

146 Porter (1997, p. 56).

147 Porter (1997, pp. 179–181).

148 Morgagni (1769).

post-mortem observations and thinking in understanding the anatomic correlates of many illnesses, and laid waste to centuries of unfounded speculation.[149]

But correlating symptoms with the visible manifestations of diseases, while a necessary and major advance, was only one piece of the loom. Knowledge of *how the body works* is indispensable for extending the effective domain of the healing arts. Piercing the veil of the dynamic interior of living stuff takes more than cultural and conceptual leaps—sophisticated physical tools were also required. A prime article of modern biology—cell theory (which identifies the cell as the basic functional unit of tissues)—was not written until 1833–1840, in part because, while reasonably powerful microscopes date back to the early 1600s, methods of preparing tissue to enhance visualization were developed much later.[150] Many of the instruments needed for physiologic investigations, including devices to measure blood pressure, the kymograph (for recording physiological variables), the galvanometer and the rheotome (for investigating electrical phenomena in organisms), a device for measuring oxygen and carbon dioxide in the blood, and X-ray imaging, are all nineteenth century inventions. Given the paucity of measuring devices and imaging prior to the mid-1800s, it is no surprise that physiology (the study of how organisms work) hit its stride only then.[151] Indeed, it amazes me how much was known at that time, since many of the most powerful tools for biological discovery (electron microscopy; methods of reading and modifying DNA; ways to visualize proteins in individual cells; and imaging of tissues and organs using CT and MRI, to name only a few) were not invented until deep into the twentieth century.

But medical innovators were not alone in having to create in the face of inadequate knowledge—ancient engineering artifacts were achieved despite only a limited knowledge of the system of interest. Knowing how materials behave—how they react to compression, stretch, shear (sideways), and bending forces—is fundamental to designing and building stuff. But the designers of ancient aqueducts, churches, and other artifacts had no such knowledge, at least in the quantitative sense. Engineer Stephen Timoshenko's *History of Strength of Materials* devotes only six pages out of over 450 to what engineers knew about the strength of materials prior to Galileo's seminal *Two New Sciences* (1638). This great Italian mathematician and scientist was the first to publish relevant investigations (if not entirely correct),[152] but it was Robert Hooke who made the first major contribution (1676), observing that the deflection (strain) of a solid is proportional to the amount of force (stress) applied. This foundational step notwithstanding, clear expression of the fundamental concepts of stress and strain hung fire until 1822, and dissemination of these ideas to most working engineers lagged behind for another 30 years.[153] It was only starting in the mid-eighteenth century that engineers developed a quantitative

[149] Ventura (2009), Hurst et al. (2003, pp. 41–43), Nuland (1989, pp. 145–170), and Ghosh (2017).

[150] Porter (1997, pp. 320–330) and Mazzarello (1999).

[151] Fishman and Richards (1964, pp. 48–56, 80–85, 281–285).

[152] Timoshenko (1983, pp. 7–13) and Kirby et al. (1990, p. 127).

[153] Gordon (1978, pp. 28–61).

catalogue of material properties and a formal understanding of how loads and other forces should be managed.[154]

Engineer and historian Henry Petroski (and many others) pointed out that pyramids and medieval cathedrals were constructed in the "pre-rational" age of engineering.[155] Gothic engineers used no numerical calculations: "[G]eometric proportion, not calculations of material strengths or deflections, was central to the design of stone masonry structures that were stable and safe. The compass and square were the essential tools with which the architect-engineer applied his deep geometrical knowledge to create a cathedral."[156] Trial and error, intuition, and practical experience, not "science," are what informed these masterpieces.[157] And even years later, these types of knowing were at the root of countless successful designs. Scotsman Thomas Telford (1757–1834) was a civil engineer's civil engineer who decorated the landscape with many successful roads, bridges, and canals. His engineering prowess was legendary despite the fact that this "Colossus of Roads" had little regard for mathematical studies, nor even bothered to learn elements of geometry.[158]

In fact, many groundbreaking inventions ran ahead of a deep comprehension of the underlying phenomena: The first aircraft cleared terra firma far in advance of any sophisticated theoretical—or much practical—knowledge of how to design efficient wings. Steam engines were contrived long before the science of thermodynamics, which was formalized only in the mid-1800s. Indeed, the invention of that artifact was a powerful driver of the development of thermodynamics, not vice versa. Much more recently, the very first design for a transistor preceded the theoretical knowledge needed to advance the field very far.[159]

That new stuff can be created despite imperfect knowledge is, of course, easily enough explained: The inventor doesn't need to know everything, only enough for the project at hand. Early internal combustion engines propelled horseless carriages even though people had a lot to learn about the intricacies of engine design. The same is true for the medical innovator, as the problem of a fractured arm exemplifies. Informal observations (immobilized broken arms hurt less and heal quicker) must have informed the invention of casting as a therapy, even though the biology of the healing process was a black box for proto-orthopedists.

---

[154] Lewis (2004, pp. 144–164).

[155] Petroski (1992, pp. 55–56).

[156] Lewis (2004, p. 64).

[157] Lewis (2004, pp. 15, 18–19, 63–65), Gordon (1978, pp. 62–63), and Kirby et al. (1990, p. 103).

[158] Perhaps the price for leaning exclusively on intuition and experience, rather than taking comfort from numerical authority, is revealed by the following anecdote: "When heavy chains for [Telford's] Menai suspension bridge had been hoisted successfully in the presence of a large crowd, Telford was discovered, away from the cheering spectators, giving thanks on his knees" (Kirby et al. 1990, p. 62).

[159] Leinhard (2006, pp. 51–93), Lewis (2004, pp. 20, 206), Vincenti (1990, pp. 34–40), and Wikipedia (2024).

I would suggest that engineers are much closer to "perfect" knowledge of their systems of interest than medical innovators are of theirs. Even though physicists and materials scientists and engineers will surely discover new things about atoms and masses of atoms and molecules and photons into the indefinite future, they have already learned enough to astound us with their achievements. Bioscience investigators have also accrued an amazing cache of knowledge but given the human machine's massive number of parts and layers of connections, its catalogue suffers in relative comparison to the engineer's.

## Testing

Except for the simplest stuff, inventions rarely work the way you want the first time around. While experience and knowledge increase the odds that an artifact will perform properly straight off the drawing board, a considerable amount of fiddling around usually separates the conception from the final expression. Engineer E.E. Lewis crystallized this process: "The exhilaration is palpable when the prototype performs well. But exaltation is usually short-lived, for surprises inevitably turn up between drawings and hardware. The prototype tests make apparent the oversimplifications in the computer models, the inadequacies of the parts' tests, and the inability of designers to anticipate every nuance of behavior. Thus, still to come are *extensive periods to test, fix, and redesign*, as unforgiving reality reveals design flaws and construction shortcomings. Many tests lie ahead."[160] This iterative process is testing.[161]

If testing is the backbone of engineering artifact development, exactly the same can be said for therapy creation. Examining its role in medical creation reveals the crucial reason that medical innovation has lagged behind technological advances: The engineering-medicine testing differential is—to understate it—enormous, with engineers occupying the catbird seat.

Using testing to develop and optimize technological artifacts must extend back into pre-history, and we have ancient accounts of the methodical use of this invaluable tool. The Greeks, for example, improved their catapults by systematically changing the dimensions of key components and measuring the effect on catapult performance.[162] In the 1800s, water-driven turbine development was facilitated by

[160] Lewis (2004, p. 24); emphasis mine. Consider also James Watt's challenge in perfecting his steam engine. He needed to create a piston/cylinder configuration which would maintain pressure yet operate with low friction. To do so, Watt contemplated using round, square, and flexible pistons; tried tin, copper, wood, and cast iron for the cylinders and pistons; experimented with piston discs and rings of leather, pasteboard, cloth, cork, oakum, hemp, asbestos, a lead-tin alloy, and a copper-lead alloy, as well as using mercury, oil, graphite, tallow, horse dung, vegetable oil, and other substances to improve the piston/cylinder seal (Scherer 1965, pp. 177–178).

[161] Staudenmaier (1985, p. 45).

[162] Hacker (1968).

the invention of the Prony brake, a device to measure power output.[163] As engineers learned more about the properties of materials and developed a theoretical understanding of how their devices worked, they became better at conjuring up designs with less need for development,[164] but testing remains a vital part of any development program.

An important modern development is *computer simulation*, which predicts how materials and parts will behave under specified conditions, reducing the number of physical iterations needed to perfect a device. Computer-aided design of large, extremely complex objects (such as aircraft) also simplifies artifact creation by assuring that a component configured by one team of engineers (say, a hydraulic line) does not occupy the same space as a part (e.g., an electrical cable) penned-in by another team.

All that said, physical testing of the actual artifact, or physical models of the same, remains indispensable. There are different ways of testing artifacts or their physical surrogates. It may be possible to test a *prototype* of the desired device, and testing often continues even after the device has matured from prototype to final configuration. Some objects too large to prototype (say, a bridge or skyscraper) have their performance characteristics evaluated by computer simulation and scale models.[165] Studying a model of an airplane in a wind tunnel to determine its aerodynamic characteristics is a classic example.[166]

But the ultimate test is the actual artifact's performance, whether it be a slingshot or an aircraft. Christopher Orlebar, a former Concorde pilot and instructor, related how, early in the airplane's life, it was dispatched on a demonstration run with the Shah of Iran. During the flight, the Concorde, upon encountering a change in atmospheric conditions, "shot into a barely controllable climb," revealing a nasty characteristic which had to be eliminated before the aircraft could enter into service.[167] Goodness knows how many hours of wind tunnel testing were used to design this artifact, yet only actual flight experience exposed a potentially serious design weakness.

While creating new engineering objects can be exceedingly challenging, at least inanimate materials don't mind being cut, hammered, drilled, and otherwise fashioned into stuff. Nor do prototypes mind being deconstructed, sometimes violently. Bugs can be worked out over the course of many trials, with successive modifications ultimately culminating in a successful artifact.

---

[163] Constant II (1980, pp. 41, 44, 56, 64).

[164] Vincenti (1990, p. 256).

[165] See Vincenti (1990, pp. 138–140), for a brief summary of some historical aspects of the use of scale models in engineering, with useful references.

[166] Results obtained from models cannot always be directly applied to the full-scale object; "scale effects" limit extrapolation of results derived from studying models to the real thing. For a detailed discussion of scale effects, see Vincenti (1990), especially pp. 139–141, 149–151, 164–165.

[167] Orlebar (1997, p. 56).

The strategy of building a prototype, testing it, modifying it, re-testing and re-modifying again and again is largely unavailable to the medical innovator, since the opportunity to try out a new therapy, then altering it in this way or that, is extremely limited if human beings serve as the test bed. Imagine a surgeon conceiving of a new procedure, performing it in a patient, and when the results were unsatisfactory, re-operating with modifications again and again in the same patient until it worked properly—clearly unethical and biologically unsustainable. Developing a surgical procedure by serially operating on many *different* patients and refining the operation on the basis of observed results is a way that therapy is improved—in fact, successful therapy for mitral valve stenosis was partly developed in that way. But this takes time and faith, and because practitioners and potential patients are discouraged by unsuccessful therapeutic experiments, it's difficult to try variations on a theme multiple times unless it proves successful early on, as Charles Bailey (Chap. 7) experienced.

You may be thinking, but medical inventors can test their ideas in non-human settings and apply them to people only after they have been perfected. Indeed, medical innovators do use models, just like engineers. The first successful cardiac operation of some complexity—surgical closure of a ductus arteriosus—followed a program of preclinical investigation, using dogs and human cadavers as models.[168] The same is true for the even more impactful Blalock-Taussig-Thomas shunt,[169] as well as for another foundational operation for single ventricle patients, the Glenn shunt.[170] Indeed, surgery has advanced in great part on the backs of models, usually animal, which inform technique and assess function: Surgeons learn how to rearrange tissue and then observe the physiological and outcome effects of the reconstruction. The importance of animal models in developing novel surgical procedures is hard to overstate.

But such models can be misleading. Situated at the top of the current hierarchy of single ventricle surgical palliation is the Fontan operation. Francis Fontan conceived of this breakthrough operation, then used a canine model to test it: "Experimental research on dogs enabled us to check the technical feasibility of this procedure, but there were no survivals for more than a few hours, perhaps… because the right atrium of the normal heart could not provide the required work, whereas a hypertrophied (thickened) right atrium, as in tricuspid atresia (the actual human disease), could supply the additional work (needed to propel the blood through the lungs)."[171] Assuming that his model inadequately modeled the human condition, Fontan forged ahead and applied his operation to humans, and the rest is history

[168] Gross (1939).

[169] Thomas (1985, pp. 36, 70–72, 88–92).

[170] Glenn (1989).

[171] Fontan and Baudet (1971). Other surgeons had also created experimental models of a Fontan-like circulation with uniformly discouraging results (Robicsek and Watts 2007). Alex Haller had reported "chronic" survivors in 1966, but only 3 dogs of 20 operated upon had complete exclusion of the right ventricle, and the duration of survival was not reported (Haller et al. 1966).

(Chap. 9). We know now that it wasn't a too thin right atrial wall that got in the way, but whatever the explanation for the dog's poor survival, the Fontan operation was invented because the surgeon's hunch trumped the surgeon's model. In a similar vein, laboratory experiments aimed at perfecting an operation to relieve narrowing (coarctation) of the aorta were also complicated by the imperfection of the animal model: Healthy dogs were often paralyzed after operation, while people with coarctation run a much smaller risk.[172] And because practical concerns limit the amount of time that an animal can be observed after operation, long-term complications related to a new artifact may not be manifest; it was clinical, not laboratory-based experience that identified liver dysfunction and arrhythmias as significant issues after Fontan palliation.

The lack of good models is a big problem for creation of new medications. Animals are used extensively to evaluate compounds that might prove to be effective drugs, but such models are notoriously poor at predicting whether a candidate medication will actually be useful in humans. They may also fail to reveal toxicity in humans, a potentially even bigger problem.[173] The poor reliability of available models is reflected in the percentage of candidate drugs which are ultimately approved for use by the FDA. One study found that the overall success rate in clinical trials from 2001 to 2015 was only 13.8%; even if the sorry success rate of oncology trials (3.4%) is neglected, only 20.9% of medications clinically tested secured FDA approval.[174] There are reasons unrelated to faulty preclinical models which explain some fraction of failed clinical trials, but surely the success rate would be far higher if experimental prediction was much more reliable.

Many factors explain the poor performance of preclinical studies, the most obvious being that animals are not humans, nor—in many cases—are the diseases they model identical to the human disease of interest. Also, measuring relevant therapeutic endpoints in animals may not be possible, and modeling diseases with slow onset and long duration may be compromised by the short life spans of most animals used for such experiments.

That's not to declare animal models always useless; indeed, there are innumerable examples of such studies proving invaluable in therapy creation.[175] A recent example: A mouse model of Marfan syndrome led to a new pharmacologic means (losartan) of slowing the rate of progression of aortic dilation.[176] And novel techniques, such as studying mice expressing human genes, and experiments utilizing human pluripotent stem cells, may open new avenues for therapy development.[177] But the all too often disconnect between how a therapeutic artifact performs in the

[172] Shumacker Jr. (1992, pp. 50–51).

[173] McGonigle and Ruggeri (2014).

[174] Wong et al. (2019).

[175] Cooter and Pickstone (2000).

[176] Lacro et al. (2007) and Milewicz et al. (2017).

[177] McGonigle and Ruggeri (2014), Walsh et al. (2017), and Avior et al. (2016).

laboratory versus the real world leaves the medical innovator at a disadvantage relative to his engineering colleagues.

And so we are often left with testing poorly vetted—despite our best efforts—agents in humans. The very term used to describe the way that new therapies are tested—"*clinical trials*"—properly implies that jeopardy is involved, for both the prospective treatment and the participating patients. Ethical and moral constraints have been amplified and codified by legal and administrative structures and regulations which complicate therapeutic trials, making them very expensive in time and money.[178] Even prospectively gathering data on patients for research purposes—not performing extra tests or giving experimental therapy, *just keeping track* of the test results and outcomes of therapy that is provided for ordinary clinical care—requires specific permission from the patient.

While rules regulating clinical studies are necessary and important, these requirements make therapy creation a much thornier problem than simply hauling insights from the lab into the clinic. And recruiting an adequate number of subjects, especially for uncommon ailments, can prove to be a nightmare. Medical testing is therefore limited to the most promising ideas, and unless a therapy is successful pretty much from the get-go, it often gets consigned to the back shelf. Even more important, there is seldom an opportunity to make successive modifications to a medicine or other intervention in hopes of improving its function, at least once it has reached the point of human trials. (Before clinical testing, many iterations and modifications may be made in developing a particular therapy, surgical or medical, but once applied in humans, the clock is ticking.)

But overlooking the risks and rules and regulations and setting aside that it would be great if clinical trials were more confirmatory (of preliminary modeling) rather than exploratory, there are other reasons why evaluating the safety and efficacy of medical artifacts is a tough haul.

When engineering artifacts work well, this is easily appreciated, and when they fail (or work poorly), this is also pretty obvious. That is not to say that failure always occurs early, although it often does; bridges and dams collapse months or years after construction, ships' hulls crack long after being launched, premature failure can occur in any technological device. And, with a large number of essentially identical objects—say, automobile air bags—some will fail while others do not. But ultimately, engineering artifacts are pretty transparent in their excellence or their imperfection.

Some medical artifacts also have a clear-cut, easily perceived and even quantifiable effect. For example, as noted in the Introduction, babies with hypoplastic left heart syndrome suffer a statistically predictable fate (almost all die soon after birth), and while a few survive without surgery, this is very unusual.

When effective surgical treatment for this condition was finally developed, the likelihood of infant survival was vastly increased, which became apparent after only

[178] Martin et al. (2017).

a few patients had been operated upon. When the survival rate goes from less than one in ten without operation to eight in ten with surgery, the treatment is obviously effective, at least in the short-term.

But many other types of therapeutic artifacts are far harder to evaluate. Shortly after the Fontan procedure was invented, when follow-up information was sparse, cardiologists following single ventricle patients who had survived thus far without a "Fontan" needed to decide whether to refer their patients for this new artifact. Physiology after the Fontan is in some ways closer to normal, presumably conferring better exercise capacity, fewer complications, and longer survival. But there was a lot of uncertainty involved:

The patient will survive for an indeterminate time if nothing is done, and although the operation offers theoretical advantages, it also carries the risk of early death, and there was no way of knowing for the first many years in the Fontan experience whether it actually conferred a long-term survival benefit. (In other words, which periods of time are longer, the blue t's or the red t's. What did cardiologists recommend? In fact, until enough patients had been treated with the new therapy, and enough time has elapsed, many cardiologists were reluctant to recommend the Fontan operation. Innovation can proceed in the face of this type of uncertainty, but when the unsettling possibility that it is more harmful than helpful lingers, widespread adoption—the goal for almost any new artifact—is inhibited. This is one species of therapeutic indeterminacy—not knowing whether a new therapy is better, the same, or worse than the natural history of the disease because the effects of the treatment are only reckoned over considerable time. (This is especially problematic in pediatrics, where we hope to optimize the patient's health for decades.)

And there are other reasons that evaluation of medical therapy is often problematic. For diseases which spontaneously resolve (the common cold, for example) or *wax and wane* (some inflammatory diseases), it can be hard to know if a treatment alters the course of the disease. Accurate measurement of the relevant endpoints (for example, time to resolution or some measure of how badly the patient is affected), can be challenging, and often many subjects are required. The inclusion of control subjects, ideally with the identical characteristics as the treated patients and who receive a placebo, is usually required to draw conclusions about efficacy. As one might imagine, this is difficult to do in surgery; the trial (test) procedure and the (control) standard procedure have to be considered to have equipoise—assumed equal "value" based on published medical literature, experience, and animal experiments if relevant and feasible.

*Variability in patients, their disease, and their response* to therapy also complicates therapy evaluation, especially since treatments often have only a modest effect. The way around this is to enroll a lot of patients. For the SOLVD study (a clinical trial of enalapril versus placebo for heart failure; see Appendix 1), 2569 subjects were enrolled; in the sacubitril/valsartan trial, 8399 subjects were included.

While not all clinical trials require this many subjects, some are far larger,[179] and most enroll subjects in at least the hundreds. Lots of subjects means lots of expense, and—especially for rare diseases and some pediatric disorders—enrolling enough subjects may be difficult or impossible.

*Flawed study design* can also lead to incorrect conclusions about therapy efficacy. One could quickly get into deep weeds regarding the intricacies of trial design but suffice it to say that problems with patient selection and randomization (treatment vs. control), the endpoints used, opportunities for investigator bias to affect study results, and a host of other factors can easily lead to misleading or frankly incorrect conclusions about the utility of medical artifacts.

The pediatric carvedilol trial for heart failure illustrates some of the difficulties encountered in testing medications, especially in children who (thankfully) are less often afflicted by most diseases than adults, and therefore present fewer study subjects. Although, as mentioned previously, beta blockers were well-established therapy for adults with heart failure, no rigorous clinical trials had been conducted in pediatric patients by the 2000s. It was high time to study these medications in children, so some of the smartest and most experienced people in the field devised a clinical trial of the most sophisticated design: prospective, randomized, placebo-controlled, double-blinded (neither investigators nor subjects knew who was given test drug versus placebo). Consuming several years and millions of dollars, the study would presumably provide a strong "evidenced-based" justification for beta blockers in children.

It turned out that carvedilol had *no* apparent effect on the patients' condition, the primary outcome variable of interest. The tone of the paper reporting the results of the trial suggests that this both surprised and disappointed the investigators.[180] They cursorily admitted that their findings *could* indicate that the drug was, in fact, ineffective, while devoting far more attention to reasons why their results might be *falsely* negative: the primary endpoint poorly reflected the patients' true clinical status; more children spontaneously (on placebo) got better than had been assumed, so more patients were needed to show any positive effect; the fact that a heterogeneous group of patients was enrolled (which was needed, however, to gather enough subjects); the doses of carvedilol used may have been sub-optimal. This is quite the opposite of most such reports, where the authors mount a vigorous defense of the validity of their findings, even if dubious, rather than articulating a raft of reasons to discount them. Concern about these possible confounders, combined with (weak) evidence that cardiac function was improved by the drug and strong evidence of efficacy in adults led clinicians to reject the implications of what was intended to be a practice-defining study: Beta blockers are currently considered standard of care

[179] For example, the GUSTO trial compared four thrombolytic strategies for treating acute myocardial infarction and enrolled 41,021 patients (GUSTO Investigators 1993).

[180] Shaddy et al. (2007).

for pediatric heart failure patients, despite the findings of the most rigorous study of these medications yet conducted.[181]

We do not know enough, and likely never will, to reliably design effective and safe artifacts without human testing. We toss therapies against the wall and see what sticks (and doesn't dissolve the paint). The time, risk, uncertainty, and expense of seeing what works greatly reduces the number of therapeutic artifacts that can be evaluated, and therefore the number invented. And, even more discouraging, clinical testing may not be definitive despite its heavy cost and its status as the "evidence based" therapeutic standard.

Considering the medical innovator's technical challenges and testing constraints, it seems almost a miracle that safe and effective therapy *ever* gets invented. But it does, which brings us to the second main idea of this appendix: What substitutes for miracles are powerful *therapy facilitators*—properties inherent in the human body, or in other organisms—that innovators exploit when creating otherwise impossible therapies. These facilitators are homeostasis and adaptation, spare capacity, self-healing, and nature-derived medications.

## Homeostasis and Adaptation

Physiologist James Houk concisely summarized, and accurately assessed the significance of one of physiology's root concepts thusly: "One of the great events of the history of physiology occurred in 1878 when Claude Bernard enunciated the general principle of the constancy of the 'milieu intérieur' … [that is,] the internal environment of the body is closely regulated. This regulated environment is characterized by a constancy of certain biophysical variables, for example, temperature, blood pressure, the concentrations of many substances in body fluids, the volumes of fluids in body compartments, and the density of red cells in the blood."[182] Many others studied the mechanisms of such regulation, including Walter Cannon, chair of the Department of Physiology at Harvard Medical School, whose classic *The Wisdom of the Body* (1932) presented a wide-ranging review of how the body maintains an even keel despite changes in the external and internal environment. Cannon coined the term "homeostasis" to shorthand the concept that the body can automatically adjust a variety of parameters (such as cardiac output, blood pressure, respiration, neural impulses, urine output, and other substances in the blood) to maintain stability in the face of ever-changing conditions. This exquisite capacity for dynamically adjusting their physiology is *de rigueur* for the survival of complex organisms.[183]

These complex regulatory mechanisms are also a big part of why the biology of the organism is so difficult to tease apart, since part of their charge is warding off the

[181] Personal communication with Elizabeth D. Blume, MD (June 8, 2018).

[182] Houk in Mountcastle (1980, p. 246).

[183] Cannon (1932).

dangerous environment players of everyday living, such as external intruders who stimulate the body's immunological weapons. But consider the other side of the fabric: Many therapies are *possible only because of* homeostasis and its kissing cousin, adaptation. Though they seldom articulate it, medical innovators are often beholden to the body's ready assistance in creating effective therapies. Let's consider an example of adaptation before seeing how it and homeostasis play key roles in single ventricle therapy.

One of the difficulties inherent in extreme altitude climbing is, well, the altitude. Because the barometric pressure at 8000 m (about 26,000 feet) is roughly 35% of that at sea level, air offers too little oxygen for humans acutely exposed to this elevation. Mountain climbers who tackle extreme altitudes in the Himalaya adapt to thin air by spending weeks at elevation before the actual climb. In 2007, the Caudwell Xtreme Everest Research Group studied this adaptation: Physiological measurements of volunteer mountaineers were made at sea level, after 60 days of acclimatization (at higher than 8000 feet), and while high on Mt. Everest. They found that each gram of hemoglobin (the protein that carries almost all the oxygen in the blood) carried only a little more than half as much oxygen at 27,559 feet as at sea level, but because the *amount* of hemoglobin in the blood had increased by about 35% during the acclimatization and the climb, the blood's oxygen *content* was only reduced by about 25% relative to normal.[184] Since the quantity of oxygen delivered to the tissues is hugely impacted by oxygen content, the increased hemoglobin substantially offset the oxygen-denying effect of altitude. The partial pressure of oxygen in arterial blood at this extreme altitude was only 30 mmHg (it is nearly 100 at sea level), a life-threatening value in an acutely ill patient in Boston, but tolerated surprisingly well on Everest in these well-adapted climbers. The body makes multiple adjustments to high altitude—increased hemoglobin is only one—and the obliging result is a mountaineer now equipped for an otherwise disabling or even fatal environment.[185] The organism is not fixed in a rigid physiological straitjacket, but has generous latitude to adapt to adverse circumstances, both external and internal.

Interventions which change one aspect of a patient's physiology often mandate alterations in others. Practitioners can only tend to these adjustments in a very limited way. Were the body unable to dynamically fine-tune its physiology in response to otherwise salutary medical and surgical modifications, some therapeutic artifacts would prove more calamitous than beneficial. Like high-altitude climbers, but for a different reason, single ventricle patients need to adapt to hypoxia, at least for a period of their early lives.[186] Later, as Fontan patients, they adjust their circulatory system to maintain the higher than normal venous pressure needed for adequate cardiac output, and their small blood vessels become more resistant to leakage of

[184] These measurements were made with the climbers at rest and breathing only air, but while climbing, they used supplemental oxygen. A few mountaineers have summited Everest without supplemental oxygen (Grocott et al. 2009; Murray et al. 2018).

[185] Grocott et al. (2009) and Murray et al. (2018).

[186] Migliavacca et al. (2001) and Magee et al. (1996).

fluid at the increased venous pressure.[187] The body—not the doctor—makes these necessary accommodations to the therapeutic artifact that is the Fontan.

The organism looks after its biochemical milieu as well, including disposing of unwelcome substances which find their way into the blood. Medicines would be difficult and hazardous to use if, having taken a dose, the drug were to stick around indefinitely. The simple fact that the body eliminates medications, while inconvenient in the sense that repeated doses are required, greatly facilitates adjusting the amount of drug given to achieve the desired effect. It also makes it possible to discontinue the medication when no longer needed, or if it proves ineffective or harmful.

## Spare Capacity

At the Harvey Society lecture of 1906, Samuel Meltzer formally addressed, apparently for the first time, the notion of "factors of safety"[188]—I find "spare capacity" more congenial—in animals. This Rockefeller Medical Research Institute physiologist presented many examples of spare capacity, only a few of which include bones that are stronger than needed, paired organs and those which normally work at a level far below their maximum, and necessary physiologic functions performed by more than one organ. Especially relevant to our discussion, Dr. Meltzer found that "The complex apparatus of circulation is well provided with factors of safety" owing to excess capacity with respect to the amount of blood in the vascular system, the ability of the vascular system to adjust venous pressure, and the heart's facility in increasing its output.[189] Spare capacity, which lies cheek by jowl alongside adaptation, can be pretty obvious, as Meltzer pointed out—one can lose a lung, or donate a kidney or part of the liver, and still function at a high level.

But spare capacity can also be more subtle. As we will see, some single ventricle surgeries work only because of the incredible efficiency of the vascular system, an efficiency exceeding that needed for two ventricles. The adult heart, with its owner at rest, generates only about 1 watt of power propelling blood throughout the circulation, roughly the amount consumed by the tiny incandescent light bulb in a flashlight.[190] As noted by Willems, the power generated by the heart pumping blood can be calculated: power (watts) = cardiac output (L/min) × mean arterial pressure (mmHg) × $2.22 \times 10^{-3}$. For a normal adult with a cardiac output of 5 L, and a mean

[187] Krishnan et al. (2009).

[188] In engineering, *factor of safety* refers to the practice of engineers designing artifacts to be stronger than calculations require to provide a margin of error to cover for unknown factors that could impact its integrity (Petroski 1992, pp. 98–106).

[189] Meltzer (1907).

[190] This flashlight light bulb consumes about the same amount of power as a human heart generates while pumping blood. From Amazon, accessed November 23, 2024.

arterial pressure of 100 mmHg = 1.1 watts.[191] That's how good the body is at directing blood—and therefore oxygen and nutrients and other critical substances—to every single cell in its domain. Were the vascular system to not allow such luxuriously easy passage of blood, much of current single ventricle surgical therapy would be impossible.

## Self-Healing

The body's capacity for self-healing gets the innovator off the hook for providing a component of surgical therapy which is both absolutely necessary and well beyond her ken. Surgical procedures disrupt tissues and organs, and these cuts and rents must heal. When the body is incised, cells multiply and produce "connective tissue," mending the wound. Stitches placed by the surgeon hold tissues in place during the healing process, but without the body's reconstructive efforts, these bits of suture will ultimately fail, and the tissue will fall apart. Surgical procedures are partnerships, as they have been for thousands of years, between the surgeon and the patient's body, not independent interventions.

## Nature-Derived Medications

Engineering artifacts spring from the hand of man, while therapeutic artifacts often do not. Engineers massage materials to create stuff, and seldom solve a problem using an unmodified naturally occurring object. That is not to say that nature's stuff (both animate and inanimate) hasn't helped inform the design of technological devices, but such artifacts are not found objects; their design springs from the brow of an engineer. In contrast, many of our most powerful medications hail from the natural world. Substances produced in bacteria (e.g., botulinum toxin), molds (e.g., penicillin), and plants (e.g., digitalis) are commonly employed as drugs, and there are many others. In fact, one estimate has over 60% of all medicines in industrialized nations as either natural products or their secondary metabolites.[192] Even when medicines cannot be lifted directly from their natural source, new drug discovery strategies based on natural substances have an inherent advantage, since their biological effects have been optimized through eons of evolution.[193]

How did we get so lucky? Why is it that organisms ranging from microbes and molds to trees synthesize molecules that humans can hijack for drugs? The answer is open to debate, but one persuasive view holds that the capacity to produce such molecules evolved by various organisms for self-protection from nearby competing

[191] Williams et al. (2001). Note that the total amount of power consumed by the heart to generate this propulsive force exceeds this number, since the heart is not perfectly efficient.

[192] Mathur and Hoskins (2017) and Newman et al. in Wermuth et al. (2015, p. 102).

[193] Swinney and Anthony (2011).

organisms (for example, mold producing antibacterials). In some cases, microbe-synthesized molecules which interact with higher vertebrates (such as certain hormones) may have actually first evolved in simple organisms, and only later were later added to the repertoire of more complex species.[194]

But nature-derived drugs are not exactly manna from heaven, since transforming a naturally occurring substance into a useful medicine is a creative act in itself. Identifying the salutary properties of, say, a medicinally useful plant substance takes observation and insight, and working out the pharmacologic profile of the drug (appropriate doses, adverse effects, contraindications, and so on) is a big project. Purification and mass production may pose difficult challenges. Even so, the medical innovator's power to adjust human physiology would be a tiny fraction of what it is if every therapeutic agent had to be invented from scratch.

In Appendix 3, I suggested that engineering invention has been more effective than medical invention, and I used this idea here to explore the nature of medical artifact creation. To summarize here, four factors explain, to varying degree, why inventing therapy is so tough: There are many ways that well-intentioned therapy can seriously annoy the body; there is difficulty getting therapeutic artifacts to the required location in the body; our limited knowledge of the body dynamic means that we often don't know what is wrong or how to fix it; and most importantly, opportunities for testing therapies are infinitely fewer—that's only a tiny overstatement—than for engineering artifacts. Finally, we've also appreciated rather the converse; how therapy often works by exploiting marvelous qualities inherent in the body. For some therapeutic interventions, the body fills in lacunae that imperfect knowledge, or technique, leaves behind. The body's willingness to participate in the therapeutic process helps level the lopsided engineering-medical playing field.

## References for Appendix 4

Avior Y, Sagi I, Benvenisty N (2016) Pluripotent stem cells in disease modelling and drug discovery. Nat Rev. Mol Cell Biol 17:170–182

Cannon WB (1932) The wisdom of the body. W.W. Norton & Company, New York

Constant EW II. (1980) The origins of the turbojet revolution. Johns Hopkins University Press, Baltimore

Cooter R, Pickstone J (eds) (2000) Medicine in the twentieth century. Harwood Academic Publishers, Amsterdam

Demirci S, Uchida N, Tisdale JF (2018) Gene therapy for sickle cell disease: an update. Cytotherapy 20(7):899–910

Fishman AP, Richards DW (1964) Circulation of the blood. Men and ideas. Oxford University Press, New York

Fontan F, Baudet E (1971) Surgical repair of tricuspid atresia. Thorax 26(3):240–248

Ghosh SK (2017) Giovanni Battista Morgagni (1682–1771): father of pathologic anatomy and pioneer of modern medicine. Anat Sci Int 92:305–312

Glenn WWL (1989) Superior vena cava-pulmonary artery shunt. Ann Thorac Surg 47:62–64

[194] Williams et al. (1989) and Newman et al. in Wermuth et al. (2015).

Gordon JE (1978) Structures: why things don't fall down. Da Capo Press, Cambridge
Grocott MPW, Martin DS, Levett DZH et al (2009) Arterial blood gases and oxygen content in climbers on Mount Everest. N Engl J Med 360:140–149
Gross RE (1939) Surgical management of the patent arteriosus. Ann Surg 110:321–351
GUSTO Investigators (1993) An international randomized trial comparing four thrombolytic strategies for acute myocardial infarction. N Engl J Med 329:673–682
Hacker BC (1968) Science, technology, and war in the ancient world. Technol Cult 9:34–50
Haller JA, Adkins JC, Worthington M, Rauenhorst J (1966) Experimental studies on permanent bypass of the right heart. Surgery 59:1128–1132
Harvey W (1628/2016) Exercitatio anatomica de motu cordis et sanguinis in animalibus [On the motion of the heart and blood in animals]. Carty JA (ed), Willis R (trans.). Resource Publications, Eugene
Hurst JW, Conti CR, Fye WB (2003) Profiles in cardiology. Foundation for Advances in Medicine and Science, Mahwah
Kirby RS, Withington S, Darling AB, Kilgour FG (1990) Engineering in history. Dover Publications, New York
Krishnan US, Taneja I, Gewitz M et al (2009) Peripheral vascular adaptation and orthostatic tolerance in Fontan physiology. Circulation 120:1775–1783
Lacro RV, Dietz HC, Wruck LM, et. Al. (2007) Rationale and design of a randomized clinical trial of β-blocker therapy (atenolol) versus angiotensin II receptor blocker therapy (losartan) in individuals with Marfan syndrome. Am Heart J 154:624–631
Leinhard JH (2006) How invention begins: echoes of new voices in the rise of new machines. Oxford University Press, Oxford
Lewis EE (2004) Masterworks of technology: the story of creative engineering, architecture, and design. Prometheus Books, Amherst
Magee A, Sim E, Benson LN et al (1996) Augmentation of pulmonary blood flow with an axillary arteriovenous fistula after a cavopulmonary shunt. J Thorac Cardiovasc Surg 111:176–180
Martin M, Hutchens M, Hawkins C, Radnov A (2017) How much do clinical trials cost? Nat Rev. Drug Discov 16:381–382
Mathur S, Hoskins C (2017) Drug development: lessons from nature (review). Biomed Rep 6:612–614
Mazzarello P (1999) A unifying concept: the history of cell theory. Nat Cell Biol 1(1):E13–E15
McClellan JE III, Dorn H (2015) Science and technology in world history: an introduction, 3rd edn. Johns Hopkins University Press, Baltimore
McGonigle P, Ruggeri B (2014) Animal models of human disease: challenges in enabling translation. Biochem Pharmacol 87:162–171
Meltzer SJ (1907) The factors of safety in animal structure and animal economy. Science 25:481–498
Migliavacca F, Pennati G, Dubini G et al (2001) Modeling of the Norwood circulation: effects of shunt size, vascular resistances, and heart rate. Am J Phys 280:H2076–H2086
Milewicz DM, Prakash SK, Ramirez F (2017) Therapeutic targeting drivers of thoracic aortic aneurysms and acute aortic dissections: insights from predisposing genes and mouse models. Ann Rev Med 68:51–67
Morgagni JB (1769) The seats and causes of diseases investigated by anatomy in five books, vol I (trans: Alexander B). A. Millar and T. Cadell, Johnson and Payne, London
Mountcastle VB (ed) (1980) Medical physiology, vol 1, 14th edn. C.V. Mosby Company, St. Louis
Murray AJ, Montgomery HE, Feelisch M et al (2018) Metabolic adjustment to high-altitude hypoxia: from genetic signals to physiological implications. Biochem Soc Trans 46:599–607
Nuland SB (1989) Doctors: the biography of medicine. Knopf, New York
Orlebar C (1997) The concorde story. Osprey Publishing, London
Parenti G, Pignata C, Vajro P, Salerno M (2013) New strategies for treatment of lysosomal storage diseases (review). Int J Mol Med 31:11–20
Petroski H (1992) To engineer is human: the role of failure in successful design. Vintage, New York

Porter R (1997) The greatest benefit to mankind: a medical history of humanity. W.W. Norton & Co., New York

Porter R (ed) (2006) The Cambridge history of medicine. Cambridge University Press, Cambridge

Robicsek F, Watts LT (2007) A prelude to Fontan. Pediatr Cardiol 28:422–425

Scherer FM (1965) Invention and innovation in the Watt-Boulton steam engine. Technol Cult 6:165–187

Shaddy RE, Boucek MM, Hsu DT et al (2007) Carvedilol for children and adolescents with heart failure: a randomized controlled trial. JAMA 298:1171–1179

Shumacker HB Jr (1992) The evolution of cardiac surgery. Indiana University Press, Bloomington

Staudenmaier JM (1985) Technology's storytellers: reweaving the human fabric. The Society for the History of Technology and The MIT Press, Cambridge

Swinney DC, Anthony J (2011) How were new medicines discovered? Nat Rev. Drug Discov 10:507–519

Thomas VT (1985) Pioneering research in surgical shock and cardiovascular surgery: Vivien Thomas and his work with Alfred Blalock. University of Pennsylvania Press, Philadelphia

Timoshenko SP (1983) History of strength of materials. Dover Publications, New York

Ventura HO (2009) Giovanni Battista Morgagni and the foundation of modern medicine. Clin Cardiol 23(10):792–794

Vincenti WG (1990) What engineers know and how they know it: analytical studies from aeronautical history. The Johns Hopkins University Press, Baltimore

Walsh N, Kenney L, Jangalwe S et al (2017) Humanized mouse models of human disease. Annu Rev. Pathol 12:187–215

Wermuth CG, Aldous D, Raboisson P, Rognan D (eds) (2015) The practice of medicinal chemistry, 4th edn. Academic Press, London

Wikipedia. The history of the transistor. Accessed 25 Nov 2024. https://en.wikipedia.org/wiki/History_of_the_transistor

Williams DH, Stone MJ, Hauck PR, Rahman SK (1989) Why are secondary metabolites (natural products) biosynthesized? J Nat Prod 52:1189–1208

Williams SG, Cooke GA, Wright DJ et al (2001) Peak exercise cardiac power output: a direct indicator of cardiac function strongly predictive of prognosis in chronic heart failure. Eur Heart J 22:1496–1503

Wilson JM (2009) Lessons learned from the gene therapy trial for ornithine transcarbamylase deficiency. Mol Genet Metab 96:151–157

Wong CH, Siah KW, Lo AW (2019) Estimation of clinical trial success rates and related parameters. Biostatistics 20(2):273–286

# Index




T. J. Kulik, M. Dick, *Reimagining a Child's Heart*,
https://doi.org/10.1007/978-3-031-88608-9

MIX
Papier aus verantwortungsvollen Quellen
Paper from responsible sources
FSC® C105338

If you have any concerns about our products,
you can contact us on
**ProductSafety@springernature.com**

In case Publisher is established outside the EU,
the EU authorized representative is:
**Springer Nature Customer Service Center GmbH**
**Europaplatz 3, 69115 Heidelberg, Germany**

Printed by Libri Plureos GmbH
in Hamburg, Germany